Cardiology: A Clinical Guide

Cardiology: A Clinical Guide

Edited by **Jeff Wilson**

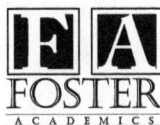

FA
FOSTER
A C A D E M I C S

New Jersey

Published by Foster Academics,
61 Van Reypen Street,
Jersey City, NJ 07306, USA
www.fosteracademics.com

Cardiology: A Clinical Guide
Edited by Jeff Wilson

International Standard Book Number: 978-1-63242-463-1 (Hardback)

Printed in the United States of America.

Contents

Preface

This book has been an outcome of determined endeavour from a group of educationists in the field. The primary objective was to involve a broad spectrum of professionals from diverse cultural background involved in the field for developing new researches. The book not only targets students but also scholars pursuing higher research for further enhancement of the theoretical and practical applications of the subject.

Cardiology is a part of medical sciences which deals with the disorders related to heart. There are two sub-divisions of cardiology, namely, adult cardiology which incorporates cardiac electrophysiology, echocardiography, interventional cardiology, nuclear cardiology, etc. and paediatric cardiology which is the study of heart diseases in children and infants. Cardiologists use techniques like electrocardiography (ECG), cardiac stress testing, coronary catheterization, echocardiogram, intravascular ultrasound, etc. to diagnose and treat the diseases. This book provides comprehensive insights into this field and highlights some of its key concepts. It discusses the fundamental and modern approaches of this area. Coherent flow of topics, reader-friendly language and extensive use of case studies from across the globe make this book an invaluable source of knowledge. It will serve as a beneficial guide of reference for students and researchers alike.

It was an honour to edit such a profound book and also a challenging task to compile and examine all the relevant data for accuracy and originality. I wish to acknowledge the efforts of the contributors for submitting such brilliant and diverse chapters in the field and for endlessly working for the completion of the book. Last, but not the least; I thank my family for being a constant source of support in all my research endeavours.

Editor

Acute Myocarditis in a Patient with Newly Diagnosed Granulomatosis with Polyangiitis

Anne Munch,[1] **Jens Sundbøll,**[2] **Søren Høyer,**[3] **and Manan Pareek**[4]

[1]*Department of Oncology, Aarhus University, Nørrebrogade 44, 8000 Aarhus C, Denmark*
[2]*Department of Cardiology, Aarhus University Hospital, Palle Juul Jensens Boulevard 99, 8200 Aarhus N, Denmark*
[3]*Institute of Pathology, Aarhus University Hospital, Nørrebrogade 44, 8000 Aarhus C, Denmark*
[4]*The Cardiovascular and Metabolic Preventive Clinic, Department of Endocrinology, Centre for Individualized Medicine in Arterial Diseases, Odense University Hospital, 5000 Odense C, Denmark*

Correspondence should be addressed to Anne Munch; annemunch00@gmail.com

Academic Editor: Monvadi Barbara Srichai

A 22-year-old woman recently diagnosed with granulomatosis with polyangiitis (GPA) was admitted to the department of cardiology due to chest pain and shortness of breath. The ECG showed widespread mild PR-segment depression, upwardly convex ST-segment elevation, and T-wave inversion. The troponin T level was elevated at 550 ng/L. Transthoracic echocardiography showed basal inferoseptal thinning and hypokinesis, mild pericardial effusion, and an overall preserved left ventricular ejection fraction of 55%. Global longitudinal strain, however, was clearly reduced. Cardiac magnetic resonance imaging (MRI) showed findings consistent with myocarditis but the etiology of the apical hypokinesis could not be determined with certainty and may well have been due to a myocardial infarction, a notion supported by a coronary angiogram displaying slow flow in the territory of the left anterior descending artery. Finally, an endomyocardial biopsy confirmed the diagnosis of myocarditis. The cardiac symptoms subsided upon treatment with high-dose prednisolone and rituximab.

1. Introduction

GPA, formerly known as Wegener's granulomatosis, is a primary systemic small-vessel vasculitis, which typically produces granulomatous inflammation of the upper and lower airways, necrotizing glomerulonephritis in the kidneys, and is associated with a cytoplasmic pattern of antineutrophil cytoplasmic antibodies (cANCA), with specificity against proteinase-3 (PR3). Although clinically overt cardiac involvement in GPA is relatively rare, it is important to recognize, as adjunctive immunosuppression may be indicated. Furthermore, it is essential to determine the nature of the cardiac condition to ensure appropriately targeted treatment [1–3].

2. Case Presentation

A 22-year-old woman was admitted to the department of cardiology due to episodic pressure-like chest pain and shortness of breath. She had received a diagnosis of GPA only a few days earlier, based on cutaneous vasculitis and neuropathy in the lower legs, sinusitis, pulmonary nodules, bilateral wrist arthritis, a markedly elevated PR3-ANCA level > 100 IU/mL (normal range 0–10 IU/mL), and histological findings from the nasal mucosa and lungs supportive of the disease. Vital parameters recorded at admission included a normal blood pressure at 116/83 mm Hg, heart rate at 95 beats per minute, a respiratory rate of 20 breaths per minute, and SpO2 at 97%.

An ECG recorded at admission showed widespread mild PR-segment depression consistent with pericarditis and upward convex ST-segment elevation and T-wave inversion, somewhat more indicative of acute myocardial ischaemia (Figure 1). The troponin T level was elevated at 550 ng/L (normal range 0–13 ng/L), and transthoracic echocardiography showed basal inferoseptal thinning, hypokinesis, and minimal pericardial effusion. The left ventricular ejection

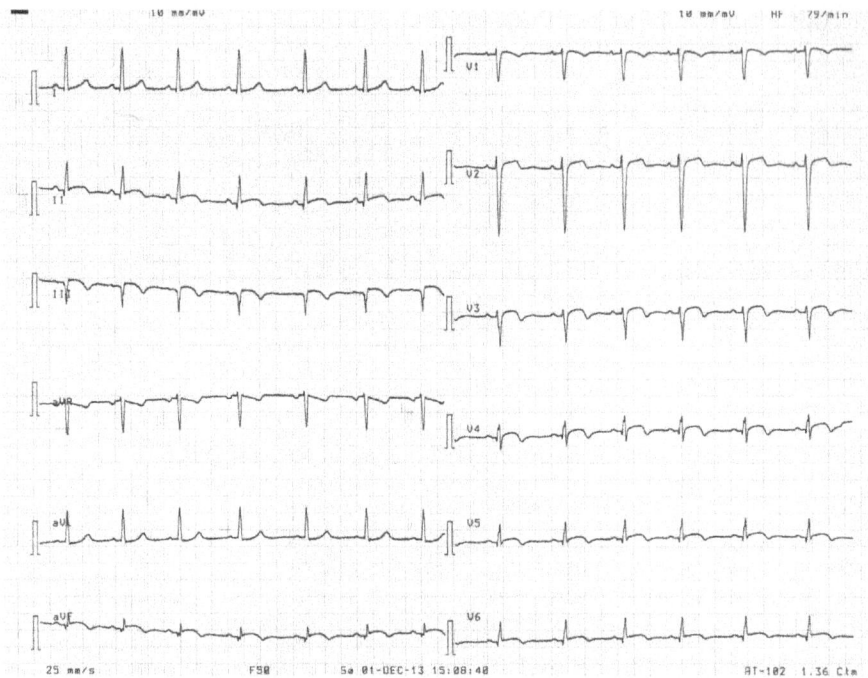

FIGURE 1: Upward convex ST-segment elevation and T-wave inversion in inferior and precordial leads suggestive of acute ischaemia and mild widespread PR-segment depression suggestive of pericarditis (although nearly subsided in this ECG).

fraction was overall preserved at 55%; however, the longitudinal function was clearly reduced as evaluated by both Doppler-based tissue velocity tracking and speckle-tracking based midwall global longitudinal strain. Cardiac magnetic resonance imaging (MRI) showed findings consistent with myocarditis with myocardial hyperaemia and capillary leak in the basal inferoseptal region (Figure 2). Moreover, thinning as well as late gadolinium enhancement was found apically, indicative of transmural infarction. Coronary angiography demonstrated slow flow in the distal LAD but no culprit lesion. Finally, an endomyocardial biopsy from the right ventricle showed fibrosis, degenerated myocytes, and lymphocyte infiltration consistent with active myocarditis (Figure 3).

The patient's GPA was treated with a standard induction regimen of high-dose prednisolone. This was supplemented with rituximab. Shortly after treatment initiation, the symptoms subsided, and troponin T levels declined.

The patient was discharged after a couple of weeks and was followed up in the outpatient clinic one month later at which point she was in clinical and serological remission and no longer had any symptoms consistent with cardiac disease. The ECG revealed persistent, albeit mild, ST-segment elevation in the lateral leads, and the echocardiogram was normal except for persistent apical hypokinesis. At follow-up one year later, the ECG had normalized, and the echocardiogram was unaltered. Therefore, repeat cardiac MRI was not performed.

3. Differential Diagnoses

GPA should be considered as a differential diagnosis, whenever a patient presents with multiple organ involvement.

The diagnosis is primarily based on characteristic clinical features, specific organ involvement, and histological findings. In this particular case, the findings on cardiac MRI could themselves have warranted a differential diagnosis of sarcoidosis; however, the patient had very recently received a histologically confirmed diagnosis of GPA.

Pulmonary embolism and acute coronary syndrome were suspected at admission, since the patient presented with acute dyspnea, chest pain, and moderately elevated heart rate. The initial suspicion of acute coronary syndrome was supported by the ECG changes (ST-segment elevations) and the elevated troponin T levels. However, as the troponin T levels in the acute phase were fixed at around 550 ng/L without significant fluctuations, and echocardiography did not show signs of right ventricular dysfunction or elevated pulmonary artery pressure, a diagnosis of myocarditis was more plausible [4].

4. Discussion

This case report describes a case of GPA with clinically overt cardiac involvement. The diagnosis of myocarditis was supported by complementary imaging modalities and histology. Although we cannot be entirely certain that a causal relationship exists, the close temporal association between the diagnosis of GPA and the onset of cardiac symptoms in an otherwise healthy 22-year-old woman suggests that GPA was responsible for the histologically verified myocarditis. Although the nature of the apical lesion could not be completely determined, we speculate that the active myocarditis somehow resulted in decreased flow in the terminal part of the left anterior descending artery, causing transmural

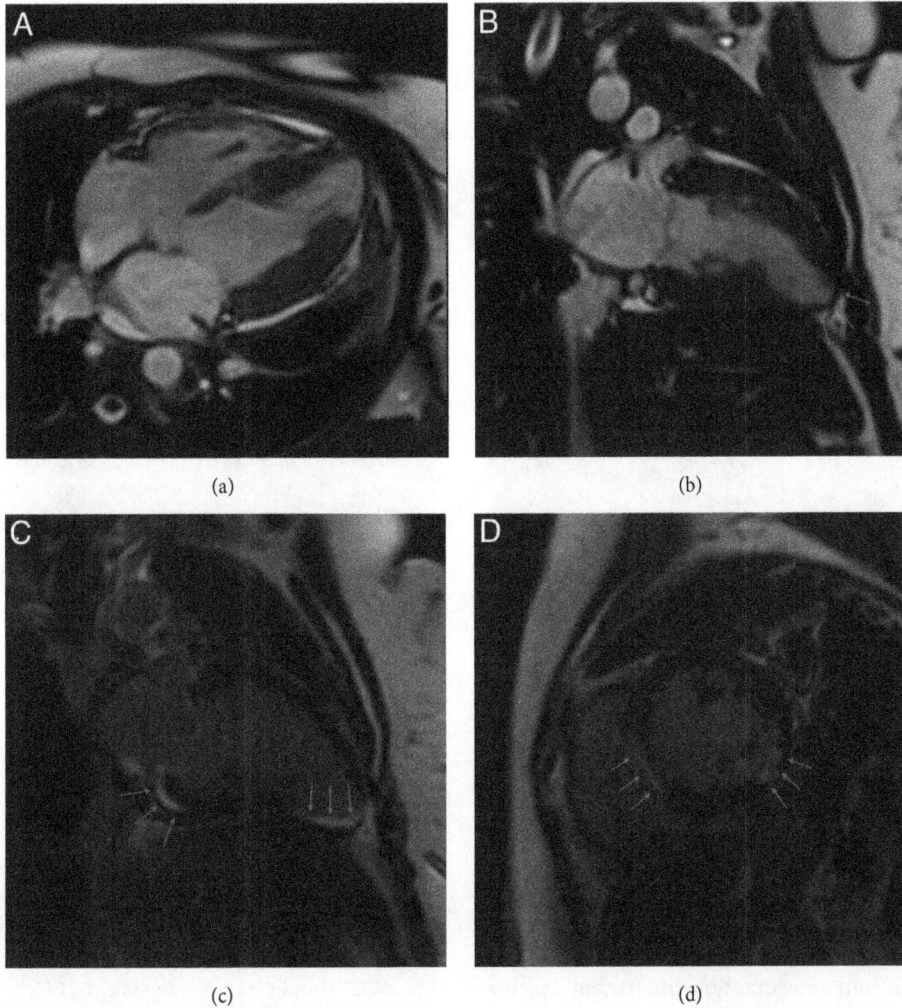

FIGURE 2: MRI scan with apical thinning of the myocardium (arrows) in 4-chamber view (a) and 2-chamber view (b). Late gadolinium enhancement (arrows) of the apical and inferobasal segments in 2-chamber view (c) and of the inferolateral and septal segments in short axis view (d).

infarction in the most distal part of its supplied territory, that is, the inferior part of the apex.

GPA is a systemic autoimmune disease of unknown etiology. The clinical presentation may vary, but its hallmark features include necrotizing vasculitis in small- and medium-sized blood vessels and granuloma formation, primarily in the respiratory tract and kidneys. Clinically evident cardiac manifestations are rare, but subclinical cardiac involvement may occur in up to 90% of cases, depending on case selection and diagnostic methods. In addition, previous studies have indicated that cardiac involvement may be associated with initial treatment resistance, increased risk of disease relapse, and increased mortality [2, 3, 5].

In symptomatic patients, pericarditis is the most common finding, but coronary artery disease, cardiomyopathy/myocarditis, valvulitis, endocarditis, and conduction abnormalities may be seen as well [6]. Only few reports exist on myocarditis caused by GPA [7]. In these cases, myocardial involvement was most often focal with the basal part of

the septum as predilection site, which was in accordance with the findings in our case.

Our case report underscores the fact that GPA truly is a systemic condition that can involve almost every organ in the body. Symptoms suggestive of cardiac disease must entail thorough investigations before cardiac involvement can be ruled out. In the present case, the presence of cardiac involvement was assessed using an integral approach with several complementary imaging modalities, including echocardiography, MRI, and coronary angiography. Cardiac MRI was the most comprehensive imaging modality and has emerged as a leading technique in the noninvasive diagnosis of myocarditis, as it allows for a safe and reproducible description of affected sites, quantification of ventricular volumes, and function and can assess myocardial morphology as well as identify ongoing myocarditis, which is useful not only in the diagnostic process, but also in the follow-up of the patient [8, 9]. However, despite its invasive nature and limited sensitivity, endomyocardial biopsy is still considered the gold

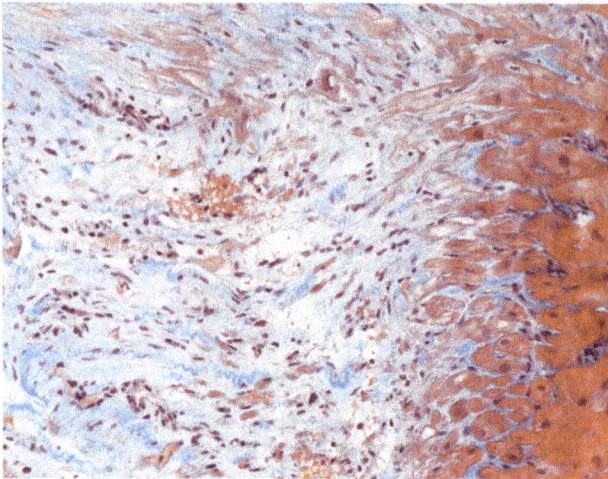

FIGURE 3: Endomyocardial biopsy showing a large collagenous scar, including several degenerated myocytes. There is a marked vascular proliferation and scanty nongranulomatous chronic inflammation. There is no evidence of vasculitis (Masson Trichrome).

standard for the diagnosis of myocarditis caused by GPA and was therefore also performed (Figure 3) [10].

Cyclophosphamide and corticosteroids constitute the classical induction regimen in the treatment of GPA and most often result in clinical remission after 6 months of therapy [11]. However, rituximab is an effective alternative to cyclophosphamide, especially in patients with concerns about fertility or a high risk of malignancy. In this case, initial therapy with rituximab instead of cyclophosphamide was chosen having taken into consideration the patient's young age and thus fertility, and she responded well to the therapy.

In conclusion, in patients recently diagnosed with GPA, it is important to consider the possibility of cardiac involvement and provide a thorough workup when cardiopulmonary symptoms are present. Cardiac MRI may be particularly useful when the initial presentation mimics that of an acute coronary syndrome, as it allows differentiating between acute myocarditis and manifestations of ischemia [9, 12].

5. Learning Points

(i) Granulomatosis with polyangiitis is a systemic vasculitis of the small- and medium-sized blood vessels characterized by granulomatous inflammation of both upper and lower respiratory tracts as well as necrotizing glomerulonephritis in the kidneys.

(ii) Symptomatic cardiac involvement is rare and usually presents as pericarditis. However, coronary artery disease, myocarditis, valvulitis, and conduction abnormalities may be seen as well.

(iii) Cardiac magnetic resonance imaging has emerged as a leading modality in the noninvasive diagnosis of myocarditis and is able to discriminate acute myocarditis from acute myocardial infarction.

Conflict of Interests

The authors declare that there is no conflict of interests regarding the publication of this paper.

References

[1] C. Comarmond and P. Cacoub, "Granulomatosis with polyangiitis (Wegener): clinical aspects and treatment," *Autoimmunity Reviews*, vol. 13, no. 11, pp. 1121–1125, 2014.

[2] M. R. Hazebroek, M. J. Kemna, S. Schalla et al., "Prevalence and prognostic relevance of cardiac involvement in ANCA-associated vasculitis: eosinophilic granulomatosis with polyangiitis and granulomatosis with polyangiitis," *International Journal of Cardiology*, vol. 199, pp. 170–179, 2015.

[3] L. McGeoch, S. Carette, D. Cuthbertson et al., "Cardiac involvement in granulomatosis with polyangiitis," *The Journal of Rheumatology*, vol. 42, no. 7, Article ID 141513, pp. 1209–1212, 2015.

[4] S. Korff, H. A. Katus, and E. Giannitsis, "Differential diagnosis of elevated troponins," *Heart*, vol. 92, no. 7, pp. 987–993, 2006.

[5] S. C. D. Grant, R. D. Levy, M. C. Venning, C. Ward, and N. H. Brooks, "Wegener's granulomatosis and the heart," *British Heart Journal*, vol. 71, no. 1, pp. 82–86, 1994.

[6] J. Z. Forstot, P. A. Overlie, G. K. Neufeld, C. E. Harmon, and S. L. Forstot, "Cardiac complications of Wegener granulomatosis: a case report of complete heart block and review of the literature," *Seminars in Arthritis and Rheumatism*, vol. 10, no. 2, pp. 148–154, 1980.

[7] A. Florian, M. Slavich, D. Blockmans, S. Dymarkowski, and J. Bogaert, "Cardiac involvement in granulomatosis with polyangiitis (Wegener granulomatosis)," *Circulation*, vol. 124, no. 13, pp. e342–e344, 2011.

[8] W. G. Hundley, D. A. Bluemke, J. P. Finn et al., "ACCF/ACR/AHA/NASCI/SCMR 2010 expert consensus document on cardiovascular magnetic resonance: a report of the American College of Cardiology Foundation Task Force on Expert Consensus Documents," *Journal of the American College of Cardiology*, vol. 55, no. 23, pp. 2614–2662, 2010.

[9] E. Gerbaud, E. Harcaut, P. Coste et al., "Cardiac magnetic resonance imaging for the diagnosis of patients presenting with chest pain, raised troponin, and unobstructed coronary arteries," *International Journal of Cardiovascular Imaging*, vol. 28, no. 4, pp. 783–794, 2012.

[10] A. L. P. Caforio, S. Pankuweit, E. Arbustini et al., "Current state of knowledge on aetiology, diagnosis, management, and therapy of myocarditis: a position statement of the European Society of Cardiology Working Group on Myocardial and Pericardial Diseases," *European Heart Journal*, vol. 34, no. 33, pp. 2636–2648, 2013.

[11] C. A. Langford, "Small-vessel vasculitis: therapeutic management," *Current Rheumatology Reports*, vol. 9, no. 4, pp. 328–335, 2007.

[12] G. Leurent, B. Langella, C. Fougerou et al., "Diagnostic contributions of cardiac magnetic resonance imaging in patients presenting with elevated troponin, acute chest pain syndrome and unobstructed coronary arteries," *Archives of Cardiovascular Diseases*, vol. 104, no. 3, pp. 161–170, 2011.

A Rare Case of Complete Stent Fracture, Coronary Arterial Transection, and Pseudoaneurysm Formation Induced by Repeated Stenting

Fumiaki Nakao,[1] Masashi Kanemoto,[1] Jutaro Yamada,[2] Kazuhiro Suzuki,[3] Hidetoshi Tsuboi,[3] and Takashi Fujii[1]

[1]Department of Cardiology, Yamaguchi Grand Medical Center, 77 Ohsaki, Hofu, Yamaguchi 747-8511, Japan
[2]Division of Cardiology, Department of Medicine and Clinical Science, Yamaguchi University Graduate School of Medicine, 1-1-1 Minami-kogushi, Ube, Yamaguchi 755-8505, Japan
[3]Department of Cardiovascular Surgery, Yamaguchi Grand Medical Center, 77 Ohsaki, Hofu, Yamaguchi 747-8511, Japan

Correspondence should be addressed to Fumiaki Nakao; nakao-ymghp@umin.ac.jp

Academic Editor: Mohammad R. Movahed

This report describes a rare asymptomatic case of complete stent fracture, coronary arterial transection, and pseudoaneurysm formation in response to repeated stenting. The proximal and distal ends of transected coronary artery were closed, and distal bypass was performed. Coronary arterial transection can occur in patients with repeated stenting as a long-term adverse event.

1. Introduction

Stent fracture after drug-eluting stent (DES) deployment is an important issue, because it is strongly associated with restenosis, target legion revascularization, and stent thrombosis [1]. A report of autopsy cases with DES deployment showed stent fracture in 29% of lesions and restenosis or stent thrombosis in 67% of cases with gapped stent fracture [2].

Stent fracture can also lead to coronary pseudoaneurysm formation, which can be life-threatening [3]. The incidence of coronary pseudoaneurysm formation after DES deployment is 0.3–4.5% [4]. Management strategies for coronary pseudoaneurysm include observation, surgical treatment and interventional treatment, such as coil embolization and deployment of a polytetrafluoroethylene- (PTFE-) covered stent [3–5].

2. Case Report

A 61-year-old male undergoing chronic hemodialysis had previously underwent rotational atherectomy and stenting (TAXUS Liberte, Boston Scientific Co.) for a long, severely calcified lesion of the right coronary artery (RCA) (first percutaneous coronary intervention [PCI#1], Figure 1). Six months later, the patient underwent emergent restenting (Cypher, Cordis) for probable stent thrombosis of the mid-RCA with ST elevation (second PCI [PCI#2], Figure 2). Four months later, he underwent emergent repeat stenting (Xience V, Abbott Vascular) for probable stent thrombosis of the mid-RCA with ST elevation (third PCI [PCI#3], Figure 3). Two months later, he was admitted for follow-up coronary angiography (CAG) and was noted to be asymptomatic. CAG showed pseudoaneurysm formation in the mid-RCA (see Figures 4(a), 4(b), and 4(c) and see Clip 1 in Supplementary Material available online at http://dx.doi.org/10.1155/2015/192853), and X-ray fluorography showed complete stent fracture (Figure 4(d)). Coronary transection was suspected, because of findings of complete stent fracture and contrast media oozing all around the part of stent fracture.

3. Discussion

Risk factors for stent fracture include RCA stenting, long stenting, overlapped stenting, and stenting on a hinge point [6, 7]. The present patient underwent long and overlapped

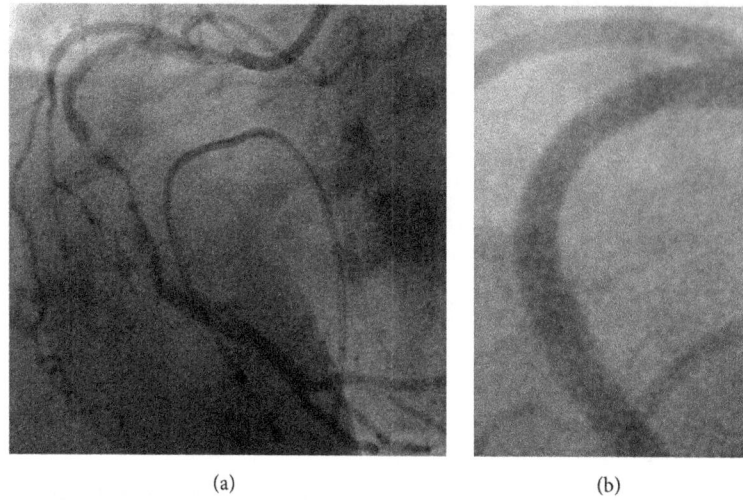

FIGURE 1: First percutaneous coronary intervention (PCI#1). (a) Baseline coronary angiography (CAG). (b) CAG after first stenting.

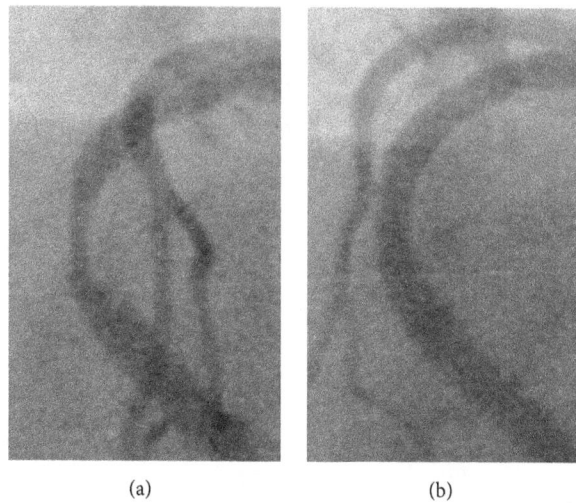

FIGURE 2: Second percutaneous coronary intervention (PCI#2). (a) Baseline coronary angiography (CAG). (b) CAG after second stenting.

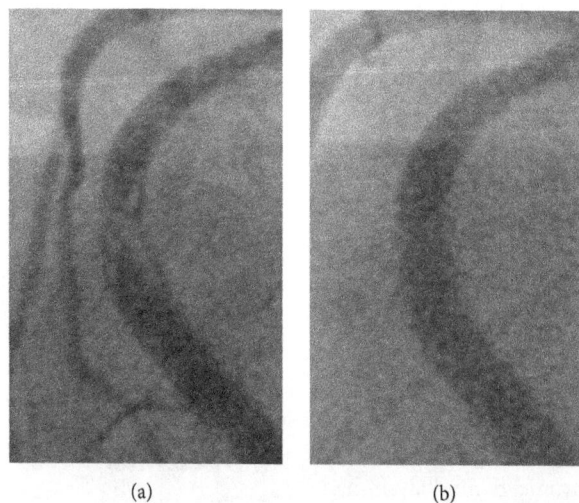

FIGURE 3: Third percutaneous coronary intervention (PCI#3). (a) Baseline coronary angiography (CAG). (b) CAG after third stenting.

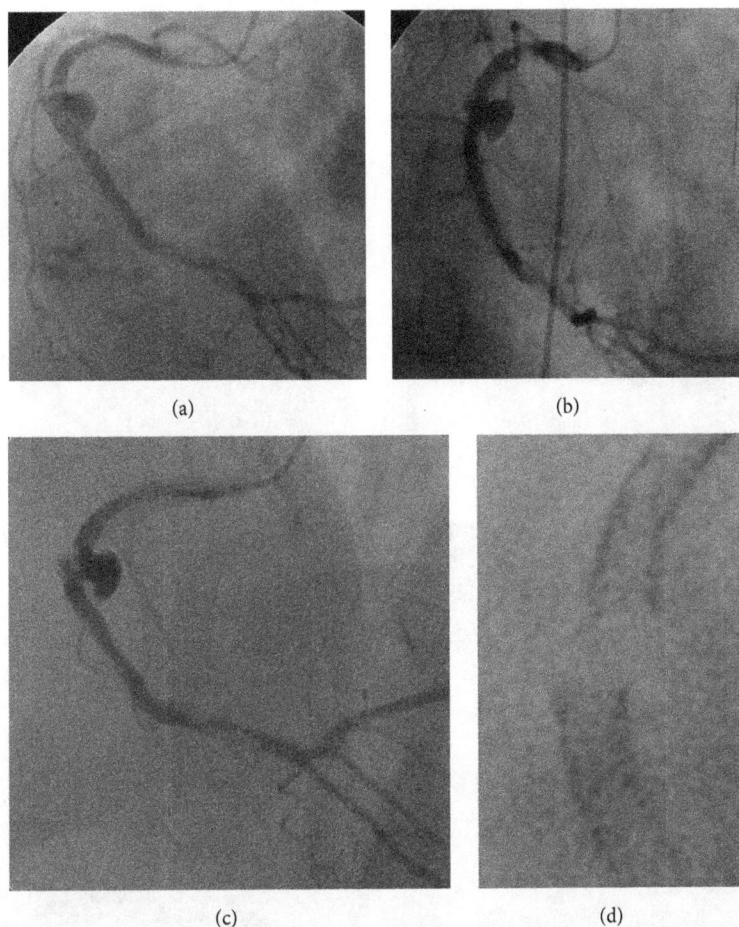

FIGURE 4: Follow-up coronary angiography showing pseudoaneurysm formation. Left anterior oblique (LAO) view (a), right anterior oblique view (b), and LAO-cranial view (c). (d) X-ray fluorography showing complete stent fracture.

stenting within the RCA and therefore was at high risk for stent fracture. Drugs and polymers of DES may induce vascular inflammation and delay vascular healing [8], and they also can contribute to pseudoaneurysm formation. In this case, the vessel wall was likely exposed to a relatively high dose of DES drug and polymer (due to three overlapping stents).

Surgical treatment and a PTFE-covered stent deployment were considered for this case. However, a guidewire could perforate the wall of the pseudoaneurysm, and deployment of the PTFE-covered stent might be difficult, because previous procedures required the mother and child (4 in 6) technique. If repeated stenting for stent fracture was performed, stent fracture might occur repeatedly, leading to lethal stent thrombosis or blow-out rupture of the pseudoaneurysm. Therefore, surgical management was selected for this case. During surgery, the pseudoaneurysm was visualized in the visceral adipose tissue (arrow heads, Figure 5(a)). After the pseudoaneurysm was opened (Figure 5(b)), coronary transection was confirmed (arrows, Figure 5(b)). The proximal and distal transected ends of the mid-RCA could not be ligated because of protrusion of the overlapped fractured

struts (arrows, Figure 5(c)). Therefore, proximal and distal transected ends of the mid-RCA were closed (Figure 5(d)), and distal bypass was performed.

In conclusion, this case report described a rare asymptomatic case of complete stent fracture, coronary arterial transection, and pseudoaneurysm formation in response to repeated stenting. Coronary arterial transection can occur in patients with repeated stenting as a long-term adverse event.

Conflict of Interests

The authors declare that there is no conflict of interests with regard to this report.

Acknowledgments

The authors thank Tooru Ueda, Takamasa Oda, and Yasuhiro Ikeda of the Department of Cardiology, Ymaguchi Grand Medical Center, for their support and thank Takayuki Okamura and Masafumi Yano of the Division of Cardiology, Department of Medicine and Clinical Science, Yamaguchi

(a)

(b)

(c)

(d)

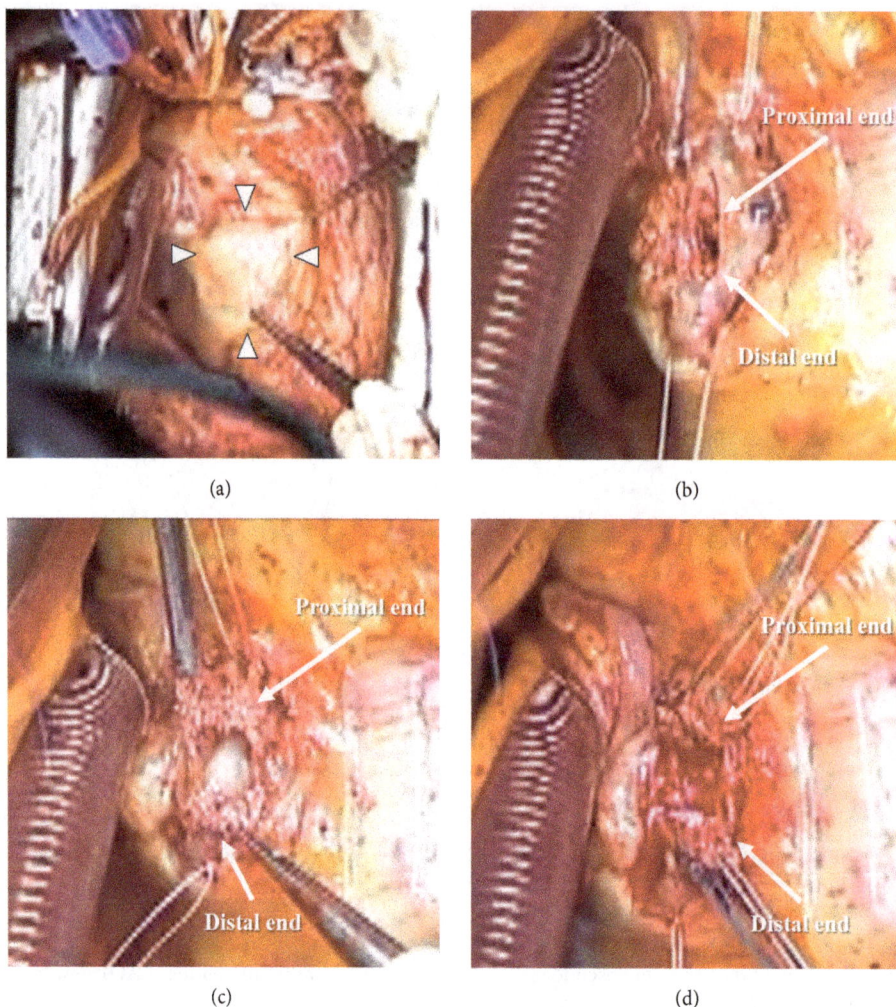

FIGURE 5: Intraoperative findings. The pseudoaneurysm is in the visceral adipose tissue (arrow heads) (a) and opened (b). (c) Coronary arterial transection. (d) Proximal and distal transected ends are closed.

University Graduate School of Medicine, for their helpful advice.

References

[1] S. E. Lee, M. H. Jeong, I. S. Kim et al., "Clinical outcomes and optimal treatment for stent fracture after drug-eluting stent implantation," *Journal of Cardiology*, vol. 53, no. 3, pp. 422–428, 2009.

[2] G. Nakazawa, A. V. Finn, M. Vorpahl et al., "Incidence and predictors of drug-eluting stent fracture in human coronary artery a pathologic analysis," *Journal of the American College of Cardiology*, vol. 54, no. 21, pp. 1924–1931, 2009.

[3] Y. Kawai, M. Kitayama, H. Akao, A. Motoyama, T. Tsuchiya, and K. Kajinami, "A case of coronary rupture and pseudoaneurysm formation after fracture of implanted paclitaxel-eluting stents," *Cardiovascular Intervention and Therapeutics*, pp. 1–7, 2015.

[4] S. Bajaj, R. Parikh, A. Hamdan, and M. Bikkina, "Covered-stent treatment of coronary aneurysm after drug-eluting stent placement," *Texas Heart Institute Journal*, vol. 37, no. 4, pp. 449–454, 2010.

[5] A. Maroo, P. A. Rasmussen, T. J. Masaryk, S. G. Ellis, A. M. Lincoff, and S. Kapadia, "Stent-assisted detachable coil embolization of pseudoaneurysms in the coronary circulation," *Catheterization and Cardiovascular Interventions*, vol. 68, no. 3, pp. 409–415, 2006.

[6] H. Doi, A. Maehara, G. S. Mintz et al., "Classification and potential mechanisms of intravascular ultrasound patterns of stent fracture," *The American Journal of Cardiology*, vol. 103, no. 6, pp. 818–823, 2009.

[7] S. Kuramitsu, M. Iwabuchi, T. Haraguchi et al., "Incidence and clinical impact of stent fracture after everolimus-eluting stent implantation," *Circulation: Cardiovascular Interventions*, vol. 5, no. 5, pp. 663–671, 2012.

[8] R. Virmani, F. Liistro, G. Stankovic et al., "Mechanism of late in-stent restenosis after implantation of a paclitaxel derivate-eluting polymer stent system in humans," *Circulation*, vol. 106, no. 21, pp. 2649–2651, 2002.

3

Aortico-Left Atrial Fistula: A Rare Complication of Bioprosthetic Aortic Valve Endocarditis Secondary to *Enterococcus faecalis*

Abhinav Agrawal,[1] Martin Miguel Amor,[1] Deepa Iyer,[2] Manan Parikh,[1] and Marc Cohen[3]

[1]*Department of Medicine, Monmouth Medical Center, Long Branch, NJ 07740, USA*
[2]*Department of Cardiology, Robert Wood Johnson University Hospital, New Brunswick, NJ 08901, USA*
[3]*Department of Cardiology, Newark Beth Israel Medical Center, Newark, NJ 07712, USA*

Correspondence should be addressed to Martin Miguel Amor; mamor@barnabashealth.org

Academic Editor: Gerard Devlin

Paravalvular aortic root abscess with intracardiac fistula formation is an exceedingly rare complication of infective endocarditis. This condition is even more rarely encountered in patients with bioprosthetic valve endocarditis. We report an unusual case of a 68-year-old Bosnian female with a bioprosthetic aortic valve, who developed an extensive aortic root abscess, complicated by an aortico-left atrial intracardiac fistula. This case illustrates that a high index of suspicion, prompt diagnosis by echocardiography, proper antibiotic therapy, and early surgical intervention are crucial to improving treatment outcomes for this rare condition.

1. Introduction

The spread of infective endocarditis from valvular structures to surrounding tissues results in periannular complications that may place patients at increased risk for adverse outcomes, including congestive heart failure, heart block, and death. Extension beyond valvular structures may result in aorto-cavitary fistulization. The incidence of this complication is estimated at 1-2% of all cases of infective endocarditis. It is seen in 3.3% of cases of prosthetic valve endocarditis and more commonly encountered with mechanical prosthetic valves compared to bioprosthetic valves [1]. We report an unusual case of a 68-year-old Bosnian female with a bioprosthetic aortic valve, who developed an extensive aortic root abscess, complicated by an aortico-left atrial intracardiac fistula.

2. Case Report

A 68-year-old Bosnian female with prior aortic valve replacement with a bioprosthetic valve for aortic regurgitation was admitted to our facility for worsening shortness of breath, fever, and lethargy. She was on a vacation in Bosnia, where she fell ill, was hospitalized for 1 month, and was treated for suspected sepsis and renal failure. Medical records from her prior hospitalization in Bosnia were not available. She had an extensive past medical history, pertinent for coronary artery disease, diastolic congestive heart failure, atrial fibrillation, chronic kidney disease, systemic hypertension, cerebrovascular accidents, and chronic urinary tract infection (UTI). Physical examination revealed neck vein distention, bibasal crackles, and bilateral pitting edema. Auscultation revealed an irregularly irregular heart rhythm, a grade 3/6 systolic ejection murmur in the left lower sternal border, and a grade 2/6 early diastolic murmur. EKG revealed atrial fibrillation with low voltage QRS, without evidence of bundle branch blocks or conduction delays. Within an hour, she became markedly hypotensive and hypoxic. She was subsequently intubated and started on a dopamine and norepinephrine infusion. The patient was treated for septic shock with intravenous vancomycin and meropenem. Two sets of blood cultures showed growth of *Enterococcus faecalis* that was sensitive to penicillin and vancomycin. A bedside transthoracic echocardiogram (TTE) revealed new paravalvular leakage around the bioprosthetic aortic valve, raising concern for an aortic root abscess. She was transferred

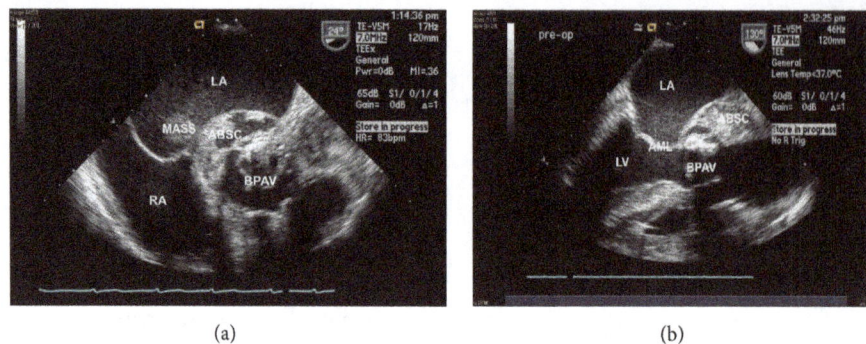

(a)   (b)

FIGURE 1: Transesophageal echocardiogram in short axis (a) and long axis (b) views, showing an extensive aortic root abscess around a bioprosthetic aortic valve, forming a fistulous communication to left atrium (legend: ABSC = abscess, LA = left atrium, MASS = mass in LA, BPAV = bioprosthetic aortic valve, RA = right atrium, AML = anterior mitral leaflet, and LV = left ventricle).

to a tertiary care facility for possible surgical intervention. A transesophageal echocardiogram (TEE) revealed an extensive aortic root abscess involving the entire root and base of the anterior mitral leaflet. The abscess had ruptured into the left atrium, which contained a 5–7 cm cystic mass, with a fistula connecting from the aortic root to the left atrial cavity, running through the mass. The abscess was located around the bioprosthetic aortic valve which had a large vegetation and paravalvular leak with severe paravalvular aortic regurgitation (Figures 1–3). She became hemodynamically unstable during the TEE and was brought to the operating room for emergent surgery. She underwent homograft aortic valve replacement, aortic root replacement, VSD repair, and ligation of the aortico-left atrial fistula. Tissue samples from the excised aortic root and bioprosthetic valve also revealed growth of *Enterococcus faecalis* again found to be sensitive to penicillin and vancomycin. Postoperatively, she developed worsening septic shock. She was subsequently treated with ampicillin and gentamicin. She remained intubated and required vasopressor support with milrinone, norepinephrine, phenylephrine, and vasopressin. She became anuric and was placed on CVVHD support. Her leucocyte count as well as INR continued to increase and she progressively became more thrombocytopenic and eventually succumbed to disseminated intravascular coagulation from septic shock.

3. Discussion

Paravalvular extension of endocarditis is caused by bacterial destruction and invasion of local tissue and necrosis. In prosthetic valves, this process usually begins on the prosthesis cuff and often extends outside the valvular apparatus, resulting in valvular dehiscence, abscess formation, and myocardial involvement [2]. Left untreated, these abscesses may eventually rupture into adjacent cardiac chambers, leading to aorto-cavitary fistulae. Hemodynamic instability ensues due to intracardiac shunting. This leads to volume overload of the left ventricle, with subsequent left-sided heart failure and pulmonary edema.

Staphylococcus species are the most common bacteria implicated in aorto-cavitary fistulae, seen in 58% of cases [3].

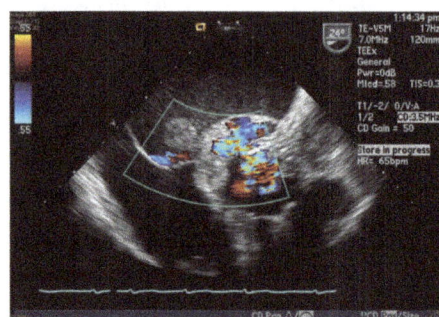

FIGURE 2: Transesophageal echocardiogram in short axis view with color flow Doppler showing blood flow from the bioprosthetic aortic valve, into the aortic root abscess, which has ruptured into the left atrium, forming an aortico-left atrial fistula.

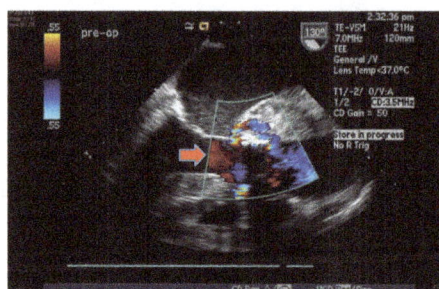

FIGURE 3: Transesophageal echocardiogram in long axis view with color flow Doppler showing severe paravalvular aortic regurgitation (indicated by red arrow), around a bioprosthetic aortic valve, around which an extensive aortic root abscess has developed.

Other bacteria implicated in the pathogenesis of this condition include *Streptococcus* spp. (28%) and *Enterococcus* spp. (7%). The remaining 7% of cases are polymicrobial. Our patient had multiple positive cultures for *Enterococcus faecalis*. Even though this bacterium is the third most common cause of infective endocarditis, it can be difficult to diagnose because the natural history of enterococcal endocarditis follows a subacute course that reminds us of other infectious and inflammatory diseases. The most common port of entry for *E. faecalis* is the urinary tract, which might also be the case in our patient suffering from chronic UTI [4].

A high index of suspicion leading to timely diagnosis and early treatment is of paramount importance in the management of aorto-cavitary fistulae. When clinically suspected, transthoracic echocardiography (TTE) is the initial technique of choice for investigation [5]. TTE is able to detect fistulous tracts in 50% of cases. This low sensitivity of detection is attributed to difficulty in characterizing abscesses at early stages, particularly when the echodensity of these lesions appears similar to contiguous tissues. With the aid of transesophageal echocardiography (TEE), overall detection rate is increased to 97%. The high rate of echocardiographic diagnosis is attributed to high-pressure differences between the aorta and the cardiac chambers. As a result of the pressure differences, flow across the fistula is highly turbulent and thus easily detectable by continuous or color Doppler monitoring. TEE also allows optimal characterization of the fistula tract, providing precise anatomic information that is invaluable for surgical planning [6]. Concern for an aortic root abscess was not entertained early on during the course of this patient's illness. This could have contributed to the delayed diagnosis of her condition.

Aortic paravalvular abscesses are associated with bundle branch blocks and first-, second-, and third-degree heart block in up to 10% of cases. These conduction defects are usually encountered when an abscess extends to the interventricular septum leading to infiltration of the nodal conduction system. Our patient did not manifest with conduction system defects on EKG. This may be explained by the course of the aorto-left atrial fistula. As shown in Figure 1, the abscess tunneled from the aortic root, posteriorly into the mitral leaflet, forming a fistulous communication with the left atrium, without infiltration of the interventricular septum.

Operative treatment remains the cornerstone of management of aorto-cavitary fistulae. Pioneering work by Ergin et al. showed that destruction and disruption of ventricular-aortic continuity in the presence of acute infective endocarditis necessitated special reconstructive techniques for treatment. Surgical treatment involved removal of all infected tissue including annular elements followed by appropriate restoration of the annulus for safe anchoring of a valve conduit [7]. Currently available conduit options for reconstruction include conventional aortic valve replacement (using a mechanical or stented biological valve), aortic valve replacement with translocation, aortic root replacement using a homograft, pulmonary autograft (Ross procedure), stentless biological valve, or a composite graft [8]. Among these options, homograft aortic root reconstruction is preferred because it offers a low recurrent infection rate and low valve-related morbidity and mortality. These aortic homografts are permeable to serum antibiotics, rendering them resistant to biofilm bacterial infection. Yankah et al. demonstrated the superiority of antibiotic-permeable cryopreserved homografts over aortic valve replacement in patient with periannular abscess [9]. The actuarial freedom from residual/recurrent infection and paravalvular leaks was 92%. Actuarial freedom from reoperation at 17 years was 75%.

Timing of operative intervention plays a pivotal role in the management of aorto-cavitary fistulae. A recent study by Kang et al. showed that as compared with conventional treatment, early surgery in patients with infective endocarditis significantly reduced mortality [10]. Our patient underwent surgical intervention after 1 month of hospitalization in Bosnia, and such delay in surgery likewise contributed to the poor outcome.

4. Conclusion

Aorto-cavitary fistulization is a rare and particularly problematic complication of periannular spread of infective endocarditis, with high mortality despite adequate therapy. This case illustrates that a high index of suspicion, prompt diagnosis by echocardiography, proper antibiotic therapy, and early surgical intervention are crucial to improving treatment outcomes for this rare condition.

Conflict of Interests

All authors have no conflict of interests to report.

References

[1] I. Anguera, J. M. Miro, J. A. S. Roman et al., "Periannular complications in infective endocarditis involving prosthetic aortic valves," *The American Journal of Cardiology*, vol. 98, no. 9, pp. 1261–1268, 2006.

[2] I. Anguera, J. M. Miro, I. Vilacosta et al., "Aorto-cavitary fistulous tract formation in infective endocarditis: clinical and echocardiographic features of 76 cases and risk factors for mortality," *European Heart Journal*, vol. 26, no. 3, pp. 288–297, 2005.

[3] N. Kang, S. Wan, S. H. Calvin, and M. J. Underwood, "Periannular extension of infective endocarditis," *Annals of Thoracic and Cardiovascular Surgery*, vol. 15, no. 2, pp. 74–81, 2009.

[4] A. Dahl and N. E. Bruun, "Enterococcus faecalis infective endocarditis: focus on clinical aspects," *Expert Review of Cardiovascular Therapy*, vol. 11, no. 9, pp. 1247–1257, 2013.

[5] F. Thuny, D. Grisoli, F. Collart, G. Habib, and D. Raoult, "Management of infective endocarditis: challenges and perspectives," *The Lancet*, vol. 379, no. 9819, pp. 965–975, 2012.

[6] E. E. Hill, P. Herijgers, P. Claus, S. Vanderschueren, W. E. Peetermans, and M.-C. Herregods, "Abscess in infective endocarditis: the value of transesophageal echocardiography and outcome: a 5-year study," *The American Heart Journal*, vol. 154, no. 5, pp. 923–928, 2007.

[7] M. A. Ergin, S. Raissi, F. Follis et al., "Annular destruction in acute bacterial endocarditis. Surgical techniques to meet the challenge," *The Journal of Thoracic and Cardiovascular Surgery*, vol. 97, no. 5, pp. 755–763, 1989.

[8] K. Okada and Y. Okita, "Surgical treatment for aortic periannular abscess/pseudoaneurysm caused by infective endocarditis," *General Thoracic and Cardiovascular Surgery*, vol. 61, no. 4, pp. 175–181, 2013.

[9] A. C. Yankah, M. Pasic, H. Klose, H. Siniawski, Y. Weng, and R. Hetzer, "Homograft reconstruction of the aortic root for endocarditis with periannular abscess: a 17-year study," *European Journal of Cardio-Thoracic Surgery*, vol. 28, no. 1, pp. 69–75, 2005.

[10] D. H. Kang, Y. J. Kim, S. H. Kim et al., "Early surgery versus conventional treatment for infective endocarditis," *The New England Journal of Medicine*, vol. 366, no. 26, pp. 2466–2473, 2012.

4

Giant Cell Myocarditis: Not Always a Presentation of Cardiogenic Shock

Rose Tompkins,[1] William J. Cole,[1] Barry P. Rosenzweig,[1] Leon Axel,[2]
Sripal Bangalore,[1] and Anuradha Lala[1]

[1]Department of Cardiology, New York University Langone Medical Center, New York, NY 10016, USA
[2]Department of Radiology, New York University School of Medicine, New York, NY 10016, USA

Correspondence should be addressed to Anuradha Lala; anu.lala@mountsinai.org

Academic Editor: Gianluca Pontone

Giant cell myocarditis is a rare and often fatal disease. The most obvious presentation often described in the literature is one of rapid hemodynamic deterioration due to cardiogenic shock necessitating urgent consideration of mechanical circulatory support and heart transplantation. We present the case of a 60-year-old man whose initial presentation was consistent with myopericarditis but who went on to develop a rapid decline in left ventricular systolic function without overt hemodynamic compromise or dramatic symptomatology. Giant cell myocarditis was confirmed via endomyocardial biopsy. Combined immunosuppression with corticosteroids and calcineurin inhibitor resulted in resolution of symptoms and sustained recovery of left ventricular function one year later. Our case highlights that giant cell myocarditis does not always present with cardiogenic shock and should be considered in the evaluation of new onset cardiomyopathy of uncertain etiology as a timely diagnosis has distinct clinical implications on management and prognosis.

1. Introduction

Giant cell myocarditis (GCM) is a rare and often fatal disease with the most obvious presentation being a rapid hemodynamic deterioration with declining left ventricular (LV) systolic function and cardiogenic shock [1]. We report the case of a patient with confirmed GCM who did not present in fulminant heart failure highlighting the variability of presentation and potential for underrecognition of GCM, which could greatly impact subsequent treatment and prognosis.

2. Case Presentation

A 60-year-old previously healthy African American man complained of progressively worsening chest pain for five days. He had no known cardiovascular risk factors. His physical examination was normal. Electrocardiogram showed diffuse ST elevations with associated cardiac troponin I of 7.6 ng/mL (reference range ≤ 0.04 ng/mL). Emergent cardiac catheterization revealed angiographically normal coronary arteries. On hospital day one, a transthoracic echocardiogram (TTE) was notable for normal left ventricular function, chamber size, and wall thickness (Figure 1(a); see Movie 1 in Supplementary Material available online at http://dx.doi.org/10.1155/2015/173826). This was followed by a contrast-enhanced cardiac magnetic resonance (CMR) imaging that showed normal left ventricular (LV) systolic function with an ejection fraction (EF) of 55% and multiple patchy areas of transmural and midwall late gadolinium enhancement (LGE) in a noncoronary distribution (Figure 2(a)). He was treated for presumed myopericarditis with nonsteroidal anti-inflammatory drugs (NSAIDs). His symptoms resolved and his troponin levels decreased.

On hospital day five, the patient complained of new dyspnea on exertion, paroxysmal nocturnal dyspnea, and recurrent chest discomfort. His blood pressure decreased from 130/80 on admission to 100/70 mmHg. His rhythm was sinus tachycardia with a heart rate (HR) of 110 bpm. The jugular venous pressure was 7 cm H_2O and hepatojugular reflux was evidenced. There was no gallop sound or murmur, the lungs

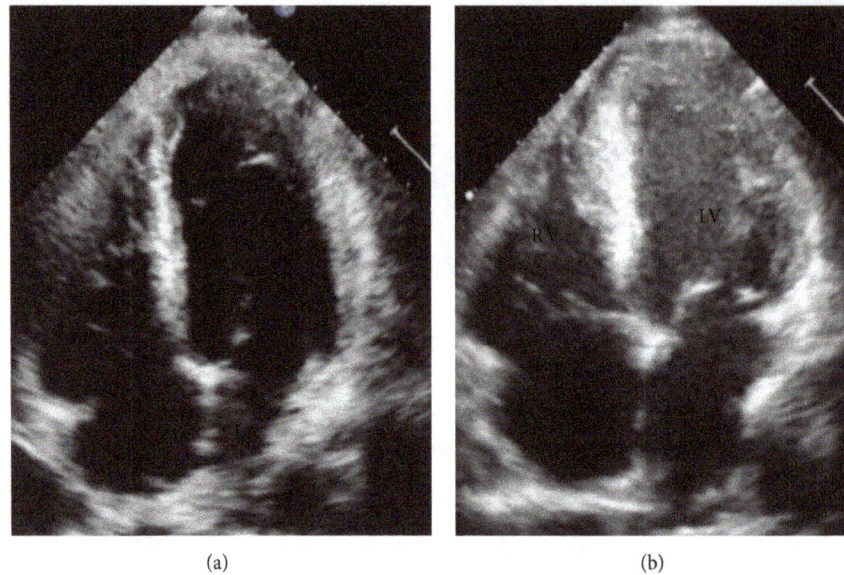

(a)   (b)

FIGURE 1: Transthoracic echocardiogram (apical four-chamber view). (a) Hospital day 1: normal ventricular function, normal wall thickness. (b) Hospital day 7: left ventricular systolic function is severely reduced, wall thickness is increased, and echocontrast is present in the left ventricle consistent with stasis of blood flow. LV: left ventricle, RV: right ventricle, LA: left atrium, and RA: right atrium.

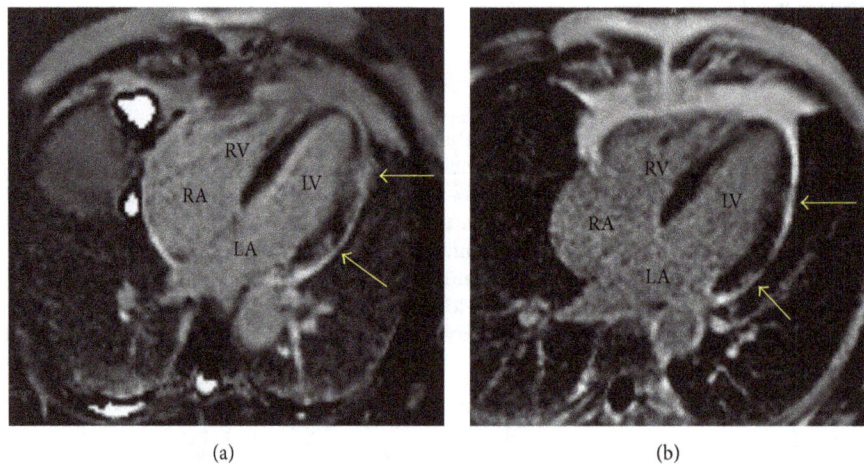

(a)   (b)

FIGURE 2: Cardiac magnetic resonance image (four-chamber view). (a) Presentation: patchy areas of late gadolinium enhancement (LGE) were detected transmurally in the mid lateral left ventricular (LV) wall and in the midwall with extension to the subepicardial in lateral and anterior LV walls near the base consistent with diffuse inflammation in a noncoronary distribution (arrows). (b) 6 weeks after presentation: markedly reduced LGE (arrows) consistent with improvement in inflammation without significant residual fibrosis. LV: left ventricle, RV: right ventricle, LA: left atrium, and RA: right atrium.

were clear, and his extremities were warm without peripheral edema. TTE now showed a mildly reduced EF of 45% with hypokinesis of the left ventricular apical anterior and apical lateral walls. Notably, the left ventricular wall motion abnormalities were in the areas of myocardium with LGE seen on CMR imaging. Low dose furosemide was initiated with improvement in his symptoms.

Over the next two days, serial TTEs showed a rapid decline in LV systolic function from 45% to 25%, increased wall thickness suggestive of myocardial edema, and spontaneous echo contrast in the left ventricle consistent with stasis of blood flow (Figure 1(b), Movie 2). Concomitantly, troponin

levels rose again to a peak of 9.6 ng/mL associated with persistence of diffuse ST elevations on electrocardiogram (Figure 3). Inflammatory markers, including erythrocyte sedimentation rate (ESR) and C-reactive protein (CRP), were elevated at 135 mm/hr and 329 mg/L, respectively. Renal function and lactate levels remained within normal limits. No significant arrhythmia or ventricular ectopy was noted. His mild symptoms were controlled with low dose oral furosemide alone.

Given the rapid and dramatic decline in LV systolic function, an endomyocardial biopsy was performed. Microscopic analysis revealed widespread necrosis and an inflammatory

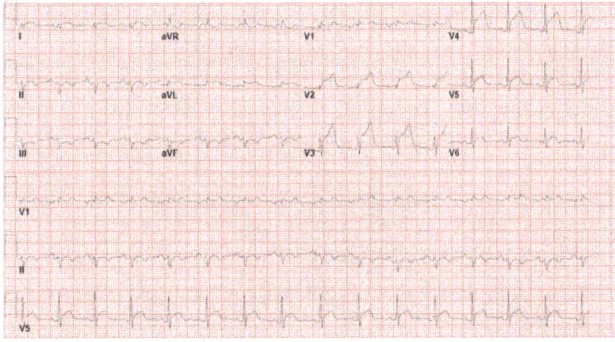

FIGURE 3: Twelve-lead electrocardiogram on hospital day 7 showed persistent diffuse ST elevation.

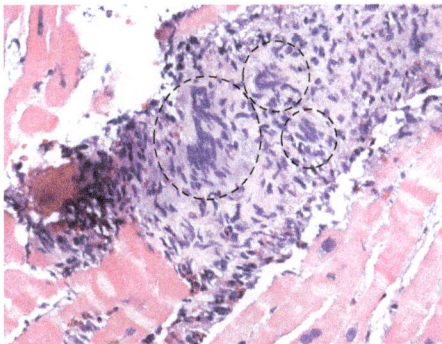

FIGURE 4: Microscopic examination from the endomyocardial biopsy of the right ventricle showing myocardial necrosis with inflammatory infiltrate containing multinucleated giant cells (within circled areas) (H&E, orig. ×40).

infiltrate comprising neutrophils, eosinophils, and multinucleated giant cells consistent with the pathological diagnosis of giant cell myocarditis (GCM) (Figure 4). Immunosuppression was initiated with intravenous methylprednisolone for three days followed by a slow oral prednisone taper. Cyclosporine was added in conjunction with low dose ACE inhibition and diuretic therapy.

Two weeks following hospital discharge, the patient was free of heart failure (HF) symptoms. TTE showed improved contractility with an EF of 45%. Repeat CMR 6 weeks later demonstrated residual patchy areas of midwall late gadolinium enhancement but the overall extent of enhancement was significantly reduced. CMR-measured EF had normalized to 55% with resolution of all wall motion abnormalities and no evidence of diastolic dysfunction (Figure 2(b)). The patient underwent stress testing with echocardiographic imaging five months after initial presentation, during which he completed 12 minutes (12.4 METS) of a Bruce protocol without exertional symptoms or ventricular ectopy. Echocardiographic imaging demonstrated an appropriate increase in myocardial contractility with exercise. Currently, nearly 12 months after his initial presentation, he remains asymptomatic on guideline-directed medical therapy (GDMT) for HF and combination immunosuppression with cyclosporine (goal trough level 100–120 ng/mL) and prednisone at a

maintenance dose of 5 mg daily. If symptoms recur, then repeat imaging with another endomyocardial biopsy may be required.

3. Discussion

Idiopathic GCM is a rare and often fatal disease [1]. Initial presentation can be one of rapidly progressive HF, ventricular arrhythmia, heart block, and/or symptoms mimicking acute coronary syndrome as seen in this case presentation [1, 2]. GCM is characterized histopathologically as a diffuse or multifocal inflammatory infiltrate with multinucleated giant cells associated with myocardial necrosis and an absence of sarcoid-like granulomas [1, 3]. Pathology remains the cornerstone of diagnosis [3]. Once the diagnosis is confirmed, there is considerable evidence to support the use of combined immunosuppression with calcineurin inhibition and corticosteroid therapy, as opposed to corticosteroids alone, in order to prolong transplant-free survival [1–4].

A rapid hemodynamic deterioration with declining LV systolic function and cardiogenic shock is the most obvious presentation of GCM requiring urgent consideration of inotropes, mechanical circulatory support, and transplant, in addition to immunotherapy [5–7]. The current report highlights the variability seen in the presentation of GCM. Our patient's initial presentation was not consistent with fulminant myocarditis, and although there was a rapid and severe decline in LV systolic function, he remained only mildly symptomatic with minimal signs of hemodynamic compromise. Such presentations can be misleading and may contribute to the underrecognition of GCM. Selected reports of GCM describe only mildly reduced LV systolic function in some patients while others had multiple admissions for HF prior to subsequent rapid ventricular deterioration [2, 5, 8, 9]. Cooper Jr. et al. reported that more than 50% of their GCM cohort had an EF > 45% at the time of diagnosis [9]. In addition, Kandolin et al. showed that 26% of their registry patients with confirmed GCM had an EF ≥ 50% [2].

A strong index of suspicion for GCM is required in the appropriate clinical context with less fulminant presentations, since the diagnosis has distinct implications for treatment and prognosis [3]. As shown in the Multicenter Giant Cell Myocarditis Registry, transplant-free survival is dismal without combined immunosuppression (1.8 months versus 33.5 months, $P < .001$) [1]. Although patients with preserved systolic function may have improved transplant-free survival compared to those patients with reduced LV function, relapse rates are high and recurrence has been described with discontinuation of immunotherapy up to 8 years following the initial diagnosis [2, 4, 9]. Current data support treatment with the combination of calcineurin inhibitors and corticosteroids, regardless of ventricular function [1–4]. Optimal treatment duration, however, remains undefined. Chronic immunosuppression is not without risks; it is associated with major adverse events and requires routine monitoring of renal function, bone density, prophylaxis for infection, and surveillance for neoplastic disease for those who survive in the long term.

4. Conclusion

GCM does not always present with rapid hemodynamic deterioration and cardiogenic shock but can also be diagnosed in patients with initially normal left ventricular function and among those with nonfulminant acute HF of uncertain etiology. Establishing the diagnosis of GCM is critical for the management and prognosis of the disease as combination immunosuppression versus corticosteroids alone significantly improves transplant-free survival [1–4, 9]. Current data suggest that GCM may be a life-long, chronic disease [2, 4]. Recommendations for long-term immunosuppression in asymptomatic patients who do not undergo cardiac transplantation remain undefined. Therefore, the risks and benefits of long-term immunotherapy should be considered and management decisions individualized.

Conflict of Interests

The authors declare that there is no conflict of interests regarding the publication of this paper.

Acknowledgment

The authors would like to thank Dr. Leslie Cooper for his expert opinion and review of this report.

References

[1] L. T. Cooper Jr., G. J. Berry, and R. Shabetai, "Idiopathic giant-cell myocarditis—natural history and treatment," *The New England Journal of Medicine*, vol. 336, no. 26, pp. 1860–1866, 1997.

[2] R. Kandolin, J. Lehtonen, K. Salmenkivi, A. Räisänen-Sokolowski, J. Lommi, and M. Kupari, "Diagnosis, treatment, and outcome of giant-cell myocarditis in the era of combined immunosuppression," *Circulation: Heart Failure*, vol. 6, no. 1, pp. 15–22, 2013.

[3] L. T. Cooper Jr. and C. Elamm, "Giant cell myocarditis: diagnosis and treatment," *Herz*, vol. 37, no. 6, pp. 632–636, 2012.

[4] L. T. Cooper, V. Orellana, J. Maleszewski, U. Kuhl, and H. P. Schultheiss, "Long term risk of death, transplantation. and disease recurrence in giant cell myocarditis," *Journal of the American College of Cardiology*, vol. 59, no. 13, supplement 1, abstract E1547, 2012.

[5] R. A. Davies, J. P. Veinot, S. Smith, C. Struthers, P. Hendry, and R. Masters, "Giant cell myocarditis: clinical presentation, bridge to transplantation with mechanical circulatory support, and long-term outcome," *Journal of Heart and Lung Transplantation*, vol. 21, no. 6, pp. 674–679, 2002.

[6] L. T. Cooper Jr., G. J. Berry, M. Rizeq, and J. S. Schroeder, "Giant cell myocarditis," *The Journal of Heart and Lung Transplantation*, vol. 14, no. 2, pp. 394–401, 1995.

[7] M. S. Nieminen, U.-S. Salminen, E. Taskinen, P. Heikkila, and J. Partanen, "Treatment of serious heart failure by transplantation in giant cell myocarditis diagnosed by endomyocardial biopsy," *The Journal of Heart and Lung Transplantation*, vol. 13, no. 3, pp. 543–545, 1994.

[8] V. V. Menghini, V. Savcenko, L. J. Olson et al., "Combined immunosuppression for the treatment of idiopathic giant cell myocarditis," *Mayo Clinic Proceedings*, vol. 74, no. 12, pp. 1221–1226, 1999.

[9] L. T. Cooper Jr., J. M. Hare, H. D. Tazelaar et al., "Usefulness of immunosuppression for giant cell myocarditis," *American Journal of Cardiology*, vol. 102, no. 11, pp. 1535–1539, 2008.

5

Malignant Course of Anomalous Left Coronary Artery Causing Sudden Cardiac Arrest: A Case Report and Review of the Literature

Mahesh Anantha Narayanan,[1] **Christopher DeZorzi,**[2] **Abhilash Akinapelli,**[3] **Toufik Mahfood Haddad,**[1] **Aiman Smer,**[2] **Janani Baskaran,**[4] **and William P. Biddle**[3]

[1]*Department of Internal Medicine, CHI Health Creighton University Medical Center, 601 North 30th Street No. 5800, Omaha, NE 68131, USA*
[2]*Creighton University School of Medicine, 2500 California Plaza, Omaha, NE 68102, USA*
[3]*Cardiac Center of Creighton University, 3006 Webster Street, Omaha, NE 68131, USA*
[4]*Sri Venkateshwaraa Medical College Hospital and Research Center, Puducherry 605102, India*

Correspondence should be addressed to Mahesh Anantha Narayanan; mahesh_maidsh@yahoo.com

Academic Editor: Expedito E. Ribeiro

Sudden cardiac arrest has been reported to occur in patients with congenital anomalous coronary artery disease. About 80% of the anomalies are benign and incidental findings at the time of catheterization. We present a case of sudden cardiac arrest caused by anomalous left anterior descending artery. 61-year-old African American female was brought to the emergency department after sudden cardiac arrest. Initial EKG showed sinus rhythm with RBBB and LAFB with nonspecific ST-T wave changes. Coronary angiogram revealed no atherosclerotic disease. The left coronary artery was found to originate from the right coronary cusp. Cardiac CAT scan revealed similar findings with interarterial and intramural course. Patient received one-vessel arterial bypass graft to her anomalous coronary vessel along with a defibrillator for secondary prevention. Sudden cardiac arrest secondary to congenital anomalous coronary artery disease is characterized by insufficient coronary flow by the anomalous left coronary artery to meet elevated left ventricular (LV) myocardial demand. High risk defects include those involved with the proximal coronary artery or coursing of the anomalous artery between the aorta and pulmonary trunk. Per guidelines, our patient received one vessel bypass graft to her anomalous vessel. It is important for clinicians to recognize such presentations of anomalous coronary artery.

1. Introduction

Sudden cardiac arrest (SCA) is a known complication of congenital coronary anomalies. In a large registry of 126,595 patients undergoing coronary angiogram, the incidence of coronary anomalies was 1.3% [1]. About 80% of coronary artery anomalies are benign and incidental findings at the time of catheterization [1]. Younger patients in their first three decades with isolated coronary artery anomalies are at risk of dying, especially with exercise [2]. Potentially serious anomalies which include ectopic coronary origin from the pulmonary artery or opposite aortic sinus, single coronary artery, and large coronary fistulae can result in angina pectoris, myocardial infarction, heart failure, arrhythmias, and SCA [1]. We hereby present a case of SCA in a middle aged female caused by anomalous coronary anatomy.

2. Case Presentation

A 61-year-old African American female with past medical history of unexplained syncope, refractory hypertension, and untreated obstructive sleep apnea was brought to the emergency room (ER) after she experienced a witnessed syncope and became unresponsive at home. When emergency medical

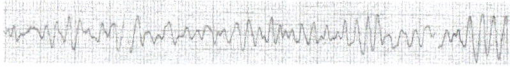

FIGURE 1: Ventricular fibrillation as the initial rhythm at presentation.

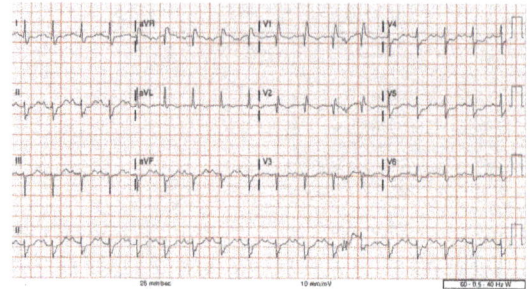

FIGURE 2: EKG showing sinus rhythm with right bundle branch block, left anterior fascicular block, and nonspecific ST-T wave changes.

service found the patient at home, the presenting rhythm was ventricular fibrillation (Figure 1) and patient was shocked twice with reversal of spontaneous circulation in less than 4 minutes. She was intubated and was taken to the ER. Her presenting blood pressure in the ER was 120/70 mmHg, and heart rate was 114/min. An electrocardiogram (EKG) showed sinus tachycardia, complete right bundle branch block (RBBB) with left anterior fascicular block (LAFB) and nonspecific ST-T wave changes (Figure 2). A bedside echocardiogram showed normal ejection fraction with severe left ventricular hypertrophy and no regional wall motion abnormalities. Initial labs drawn showed mild hypokalemia of 3.2 meq/L (normal value 3.5–5.5 meq/L), glomerular filtration rate of 47 mL/min/1.73 m^2, normal liver function tests, normal complete blood count, and a serum troponin of <0.04 ng/mL (normal value < 0.04 ng/mL). Coronary angiogram (Figure 3) revealed nonobstructive epicardial coronaries with mildly elevated left ventricular end diastolic pressure (LVEDP) of 21 mmHg. The left coronary artery (LCA) was found to originate from the right coronary sinus. Patient was started on hypothermia protocol. Her troponin started to rise peaking at 4.72 ng/mL. Computerized axial tomography (CAT) scan and magnetic resonance imaging (MRI) scan of head and electroencephalogram were normal. Patient achieved complete neurological recovery in three days. Cardiac coronary CAT scan (Figure 4) was obtained that showed anomalous left anterior descending artery (LAD) originating from the right coronary sinus sharing a common ostium with the right coronary artery (RCA). The artery then had an interarterial course between aorta and pulmonary trunk for 1.7 cm followed by an intramural course for 3.3 cm in the interventricular septum and then exited the myocardium for an epicardial course at the level of mid LAD. The intramural caliber measured 2.2 mm in cross section. The left main coronary artery had a normal origin giving rise to left circumflex and ramus intermedius. Patient underwent one vessel coronary artery bypass grafting with left internal mammary artery to the epicardial LAD at the level immediately after its intramural course. Patient then received implantable cardioverter and defibrillator (ICD) for secondary prevention and was discharged home on a stable condition.

3. Discussion

The prevalence of anomalous origin and course of coronary arteries is about 0.7–1.96% [3–5]. This includes a prevalence rate of 0.43% for the RCA branching from the left coronary sinus, the circumflex artery from the RCS or from the RCA, absence of the LMCA, and high takeoff coronary arteries [3]. Incidence of anomalous LAD artery from RCS is 0.03% which is 6 to 10 times less common than the origin of RCA from LCS [1].

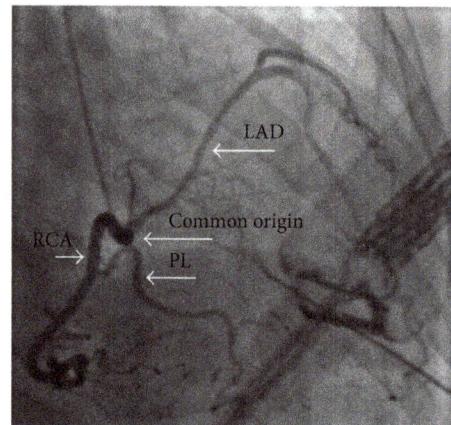

FIGURE 3: Coronary angiogram showing clear coronaries and anomalous left anterior descending artery originating from the right coronary cusp. RCA: right coronary artery; LAD: left anterior descending artery; PL: posterolateral branch.

Sudden cardiac arrest (SCA) secondary to congenital anomalous coronary artery disease occurs due to insufficient coronary flow by the anomalous LCA to meet elevated left ventricular myocardial metabolic demand, usually during exertion or exercise. In a majority of previously reported cases, SCA was triggered by exertion and most of these patients have a positive exercise stress test [6]. Contributing factors to an increased resistance in the LCA include compression between the great vessels, a slit ostium, myocardial bridging, or unfavorable geometry [7]. High risk defects include those involved with the proximal coronary artery or coursing of the anomalous artery between the aorta and pulmonary trunk [2]. Myocardial bridging refers to intramuscular course of the coronary vessels. Prevalence of myocardial bridging on coronary angiograms has been reported to be less than 5% [8], LAD being the most commonly involved artery.

In the review of 83 angiograms by Dodge Jr. et al., the left main coronary artery was found to be around 4.5 ± 0.5 mm in diameter, the proximal LAD was 3.7 ± 0.4 mm, and the distal LAD measured 1.9 ± 0.4 mm [9]. In our patient, the proximal LAD was buried in the septum with a diameter of 2.2 mm (half of its original diameter) and thus any increase in pressures in the left ventricle during exertion or stress might

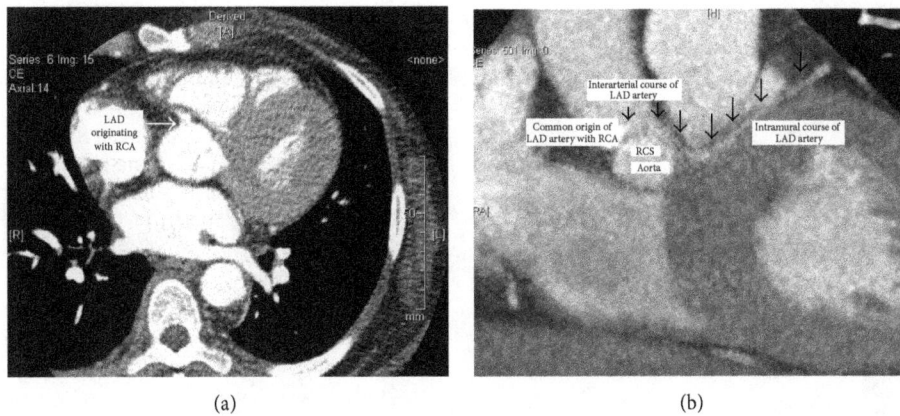

(a)   (b)

FIGURE 4: Cardiac coronary CAT scan demonstrating anomalous left coronary artery originating from the right coronary cusp and coursing between aorta and pulmonary artery followed by intramural course. LAD: left anterior descending artery; RCA: right coronary artery.

precipitate ischemia. This could be an explanation for our patient's similar episodes in the past but without sudden cardiac arrest.

Our patient's age was atypical for presentation of sudden cardiac arrest secondary anomalous coronary artery [2]. One possible explanation could be patient's uncontrolled hypertension contributing to progressive left ventricular hypertrophy, which could have caused demand ischemia, precipitating ventricular fibrillation, and SCA. We believe her LV myocardial thickness was not severe enough to precipitate ventricular fibrillation during her previous episodes, thus explaining her atypical presentation at a later age.

Quantitative scar grading with gadolinium MRI helps to assess the extent of infarction and likelihood of myocardial recovery after vascularization [10]. MRI evaluation is comparable and even better in diagnosis of subendocardial infarcts, when compared to PET scan, which is considered as the gold standard for myocardial viability evaluation [11]. In our patient, irrespective of myocardial viability assessment, a revascularization procedure was indicated, considering the episode of SCA and considering the anomalous vessel being LAD.

Documented coronary ischemia in the setting of an anomalous coronary artery coursing between aorta and pulmonary arteries is a class IB indication for surgery according to the American College of Cardiology and American Heart Association (ACC/AHA) guidelines for congenital heart diseases [12]. Exercise stress testing, though commonly employed for diagnosing coronary ischemia, is inadequate in predicting future risk of SCA in patients with anomalous coronaries [13, 14]. Guidelines also recommend surgical correction of anomalous coronary artery coursing between major vessels even in the absence of ischemia [12]. Percutaneous coronary intervention of anomalous intramural coronaries has been associated with poor durability with higher in-stent restenosis rates, coronary artery dissection/rupture, stent fracture, and stent thrombosis [15]. In a study done in pediatric population by Poynter et al., intramural course of the anomalous vessel was found in the majority of the patients who underwent surgery for anomalous coronary artery [16]. The standard surgical technique for treatment of anomalous coronary

artery is bypass grafting of the anomalous vessel alone or in combination with native vessel ligation [17], reimplantation of anomalous vessel into appropriate coronary sinus [18, 19], pulmonary artery translocation to increase the space between aorta and pulmonary artery [20], and proximal coronary artery patch enlargement [21]. Most recently, unroofing [22] of the anomalous coronary artery with or without detaching aortic valve commissure has been tried in patients without concomitant atherosclerotic coronary artery disease with favorable results. In our patient, reimplantation was not done because of the intra-arterial and intramural course of the artery, and so an end-to-side bypass of left internal mammary artery to the distal LAD was performed.

Though guidelines recommend ICD implantation in patients with SCA secondary to ventricular arrhythmias [12], there are no guidelines for ICD implantation after surgical correction of anomalous coronary vessel, especially in patients with preserved ejection fraction. In our patient, grafting cannot be done to the proximal LAD because of the long proximal interarterial and intramural course and so she received ICD for secondary prevention of malignant arrhythmias.

Since there is a possible genetic component [23, 24], a transthoracic echocardiogram has traditionally been recommended for first-degree relatives of patients with anomalous coronaries, since these patients will be asymptomatic and their EKG and physical examination will essentially be normal most of the time. Counselling was given to our patient regarding screening family members at the time of her discharge.

We reported a successful surgical repair of anomalous coronary artery causing SCA. Awareness of such presentations is essential among physicians for early recognition and treatment.

Abbreviations

SCA: Sudden cardiac arrest
LCA: Left coronary artery
LAD: Left anterior descending artery

RCA: Right coronary artery
ICD: Implantable cardioverter and defibrillator.

Conflict of Interests

The authors declare that they have no conflict of interests.

References

[1] O. Yamanaka and R. E. Hobbs, "Coronary artery anomalies in 126,595 patients undergoing coronary arteriography," *Catheterization and Cardiovascular Diagnosis*, vol. 21, no. 1, pp. 28–40, 1990.

[2] A. J. Taylor, K. M. Rogan, and R. Virmani, "Sudden cardiac death associated with isolated congenital coronary artery anomalies," *Journal of the American College of Cardiology*, vol. 20, no. 3, pp. 640–647, 1992.

[3] C. Erol and M. Seker, "Coronary artery anomalies: the prevalence of origination, course, and termination anomalies of coronary arteries detected by 64-detector computed tomography coronary angiography," *Journal of Computer Assisted Tomography*, vol. 35, no. 5, pp. 618–624, 2011.

[4] A. Yildiz, B. Okcun, T. Peker, C. Arslan, A. Olcay, and M. B. Vatan, "Prevalence of coronary artery anomalies in 12,457 adult patients who underwent coronary angiography," *Clinical Cardiology*, vol. 33, no. 12, pp. E60–E64, 2010.

[5] O. Safak, E. Gursul, M. Yesil et al., "Prevalence of coronary artery anomalies in patients undergoing coronary artery angiography: a review of 16768 patients. A retrospective, single-center study," *Minerva Cardioangiologica*, vol. 63, no. 2, pp. 113–120, 2015.

[6] C. Basso, B. J. Maron, D. Corrado, and G. Thiene, "Clinical profile of congenital coronary artery anomalies with origin from the wrong aortic sinus leading to sudden death in young competitive athletes," *Journal of the American College of Cardiology*, vol. 35, no. 6, pp. 1493–1501, 2000.

[7] C. R. Bartoli, W. B. Wead, G. A. Giridharan, S. D. Prabhu, S. C. Koenig, and R. D. Dowling, "Mechanism of myocardial ischemia with an anomalous left coronary artery from the right sinus of Valsalva," *Journal of Thoracic and Cardiovascular Surgery*, vol. 144, no. 2, pp. 402–408, 2012.

[8] S. Möhlenkamp, W. Hort, J. Ge, and R. Erbel, "Update on myocardial bridging," *Circulation*, vol. 106, no. 20, pp. 2616–2622, 2002.

[9] J. T. Dodge Jr., B. G. Brown, E. L. Bolson, and H. T. Dodge, "Lumen diameter of normal human coronary arteries. Influence of age, sex, anatomic variation, and left ventricular hypertrophy or dilation," *Circulation*, vol. 86, no. 1, pp. 232–246, 1992.

[10] S. Mavrogeni, K. Spargias, S. Karagiannis et al., "Anomalous origin of right coronary artery: magnetic resonance angiography and viability study," *International Journal of Cardiology*, vol. 109, no. 2, pp. 195–200, 2006.

[11] A. Wagner, H. Mahrholdt, T. A. Holly et al., "Contrast-enhanced MRI and routine single photon emission computed tomography (SPECT) perfusion imaging for detection of subendocardial myocardial infarcts: an imaging study," *The Lancet*, vol. 361, no. 9355, pp. 374–379, 2003.

[12] C. A. Warnes, R. G. Williams, T. M. Bashore et al., "ACC/AHA 2008 guidelines for the management of adults with congenital heart disease: a report of the American College of Cardiology/American Heart Association task force on practice guidelines (writing committee to develop guidelines on the management of adults with congenital heart disease). Developed in collaboration with the American Society of Echocardiography, Heart Rhythm Society, International Society for Adult Congenital Heart Disease, Society for Cardiovascular Angiography and Interventions, and Society of Thoracic Surgeons," *Journal of the American College of Cardiology*, vol. 52, no. 23, pp. e143–e263, 2008.

[13] P. Angelini, "Coronary artery anomalies—current clinical issues: definitions, classification, incidence, clinical relevance, and treatment guidelines," *Texas Heart Institute Journal*, vol. 29, no. 4, pp. 271–278, 2002.

[14] P. Angelini, J. A. Velasco, D. Ott, and G. R. Khoshnevis, "Anomalous coronary artery arising from the opposite sinus: descriptive features and pathophysiologic mechanisms, as documented by intravascular ultrasonography," *Journal of Invasive Cardiology*, vol. 15, no. 9, pp. 507–514, 2003.

[15] M. T. Corban, O. Y. Hung, P. Eshtehardi et al., "Myocardial bridging: contemporary understanding of pathophysiology with implications for diagnostic and therapeutic strategies," *Journal of the American College of Cardiology*, vol. 63, no. 22, pp. 2346–2355, 2014.

[16] J. A. Poynter, W. G. Williams, S. McIntyre et al., "Anomalous aortic origin of a coronary artery: a report from the congenital heart surgeons society registry," *World Journal for Pediatric and Congenital Hearth Surgery*, vol. 5, no. 1, pp. 22–30, 2014.

[17] M. Ono, D. A. Brown, and R. K. Wolf, "Two cases of anomalous origin of LAD from right coronary artery requiring coronary artery bypass," *Cardiovascular Surgery*, vol. 11, no. 1, pp. 90–92, 2003.

[18] F. Di Lello, J. F. Mnuk, R. J. Flemma, and D. C. Mullen, "Successful coronary reimplantation for anomalous origin of the right coronary artery from the left sinus of valsalva," *Journal of Thoracic and Cardiovascular Surgery*, vol. 102, no. 3, pp. 455–456, 1991.

[19] S. O. Rogers Jr., M. Leacche, T. Mihaljevic, J. D. Rawn, and J. G. Byrne, "Surgery for anomalous origin of the right coronary artery from the left aortic sinus," *Annals of Thoracic Surgery*, vol. 78, no. 5, pp. 1829–1831, 2004.

[20] M. D. Rodefeld, C. B. Culbertson, H. M. Rosenfeld, F. L. Hanley, and L. D. Thompson, "Pulmonary artery translocation: a surgical option for complex anomalous coronary artery anatomy," *Annals of Thoracic Surgery*, vol. 72, no. 6, pp. 2150–2152, 2001.

[21] P. V. Anagnostopoulos, F. A. Pigula, J. L. Myers, L. B. Beerman, R. D. Siewers, and S. K. Gandhi, "Autologous patch angioplasty of the left main coronary artery in a pediatric patient: 7-year follow-up," *Annals of Thoracic Surgery*, vol. 77, no. 4, pp. 1457–1459, 2004.

[22] J. E. Davies, H. M. Burkhart, J. A. Dearani et al., "Surgical management of anomalous aortic origin of a coronary artery," *Annals of Thoracic Surgery*, vol. 88, no. 3, pp. 844–848, 2009.

[23] J. A. Brothers, P. Stephens, J. W. Gaynor, R. Lorber, L. A. Vricella, and S. M. Paridon, "Anomalous aortic origin of a coronary artery with an interarterial course: should family screening be routine?" *Journal of the American College of Cardiology*, vol. 51, no. 21, pp. 2062–2064, 2008.

[24] J. M. Laureti, K. Singh, and J. Blankenship, "Anomalous coronary arteries: a familial clustering," *Clinical Cardiology*, vol. 28, no. 10, pp. 488–490, 2005.

6

Pulmonic Valve Repair in a Patient with Isolated Pulmonic Valve Endocarditis and Sickle Cell Disease

Timothy Glew,[1] Migdalia Feliciano,[2] Dennis Finkielstein,[1] Susan Hecht,[1] and Daryl Hoffman[3]

[1]*Department of Cardiology, Mount Sinai Beth Israel, New York, NY 10003, USA*
[2]*Department of Medicine, Mount Sinai Beth Israel, New York, NY 10003, USA*
[3]*Department of Cardiothoracic Surgery, Mount Sinai Beth Israel, New York, NY 10003, USA*

Correspondence should be addressed to Timothy Glew; tglew@chpnet.org

Academic Editor: Ramazan Akdemir

A 49-year-old woman with sickle cell disease presented with one month of exertional dyspnea, weakness, and fever and was diagnosed with isolated pulmonic valve endocarditis secondary to methicillin-resistant *Staphylococcus* bacteremia in the setting of a peripherally inserted central venous catheter. Chest computerized tomography showed multiple bilateral pulmonary nodular opacities consistent with septic emboli. Transthoracic and transesophageal echocardiograms revealed a large echodensity on the pulmonic valve requiring vegetation excision and pulmonic valve repair. In conclusion, isolated pulmonic valve endocarditis is a rare cause of infective endocarditis that warrants a high index of clinical suspicion. Furthermore the management of patients with sickle cell disease and endocarditis requires special consideration.

1. Introduction

Pulmonic valve infective endocarditis is uncommon, accounting for less than 1.5–2% of patients diagnosed with infective endocarditis [1]. Isolated pulmonic valve endocarditis even in the presence of structural heart disease is rare, with fewer than 90 cases previously reported. Risk factors for right sided endocarditis include intravenous drug abuse and central venous catheter or pacemaker implantation. We describe the first reported case of isolated pulmonic valve endocarditis requiring pulmonic valve repair in a patient with sickle cell disease.

2. Case Description

A 49-year-old African American woman with past medical history of sickle cell disease (Hgb SS) hypertension and transient ischemic attack was admitted to a community hospital for evaluation of shortness of breath, dyspnea on exertion, weakness, and fever of one-month duration.

Four months prior to admission the patient was found to have methicillin-resistant *Staphylococcus aureus* (MRSA) bacteremia for which a peripherally inserted central catheter (PICC) line was placed for long term intravenous (IV) vancomycin. A transthoracic echocardiogram (TTE) done at that time showed no evidence of endocarditis or significant valvular disease. Surveillance blood cultures were negative, she was transitioned to oral rifampin, and her PICC line was removed.

On the index admission to a community hospital, she presented with shortness of breath and fever to 102.4°F. A complete blood count showed leukocytosis (38,000 cells/mm^3), 92% neutrophils, and a microcytic anemia (Hgb 8.2 g/dL). She was found to be in sickle cell crisis. Two sets of blood cultures drawn on the day of admission grew MRSA and she was started on a sepsis protocol with intravenous vancomycin and aztreonam. An electrocardiogram (ECG) obtained revealed sinus tachycardia with nonspecific T wave abnormalities in the inferior leads. Her chest X-ray showed bilateral reticulonodular opacities in the mid to lower lung

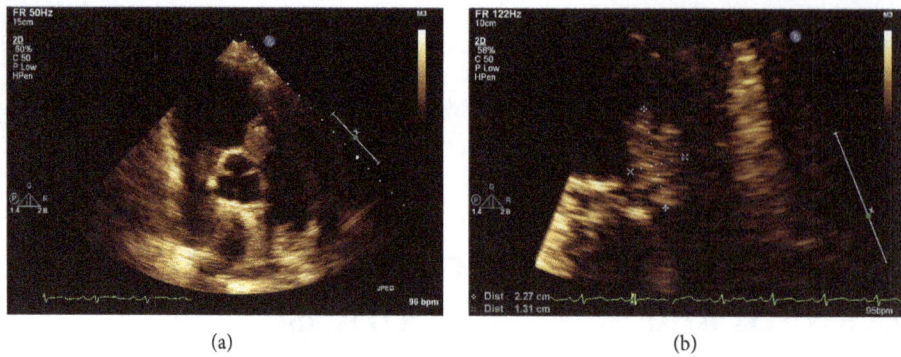

FIGURE 1: Transthoracic echocardiogram parasternal short axis showing a 2.2 × 1.31 cm echodensity on the pulmonic valve.

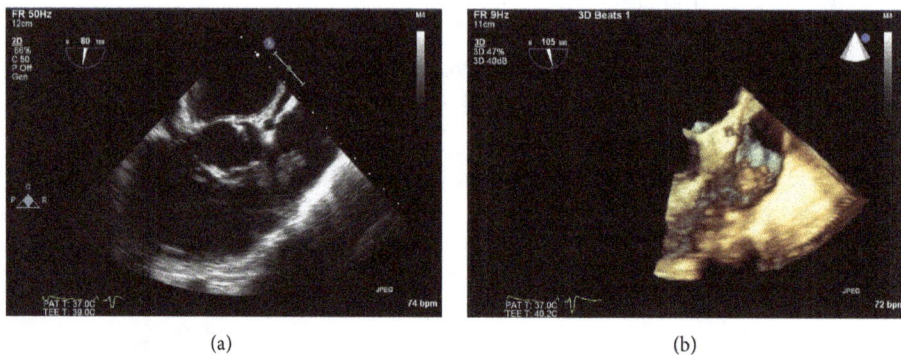

FIGURE 2: Transesophageal echocardiogram with a 2.4 × 1.8 cm echodense mobile mass seen on the pulmonic valve consistent with large vegetation in 2D and 3D views.

fields. A TTE report from day four at the community hospital revealed a normal left ventricular ejection fraction, no significant valvular disease, and no obvious vegetation.

Ten days after admission the patient developed respiratory distress and required endotracheal intubation and mechanical ventilation. Chest computerized tomography (CT) showed multiple bilateral pulmonary nodular opacities, with cavitations consistent with septic emboli. The patient was stabilized and transferred to our hospital for further management.

On admission to our hospital she was afebrile and had a previously undocumented 2/6 diastolic murmur over the pulmonary area, a leukocyte count of 15,900 cells/mm^3, and 75% neutrophils. A TTE was obtained which showed large vegetation on the pulmonic valve (2.3 × 1.3 cm) and trace pulmonic regurgitation (Figures 1(a) and 1(b)). She was continued on vancomycin and rifampin and repeat blood cultures were negative. Given the large size of the vegetation a transesophageal echocardiogram (TEE) was obtained for potential surgical planning. The TEE revealed a 2.4 × 1.8 cm echogenic mobile mass on the pulmonic valve, trace pulmonic regurgitation, and no other significant valvular pathology (Figures 2(a) and 2(b)).

At this time a multispecialty heart valve team was assembled that included cardiology, cardiothoracic surgery, cardiac anesthesiology, infectious disease, and hematology. The consensus was for a trial of conservative management;

however the patient had persistent leukocytosis and ongoing hemodynamic instability suggesting that antibiotic penetration might be limited. Ultimately the heart team recommended surgery. Her course was further complicated by respiratory distress requiring reintubation and surgery was delayed. Given her history of sickle cell disease an exchange transfusion was planned prior to surgery to reduce the percentage of Hemoglobin S but ultimately was not needed as preoperative transfusion corrected her anemia and reduced the HbS percentage to 28.7%.

Twenty-five days after her initial presentation she underwent pulmonic valve repair. While on cardiopulmonary bypass normothermia was maintained and 2.5 × 2 cm pulmonic valve vegetation was excised en bloc with the left cusp of the pulmonic valve (Figures 3(a) and 3(b)). The resected leaflet was replaced with glutaraldehyde treated bovine pericardial patch shaped to match one of the other pulmonic cusps and sewn into place along the annulus with a continuous polypropylene suture. The excised pulmonic valve vegetation was sent to pathology and revealed bacterial colonies in fibrinous exudates, consistent with bacterial endocarditis.

The patient was weaned off bypass with no evidence of pulmonic regurgitation on intraoperative TEE. The patient was extubated soon after surgery and had an uneventful postoperative course. Repeat postoperative blood cultures were negative. A postoperative TTE revealed a normal left

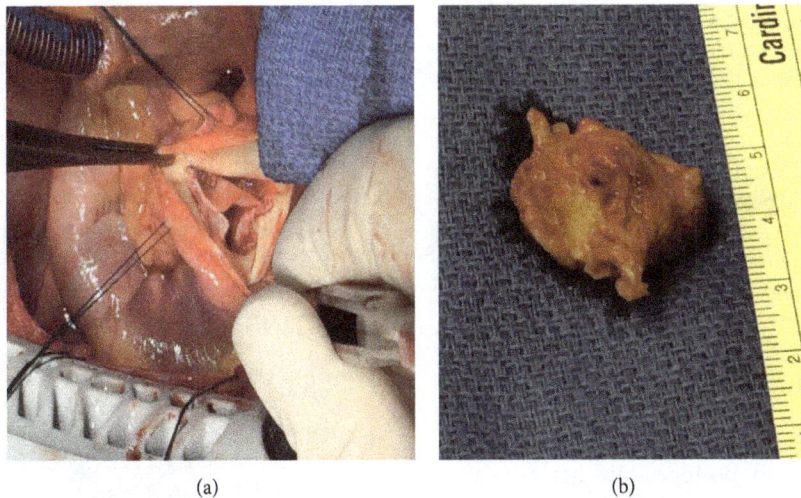

(a)   (b)

FIGURE 3: The pulmonic valve in vivo (a) and the excised valve leaflet (b).

ventricular size and systolic function and normal appearance of the pulmonic valve leaflets with trace pulmonic regurgitation. A six-week course of intravenous vancomycin was completed and her convalescence was uneventful.

3. Discussion

Right sided endocarditis is an uncommon entity, accounting for only 5–10% of all infective endocarditis cases, but the majority involve the tricuspid valve [2, 3]. Isolated pulmonic valve endocarditis is rare with as few as 45 cases reported in patients with structurally normal hearts [4, 5].

The rarity of infection of the pulmonic valve compared to other cardiac valves has been attributed to the lower pressure within the right heart, lower incidence of congenital malformations or acquired valvular abnormalities, lower oxygen content of venous blood, and the differences in the endothelial lining and vascularization of the valve [6, 7]. Risk factors for pulmonic valve endocarditis include intravenous drug abuse, alcoholism, sepsis, central venous catheter infection, pacemaker implantation with lead infection, gonorrhea, dental extraction, bowel surgery, liver or renal transplantation, and colonic angiodysplasia [3, 6, 7].

Patients present primarily with typical features of endocarditis such as fever and lethargy; the pulmonic regurgitant murmur is often a late feature [5]. Patients with right sided endocarditis may also present with pulmonary symptoms such as cough, dyspnea, and pleuritic chest pain in the setting of septic emboli. Transthoracic echocardiogram can detect pulmonic valve vegetation, but transesophageal echocardiography has higher sensitivity and specificity [5]. The most common microorganisms reported are *Staphylococcus aureus*, coagulase negative staphylococci, and group B streptococci. In the 45 reviewed cases of pulmonic valve endocarditis in a normal heart *Staphylococcus aureus* is the most common causative organism [5].

The majority of patients with pulmonic or tricuspid valve endocarditis are managed conservatively. Right sided endocarditis has a better prognosis and is more likely to respond to medical therapy than infection of the mitral and aortic valves. Parenteral antibiotic therapy is generally administered for 4–6 weeks. Results of retrospective studies suggest that vegetation less than 1 to 2 cm long in right sided endocarditis usually responds to medical treatment [8, 9]. Surgery is indicated when there is persistent bacteremia despite appropriate antimicrobial therapy, progressive valve destruction and incompetence, locally invasive infection including abscess formation, or relapsing infection after completion of a full course of antibiotic therapy. It is recommended that infection with *Staphylococcus*, the presence of vegetation larger than 2 cm long, or cardiovascular instability should prompt consideration of early surgical intervention in patients with pulmonic valve endocarditis [10]. Surgical options include debridement of the infected area, vegetation excision with either valve preservation or valve repair or valve replacement. In cases where pulmonic valve replacement is unavoidable the use of a homograft or xenograft is recommended; however small studies suggest that mechanical valve prostheses in the pulmonic position may perform well [6, 11].

It is important to note that in our case the pulmonic vegetation was not reported on the preliminary echocardiogram performed at the outside hospital. The pulmonic valve is often not well visualized on TTE making the diagnosis of pulmonic endocarditis difficult. The pulmonic valve is best visualized in the RV outflow view. This view is obtained from the parasternal long-axis position by tilting the transducer superiorly and laterally (towards the left shoulder of the patient). Making an effort to visualize the pulmonic valve is crucial in patients in whom endocarditis is suspected.

Our patient's case is unique, in that no case has ever been reported in the literature of pulmonic valve endocarditis in a patient with sickle cell disease. Patients with sickle cell disease often require long term intravenous access which is a well-recognized risk factor for right sided endocarditis. Furthermore, the operative management of patients with sickle cell disease and endocarditis requires special consideration.

Surgical interventions, especially cardiac surgery, in sickle cell disease patients are associated with high morbidity and mortality [12–16]. Specific precautions are required during the perioperative period to minimize the surgical risks. Patients with sickle cell disease who require cardiac surgery are at risk of a fatal sickling crisis, induced by acidosis, hypothermia, hypoxia, or low flow states. Low oxygen tension and acidosis can induce sickling in patients on cardiopulmonary bypass and may trigger a crisis of profound magnitude [12–16]. While performing cardiac surgery, cardiopulmonary bypass, aortic cross clamping, low flow states, hypothermia, cold cardioplegia, and use of vasoconstrictive agents may predispose a crisis state [12]. To manage sickle cell patients, it is essential to maintain adequate blood flow and oxygen tension during cardiopulmonary bypass, avoid acidosis, control intra- and postoperative hemodynamic parameters, maintain hematocrit level of 20–30%, optimize electrolytes and blood gases, and minimize postoperative pain [12–16]. It is preferable to avoid hypothermia which can cause vasoconstriction and trigger a vasoocclusive crisis; however a number of studies have employed mild to moderate cooling without adverse effects [12–16]. Partial exchange transfusions during the pre- or intraoperative period are often recommended in cardiac patients to reduce the percentage of Hemoglobin S. In our case the patient did not require an exchange transfusion and normothermia was maintained to avoid vasoconstriction and sickling.

In general the implantation of prosthetic valves in patients with sickle cell disease is particularly problematic. Mechanical prostheses require systemic anticoagulation and may cause increased hemolysis and subsequent sickle cell crises. While bioprosthetic valves are the preferred type of prosthesis, the risk of infection of prosthetic material may expose these already vulnerable patients to recurrent endocarditis. Ideally these patients should undergo valve repair if surgically feasible. Furthermore it is recommended that any patient with infective endocarditis be evaluated and managed by a multispecialty heart valve team. In consultation with our heart valve team our patient underwent successful pulmonic valve repair and had an uncomplicated postoperative course. This unique case highlights the significance of performing a complete echocardiographic evaluation in any patient with suspected endocarditis and the importance of assembling a heart valve team to help guide treatment decisions in patients with infective endocarditis.

Conflict of Interests

The authors declare that there is no conflict of interests regarding the publication of this paper.

References

[1] R. S. Cassling, W. C. Rogler, and B. M. McManus, "Isolated pulmonic valve infective endocarditis: a diagnostically elusive entity," *The American Heart Journal*, vol. 109, no. 3, pp. 558–567, 1985.

[2] F. Delahaye, V. Goulet, F. Lacassin et al., "Characteristics of infective endocarditis in France in 1991: a 1-year survey," *European Heart Journal*, vol. 16, no. 3, pp. 394–401, 1995.

[3] J. T. M. van der Meer, J. Thompson, H. A. Valkenburg, and M. F. Michel, "Epidemiology of bacterial endocarditis in the Netherlands: I. Patient characteristics," *Archives of Internal Medicine*, vol. 152, no. 9, pp. 1863–1868, 1992.

[4] K. Nishida, O. Fukuyama, and D. S. Nakamura, "Pulmonary valve endocarditis caused by right ventricular outflow obstruction in association with sinus of valsalva aneurysm: a case report," *Journal of Cardiothoracic Surgery*, vol. 3, article 46, 2008.

[5] R. A. Schroeder, "Pulmonic valve endocarditis in a normal heart," *Journal of the American Society of Echocardiography*, vol. 18, no. 2, pp. 197–198, 2005.

[6] M. P. Ranjith, K. F. Rajesh, G. Rajesh et al., "Isolated pulmonary valve endocarditis: a case report and review of literature," *Journal of Cardiology Cases*, vol. 8, no. 5, pp. 161–163, 2013.

[7] F. B. Ramadan, D. S. Beanlands, and I. G. Burwash, "Isolated pulmonic valve endocarditis in healthy hearts: a case report and review of the literature," *Canadian Journal of Cardiology*, vol. 16, no. 10, pp. 1282–1288, 2000.

[8] M. J. Robbins, R. W. M. Frater, R. Soeiro, W. H. Frishman, and J. A. Strom, "Influence of vegetation size on clinical outcome of right-sided infective endocarditis," *The American Journal of Medicine*, vol. 80, no. 2, pp. 165–171, 1986.

[9] S. R. Hecht and M. Berger, "Right-sided endocarditis in intravenous drug users: prognostic features in 102 episodes," *Annals of Internal Medicine*, vol. 117, no. 7, pp. 560–566, 1992.

[10] N. Kang, W. Smith, S. Greaves, and D. Haydock, "Pulmonary-valve endocarditis," *The New England Journal of Medicine*, vol. 356, no. 21, pp. 2224–2225, 2007.

[11] T. W. Waterbolk, E. S. Hoendermis, I. J. den Hamer, and T. Ebels, "Pulmonary valve replacement with a mechanical prosthesis. Promising results of 28 procedures in patients with congenital heart disease," *European Journal of Cardio-Thoracic Surgery*, vol. 30, no. 1, pp. 28–32, 2006.

[12] K. E. Al-Ebrahim, "Cardiac surgery and sickle cell disease," *Asian Cardiovascular and Thoracic Annals*, vol. 16, no. 6, pp. 479–482, 2008.

[13] S. M. Yousafzai, M. Ugurlucan, O. A. Al Radhwan, A. L. Al Otaibi, and C. C. Canver, "Open heart surgery in patients with sickle cell hemoglobinopathy," *Circulation*, vol. 121, no. 1, pp. 14–19, 2010.

[14] D. Métras, A. O. Coulibaly, K. Ouattara, A. Longechaud, P. Millet, and J. Chauvet, "Open-heart surgery in sickle-cell haemoglobinopathies: report of 15 cases," *Thorax*, vol. 37, no. 7, pp. 486–491, 1982.

[15] S. Balasundaram, C. G. Duran, Z. Al-Halees, and M. Kassay, "Cardiopulmonary bypass in sickle cell anaemia. Report of five cases," *Journal of Cardiovascular Surgery*, vol. 32, no. 2, pp. 271–274, 1991.

[16] K. Frimpong-Boateng, A. G. B. Amoah, H.-M. Barwasser, and C. Kallen, "Cardiopulmonary bypass in sickle cell anaemia without exchange transfusion," *European Journal of Cardio-thoracic Surgery*, vol. 14, no. 5, pp. 527–529, 1998.

7

Aneurysm of the Left Coronary Artery in Postoperative Bland-White-Garland Syndrome

Nathalie Jeanne Magioli Bravo-Valenzuela[1] and Guilherme Ricardo Nunes Silva[2]

[1]Pediatrics Department, University of Taubaté, 12020-130 Taubaté, SP, Brazil
[2]University of Taubaté, 12020-130 Taubaté, SP, Brazil

Correspondence should be addressed to Nathalie Jeanne Magioli Bravo-Valenzuela; njmbravo@cardiol.br

Academic Editor: Tayfun Sahin

We report a case of anomalous left coronary artery from the pulmonary artery (ALCAPA) or Bland-White-Garland syndrome, present the challenges of performing a differential diagnosis, and discuss the treatment of the syndrome. Although ALCAPA is a rare congenital heart disease, it is one of the most common causes of myocardial ischemia in childhood and presents a diagnostic challenge. A four-year-old girl was referred to a pediatric cardiologist for evaluation of mitral valve regurgitation murmur and heart failure. The transthoracic echocardiogram demonstrated the left coronary artery (LCA) not arising from the aorta, presence of coronary collateral circulation, and moderate mitral valve regurgitation. ALCAPA was confirmed using angiotomography. The LCA was surgically reimplanted into the aorta. After 3 years of postoperative follow-up, the patient developed an LCA aneurysm. Diagnosis of cardiac ischemia in childhood remains a challenge, and careful evaluation of coronary arteries on the echocardiogram is an important tool. In this report, we present a case of ALCAPA with an uncommon postoperative outcome.

1. Introduction

Anomalous left coronary artery from the pulmonary artery (ALCAPA) or Bland-White-Garland syndrome is a rare congenital heart disease accounting for 0.25–0.5% of all congenital heart diseases [1]. It is one of the most common causes of myocardial ischemia in childhood and, if left untreated, it is potentially fatal with a mortality rate of 80–90% within the first year of life [2].

The most common clinical presentation of ALCAPA includes paroxysm of crying, pallor, diaphoresis, and signs of heart failure in infants. Diagnosis of myocardial ischemia in childhood presents a challenge and is commonly misdiagnosed as colic in infants. In cases in which cardiac ischemia does not develop into a lethal event, it can cause dilated cardiomyopathy, heart failure, and/or mitral valve regurgitation, as in the case reported here. In 10–15% of cases, patients remain asymptomatic until a sudden lethal event occurs after intense physical activity, as a result of cardiac ischemia. The clinical course depends on the degree

of collateral vessels between the coronaries, which allows patients to survive till adulthood [3].

Dual coronary repair by direct aortic reimplantation is the treatment of choice for ALCAPA, and surgery should be performed as soon as the diagnosis is confirmed. Long-term results are satisfactory and the risk of late stenosis or occlusion of the reimplanted coronary is lower. However, the development of left coronary artery (LCA) aneurysm after surgical correction of ALCAPA is extremely rare [4].

This is a case report of a pediatric patient who presented two years after repaired ALCAPA (direct reimplantation of the LCA into the aorta) with an aneurysm of the LCA diagnosed on echocardiography, focusing on the difficulties of this diagnosis.

2. Case Presentation

A four-year-old girl was referred to a pediatric cardiologist due to low weight and heart murmur. She was born 38 weeks into gestation by cesarean section and weighed 2.915 g, with

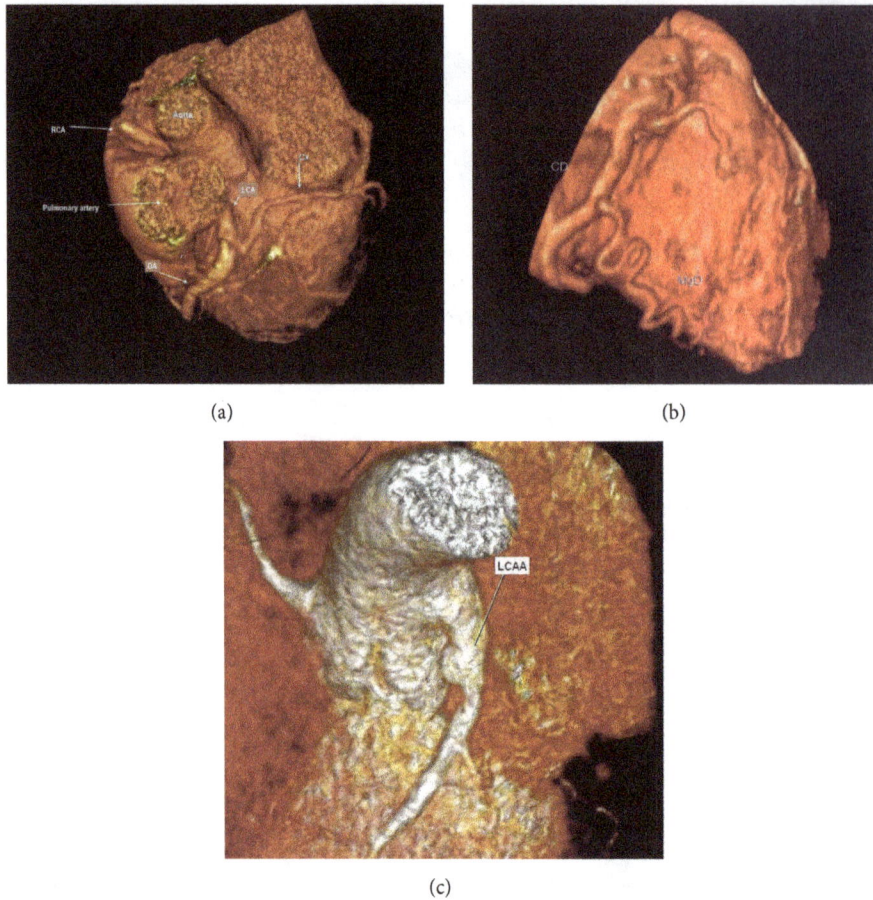

(a)

(b)

(c)

FIGURE 1: (a) Computed tomography (CT) angiography showing the left coronary artery (LC) from the pulmonary trunk (RCA: right coronary artery; AD: anterior descending artery; and Cx: circumflex artery). (b) CT angiotomography showing the coronary collateral network. (c) CT angiotomography showing the left coronary artery aneurysm.

an Apgar score of 9 at 1 min as well as at 5 min. During the first 2-3 months after birth, the parents related that she experienced episodes of pallor and irritability, which were diagnosed as infant colic.

At first evaluation, the child was acyanotic and weighed less for her age (Z-score = −2) based on WHO growth charts and presented symptoms of exercise intolerance. The heart rate was 129 beats/min, and blood pressure was 90/60 mmHg. Cardiac auscultation showed normal heart sounds (S1 and S2) and a systolic murmur (grade 3/6) at mitral area with radiation to the axilla.

The initial electrocardiogram (ECG) showed sinus rhythm at 135 beats/min, normal QTc (0.42 s), signs of left ventricular enlargement, negative and deeply inverted T waves at V4-5-6, with normal Q waves. Chest radiography demonstrated cardiomegaly. Transthoracic echocardiogram (TTE) revealed left ventricular dilatation with normal systolic function, moderate mitral valve regurgitation, flow from the LCA to the pulmonary trunk on color Doppler, and diffuse ectasia of right coronary artery (RCA) with coronary collateral circulation. ALCAPA was confirmed by coronary computed tomography (CT) angiography (Figures 1(a) and 1(b)).

The child was successfully operated on with direct reimplantation of the LCA into the aorta. The ostium of the LCA was excised with a button of surrounding pulmonary artery tissue, and the pulmonary artery was transected. The LCA was well mobilized to the left side of the aortic root, ensuring no tension or kinking of the artery. The defect in the pulmonary artery was repaired with a pericardial patch. Postoperative TTE showed LCE connected to the aorta with normal flow, mild mitral valve regurgitation, and normal left ventricle ejection fraction (Simpson's method). After a period of 6 months, the antiplatelet drug (aspirin) was discontinued. After a 3-year follow-up, the patient presented an episode of chest pain during physical activity. ECG showed T waves at V4-5-6 and normal troponin T levels (0.06; normal < 0.014). TTE revealed the presence of a saccular aneurysm of LCA (6.5×8 mm/0.4 cm^2). A coronary CT angiography showed no stenosis or thrombus and a coronary aneurysm type IV at the point of LCA-aorta anastomosis (Figure 1(c)). Tests for possible systemic diseases related to the coronary aneurysm were negative, showing normal blood cells, normal erythrocyte sedimentation rate, normal PTT, anti-DNA and anticardiolipin negatives, and normal levels of C3, C4, CH50, and C-reactive protein. Screenings for

TABLE 1: Key distinguishing features of dilated coronary arteries (LCA: left coronary artery; RCA: right coronary artery). Adapted from Peña et al. [3].

Disease	Imaging findings	Differentiating features
ALCAPA	Flow from LCA to pulmonary artery	LCA arises from the main pulmonary artery
Coronary artery dilatation related to atherosclerosis	Diffuse coronary artery dilatation	Atherosclerotic plaque
Kawasaki disease	Multiple coronary artery aneurysms	Young children with fever and exanthema
Coronary artery-coronary sinus fistula	Tortuous coronary artery plus dilated coronary veins and sinus	Arteriovenous communication
Takayasu arteritis	Coronary artery aneurysms and stenosis	Involves the aorta and great vessels

atherosclerotic diseases and genetic syndromes were also negative. In order to evaluate cardiac perfusion, a rest-exercise stress myocardial scintigraphy was obtained, which was also normal. The patient is currently asymptomatic and is taking aspirin and a beta-blocker. High-impact, competitive, and collision sports were prohibited and stress tests have been performed annually to guide recommendations for physical activities.

3. Discussion

ALCAPA or Bland-White-Garland syndrome is an extremely rare congenital heart disease with an estimated occurrence of 1 in 300.000 live births. Although it is generally an isolated defect, approximately 5% of the cases can be associated with other cardiac anomalies [5]. Similar to colic in infants, the myocardial ischemia may present as paroxysms of pallor and irritability and should be suspected when those signs are associated with heart failure, ECG changes, and cardiomegaly [3].

In pediatric patients, the TTE is considered as the main noninvasive diagnostic method of investigation [6]. Real-time 3D echocardiography represents a new approach to improve the cardiac images in the conventional TTE. Diagnostic criteria for ALCAPA using echocardiography include: a dilated RCA, a reversed color Doppler flow from the LCA to the pulmonary artery, and a prominent septal flow from collateralization. The diagnosis must be confirmed by identifying the origin of the LCA from the pulmonary trunk [3]. Other noninvasive methods include CT or magnetic resonance coronary angiography with excellent accuracy in assessing the origin of LCA anomalies [7]. Cardiac catheterization should be indicated to establish the diagnosis when other noninvasive methods fail. Furthermore, myocardial scintigraphy is the preferred method to approach myocardial viability and risk stratification in coronary artery disease. Currently, most stress myocardial scintigraphy is performed using ECG-gated single-photon emission computed tomography (SPECT) for simultaneous evaluation of myocardial perfusion and cardiac function [5, 7].

Once ALCAPA is diagnosed, early surgical treatment is critical to correct the defect and prevent complications. The preferred surgical method is restoring the dual coronary system [8]. In children, surgical repair of choice is reimplantation with translocation of the LCA from the pulmonary artery to the aorta. During ALCAPA repair, the LCA must be well mobilized to avoid tension or kinking of the coronary artery and prevent postoperative complications, such as stenosis or occlusion of the reimplanted coronary and cardiac ischemia. If direct reimplantation of the LCA is not possible, it can be connected to the aorta by an intrapulmonary tunnel such as the Takeuchi technique [9, 10]. Other surgical options include simple ligation of the LCA and bypasses using saphenous vein or arteries grafts. In general, the patients showed improvement in mitral valve regurgitation and left ventricular function after the surgical correction, mainly when the operation was performed under 1 year of age [10]. Although it has ever been described a case of a giant coronary artery in an adult patient after Takeuchi repair, the finding of coronary aneurysm in a reimplanted LCA for ALCAPA is extremely rare and unexpected [4].

Atherosclerotic aneurysms, Kawasaki disease, Takayasu arteritis, and coronary artery fistula are possible differential diagnoses with ALCAPA by dilatation of the coronary artery. Important aspects of each of these diseases are described in Table 1 [3].

Clinical management of coronary aneurysm consists of attempts to prevent thromboembolic complications. Long-term antiplatelet therapy is recommended for patients with small to medium (>3 mm but <6 mm) coronary artery aneurysm, as in the case reported. Adjunctive therapy with antithrombotic regimen is recommended for patients with large aneurysm (>6 mm) and patients in whom coronary artery contains multiple aneurysms [11]. Classification of coronary artery dilatation is described in Table 2.

The presence of a dilated LCA after surgical correction of ALCAPA could be related to stenosis at the anastomosis site (LCA-aorta) as a compensatory distal dilatation in order to provide flow to this area [5]. However, in the present case, the aneurysm of the LCA developed without proximal stenosis after a successful surgical reimplantation repair, resulting in a rare outcome [4].

TABLE 2: Group and type of dilatation of coronary arteries.

Type and group	Findings
Saccular aneurysm	Transverse > longitudinal diameter
Fusiform aneurysm	Longitudinal < transverse diameter
Type	
I	Diffuse ectasia in 2 or 3 vessels
II	Diffuse ectasia in 1 vessel and localized aneurysm in another
III	Diffuse ectasia in only 1 vessel
IV	Coronary aneurysm in 1 vessel

Conflict of Interests

The authors declare that there is no conflict of interests regarding the publication of this paper.

References

[1] E. F. Bland, P. D. White, and J. Garland, "Congenital anomalies of the coronary arteries: report of an unusual case associated with cardiac hypertrophy," *American Heart Journal*, vol. 8, no. 6, pp. 787–801, 1933.

[2] J. W. Kirklin and B. G. Barratt-Boyes, "Congenital anomalies of the coronary arteries," in *Cardiac Surgery*, J. W. Kirklin and B. G. Barratt-Boyes, Eds., pp. 945–969, John Wiley, New York, NY, USA, 1986.

[3] E. Peña, E. T. Nguyen, N. Merchant, and C. Dennie, "ALCAPA syndrome: not just a pediatric disease," *Radiographics*, vol. 29, no. 2, pp. 553–565, 2009.

[4] S. M. Dunlay, C. R. Bonnichsen, J. A. Dearani, and C. A. Warnes, "Giant coronary artery aneurysm after takeuchi repair for anomalous left coronary artery from the pulmonary artery," *The American Journal of Cardiology*, vol. 113, no. 1, pp. 193–195, 2014.

[5] M. Díaz-Zamudio, U. Bacilio-Pérez, M. C. Herrera-Zarza et al., "Coronary artery aneurysms and ectasia: role of coronary CT angiography," *Radiographics*, vol. 29, no. 7, pp. 1939–1954, 2009.

[6] D. Ropers, W. Moshage, W. G. Daniel, J. Jessl, M. Gottwik, and S. Achenbach, "Visualization of coronary artery anomalies and their anatomic course by contrast-enhanced electron beam tomography and three-dimensional reconstruction," *The American Journal of Cardiology*, vol. 87, no. 2, pp. 193–197, 2001.

[7] M. S. Cohen, R. J. Herlong, and N. H. Silverman, "Echocardiographic imaging of anomalous origin of the coronary arteries.," *Cardiology in the Young*, vol. 20, pp. 26–34, 2010.

[8] R. Bunton, R. A. Jonas, P. Lang, A. J. Rein, and A. R. Castaneda, "Anomalous origin of left coronary artery from pulmonary artery. Ligation versus establishment of a two coronary artery system," *Journal of Thoracic and Cardiovascular Surgery*, vol. 93, no. 1, pp. 103–108, 1987.

[9] S. Takeuchi, H. Imamura, K. Katsumoto et al., "New surgical method for repair of anomalous left coronary artery from pulmonary artery," *Journal of Thoracic and Cardiovascular Surgery*, vol. 78, no. 1, pp. 7–11, 1979.

[10] G. Michielon, D. Di Carlo, G. Brancaccio et al., "Anomalous coronary artery origin from the pulmonary artery: correlation between surgical timing and left ventricular function recovery," *Annals of Thoracic Surgery*, vol. 76, no. 2, pp. 581–588, 2003.

[11] J. W. Newburger, M. Takahashi, M. A. Gerber et al., "Diagnosis, treatment, and long-term management of kawasaki disease: a statement for health professionals from the Committee on Rheumatic Fever, Endocarditis and Kawasaki Disease, Council on Cardiovascular Disease in the Young, American Heart Association," *Circulation*, vol. 110, no. 11, pp. 2747–2771, 2004.

8

A Large Intra-Abdominal Hiatal Hernia as a Rare Cause of Dyspnea

Cem Sahin,[1] Fatih Akın,[2] Nesat Cullu,[3] Burak Özseker,[4] İsmail Kirli,[1] and İbrahim Altun[2]

[1]*Department of Internal Medicine, School of Medicine, Mugla Sıtkı Kocman University, Orhaniye Mahallesi İsmet Catak Caddesi, Merkez, 48000 Mugla, Turkey*

[2]*Department of Cardiology, School of Medicine, Mugla Sıtkı Kocman University, Orhaniye Mahallesi İsmet Catak Caddesi, Merkez, 48000 Mugla, Turkey*

[3]*Department of Radiology, School of Medicine, Mugla Sıtkı Kocman University, Orhaniye Mahallesi İsmet Catak Caddesi, Merkez, 48000 Mugla, Turkey*

[4]*Department of Gastroenterology, School of Medicine, Mugla Sıtkı Kocman University, Orhaniye Mahallesi İsmet Catak Caddesi, Merkez, 48000 Mugla, Turkey*

Correspondence should be addressed to Cem Sahin; cemsahin@mu.edu.tr

Academic Editor: Jesus Peteiro

Giant hiatal hernias, generally seen at advanced ages, can rarely cause cardiac symptoms such as dyspnea and chest pain. Here, we aimed to present a case with a large hiatal hernia that largely protruded to intrathoracic cavity and caused dyspnea, particularly at postprandial period, by compressing the left atrium and right pulmonary vein. We considered presenting this case as large hiatal hernia is a rare, intra-abdominal cause of dyspnea.

1. Introduction

Hiatal hernia is defined as abnormal protrusion of stomach with another intra-abdominal organ, in some cases, above diaphragm from esophageal hiatus. Its prevalence has been reported as 0.8–2.9% in upper gastrointestinal endoscopy series. Symptoms are often *related to* gastroesophageal reflux disease in the hiatal hernia which is usually asymptomatic. However, although rarely seen, a hiatal hernia can cause atypical symptoms such as chest pain or dyspnea due to the extent of hernia and organs protruded into thorax cavity. Here, we aimed to present a case with a hiatal hernia that largely protruded into thorax cavity and compressed left atrium, causing dyspnea.

2. Case Presentation

An 84-year-old woman presented to the outpatient clinic with increasing fatigue, shortness of breath, and blackening of the stool over 1 month. She noted that shortness of breath aggravated with exertion and after the ingestion of food.

The patient did not describe an underlying chronic disease and did not use any medication within the previous 6 months. On the physical examination, vital signs were stable and pallor was observed at conjunctiva. No abnormal physical examination finding was observed in the patient other than systolic murmur at apex on the cardiac examination. In the laboratory evaluations, the following results were obtained: WBC, 7400/mm^3; Hgb, 10.9 g/dL; MCV, 72.3 fL; Plt, 376.000/mm^3; iron, 18 μg/dL; iron binding capacity, 350 μg/dL; ferritin, 3,7 ng/mL. Fecal occult blood test was positive. Biochemical parameters were found to be within the normal range. On the posterioanterior chest radiograph, increased cardiothoracic index, enlarged mediastinum, and a mass appearance with an air-fluid level superposed with cardiac contours were observed (Figure 1). A thoracoabdominal CT scan including axial and coronal sections was performed in the patient because of the suspicion of a large hiatal hernia with available image. It was found that a large part of the stomach was herniated into mediastinum without any finding of incarceration and gastrointestinal obstruction and that

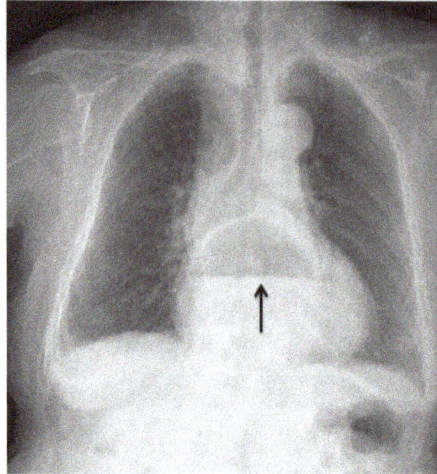

FIGURE 1: Appearance of air-fluid level superposed with cardiac contour on posterioanterior chest radiograph.

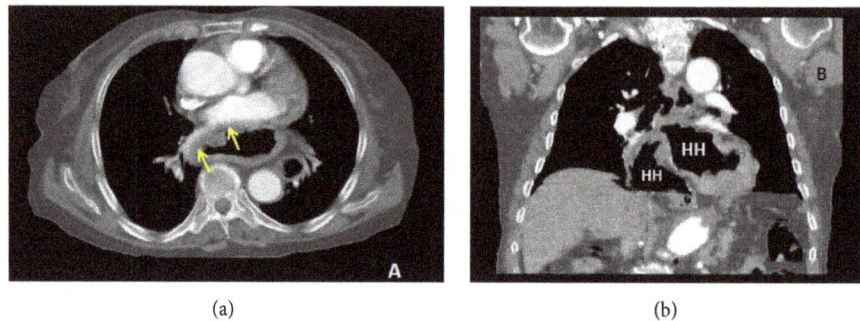

(a)   (b)

FIGURE 2: Axial and coronal images of the hiatal hernia on thoracoabdominal CT scan. (a) Compression to left atrium and right pulmonary vein by hiatal hernia on axial plane (yellow arrow); (b) herniation of majority of stomach into thorax cavity on coronal plane; HH: hiatal hernia.

hiatal hernia *compressed the* posterior wall of the left atrium and the right pulmonary vein (Figure 2).

On the upper gastrointestinal endoscopy, there were linear erosions at esophagogastric junction where hiatal hernia and diaphragmatic compression occurred. Active gastrointestinal bleeding was not observed. *Colonoscopy was considered normal,* which was performed for the etiology of iron deficiency anemia. On the transthoracic echocardiography, it was found that the left ventricle systolic and diastolic functions were normal, while the posterior wall of the left atrium was severely compressed by a large mass (Figure 3(a)). Systolic pulmonary artery pressure was estimated as high (42 mmHg) on echocardiography. As there was an increase in dyspnea after heavy meals according to anamnesis, postprandial transthoracic echocardiography was performed which revealed *an increase in the compression of the left atrium due to the hiatal hernia* (Figure 3(b)). Postprandial increase in dyspnea was attributed to the pulmonary congestion caused by the compression to the left atrium and the right pulmonary vein. Nutritional recommendations were given to the patient who denied surgical intervention due to the advanced age. A proton pump inhibitor and a motility regulator were prescribed. Hemogram was found to be normal 3 months

after iron reemplacement therapy and the patient had an uneventful course.

3. Discussion

Hiatal hernia is defined as abnormal protrusion of stomach with another intra-abdominal organ, in some cases, above diaphragm from esophageal hiatus [1]. Type I hiatal hernia (sliding type) is the most commonly observed type in which gastroesophageal junction slides together with a part of the stomach [2]. Although the cause for the development of hiatal hernia is unknown, its incidence increases by advancing age [3]. It is accepted that relaxation at diaphragmatic crura resulting from aging process is the cause for the observation of more frequent and larger hiatal hernias in elder population [4]. *Symptoms are often related to gastroesophageal reflux disease* in hiatal hernias which is usually asymptomatic. Generally, older people are unable to describe typical reflux symptoms such as burning at chest, acid regurgitation, and epigastric pain. Gastrointestinal bleeding related to ulcer or erosion, iron deficiency anemia, mucosal prolapse, incarceration, and volvulus are the main complications of hiatal

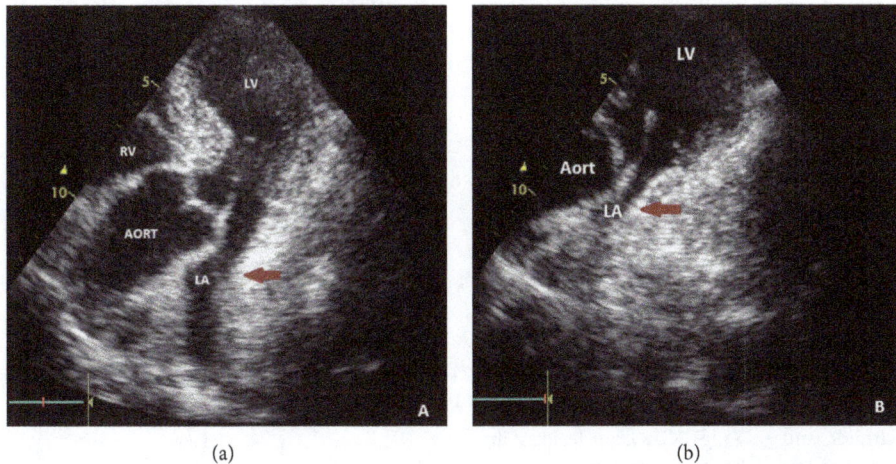

FIGURE 3: Transthoracic echocardiographic images of left atrial compression. Extrinsic compression to posterior wall of left atrium by hiatal hernia (red arrow). (a) Transthoracic echocardiographic view after fasting; (b) increased sol atrial compression on postprandial transthoracic echocardiography (red arrow); RV: right ventricle; LV: left ventricle; LA: left atrium.

hernia. Particularly, the most frightening complications are the development of incarceration or volvulus [2].

Iron deficiency anemia is one of the commonly seen complications in the setting of hiatal hernia. *Association between the* iron deficiency anemia and hiatal hernia has been known since the early 1930s [5]. *The main reason for* iron deficiency anemia in hiatal hernia is the hemorrhage resulting from linear ulcers and erosions (Cameron lesion) at mucosal folds where diaphragmatic compression occurs [6, 7]. *Bleeding is not the only factor* responsible for the anaemia in patients with hiatal hernia. *One of the reasons for iron deficiency anemia* in hiatal hernia is chronic gastritis with all the consequences. Today, although it is often missed, these lesions, one of the occult reasons for both gastrointestinal bleeding and iron deficiency anemia [8], are reported in 5% of the patients with hiatal hernia and 20% of the patients with persistent anemia and recurrent bleeding [9]. Bernardo et al. stated that Cameron lesions were not an uncommon cause of chronic gastrointestinal bleeding and should be kept in mind in the study of patients with iron deficiency anemia [10]. In our case, it was thought that chronic iron deficiency anemia had been explained by the advanced age and impaired oral ingestion in the prior examinations, resulting from occult hemorrhage secondary to hiatal hernia.

Although large hiatal hernias are infrequent, they can lead to atypical symptoms such as chest pain and dyspnea and rare complications such as pulmonary edema and cardiac failure due to the extent of hernia and the compression to heart and pulmonary veins by organs protruded into thorax cavity. Siu et al. reported that a large hiatal hernia caused cardiac failure by the compression to the left atrium in a case presenting with recurrent acute cardiac failure attacks [11]. In another case report, Chau et al. demonstrated a large hiatal hernia as the cause of chest pain in a patient that presented to emergency department with acute angina [12]. Hiatal hernia can manifest as a left atrial mass on echocardiography. It can cause pulmonary edema and cardiac failure through the pulmonary venous obstruction [13].

In our case, chronic fatigue and exertion dyspnea particularly aggravated at postprandial period. Increased pulmonary artery pressure in our case was attributed to the compression to the left atrium and the right pulmonary vein, as there was no other apparent cause. By available findings, it was thought that dyspnea aggravating after heavy meals is *due to pulmonary congestion from* the compression to the left atrium and the right pulmonary vein.

4. Conclusion

In conclusion, large hiatal hernias should be considered in the differential diagnosis as a rare intra-abdominal cause of persistent iron deficiency anemia and dyspnea. It should be kept in mind that large hiatal hernias can lead to cardiac symptoms and complications due to compression. Cases with *large hiatal hernias should be assessed by physical examination and imaging modalities such as echocardiography.*

Conflict of Interests

The authors declare that there is no conflict of interests regarding the publication of this paper.

References

[1] D. A. Johnson and W. K. Ruffin, "Hiatal hernia," *Gastrointestinal Endoscopy Clinics of North America*, vol. 6, no. 3, pp. 641–666, 1996.

[2] D. E. Maziak, T. R. J. Todd, F. G. Pearson et al., "Massive hiatus hernia: evaluation and surgical management," *Journal of Thoracic and Cardiovascular Surgery*, vol. 115, no. 1, pp. 53–62, 1998.

[3] M. Yoshimura, A. Nagahara, K. Ohtaka et al., "Presence of vertebral fractures is highly associated with hiatal hernia and

reflux esophagitis in Japanese elderly people," *Internal Medicine*, vol. 47, no. 16, pp. 1451–1455, 2008.

[4] T. J. Cole and M. A. Turner, "Manifestations of gastrointestinal disease on chest radiographs," *Radiographics*, vol. 13, no. 5, pp. 1013–1034, 1993.

[5] A. V. Bock, J. W. Dulin, and P. A. Brooke, "Diaphragmatic hernia and secondary anemia: 10 cases," *The New England Journal of Medicine*, vol. 209, article 615, 1933.

[6] C. W. Windsor and J. L. Collis, "Anaemia and hiatus hernia: experience in 450 patients," *Thorax*, vol. 22, no. 1, pp. 73–78, 1967.

[7] A. J. Cameron, "Incidence of iron deficiency anemia in patients with large diaphragmatic hernia: a controlled study," *Mayo Clinic Proceedings*, vol. 51, no. 12, pp. 767–769, 1976.

[8] N. Kimer, P. N. Schmidt, and A. Krag, "Cameron lesions: an often overlooked cause of iron deficiency anaemia in patients with large hiatal hernias," *BMJ Case Reports*, vol. 2010, 2010.

[9] A. J. Cameron and J. A. Higgins, "Linear gastric erosion. A lesion associated with large diaphragmatic hernia and chronic blood loss anemia," *Gastroenterology*, vol. 91, no. 2, pp. 338–342, 1986.

[10] R. J. Bernardo, J. P. Portocarrero, and M. Tagle, "Cameron lesions: clinical experience," *Revista de Gastroenterología del Perú*, vol. 32, no. 2, pp. 157–160, 2012.

[11] C.-W. Siu, M.-H. Jim, H.-H. Ho et al., "Recurrent acute heart failure caused by sliding hiatus hernia," *Postgraduate Medical Journal*, vol. 81, no. 954, pp. 268–269, 2005.

[12] A. M. T. Chau, R. W.-L. Ma, and D. M. Gold, "Massive hiatus hernia presenting as acute chest pain," *Internal Medicine Journal*, vol. 41, no. 9, pp. 704–705, 2011.

[13] H. S. Lim, D. P. Leong, and M. Alasady, "Massive hiatus hernia mimicking a left atrial mass," *Heart, Lung and Circulation*, vol. 22, no. 10, pp. 875–876, 2013.

9

Undifferentiated Intimal Sarcoma of the Inferior Vena Cava with Extension to the Right Atrium and Renal Vasculature

Aasim M. Afzal,[1] Jamil Alsahhar,[1] Varsha Podduturi,[2] and Jeffrey M. Schussler[3,4]

[1]Department of Internal Medicine, Baylor University Medical Center, 3600 Gaston Avenue, Dallas, TX 75246, USA
[2]Department of Pathology, Baylor University Medical Center, 3600 Gaston Avenue, Dallas, TX 75246, USA
[3]Division of Cardiology, Jack and Jane Hamilton Heart and Vascular Hospital, 621 N. Hall Street, Dallas, TX 75246, USA
[4]Department of Medicine, Texas A&M College of Medicine, Dallas Campus, 3600 Gaston Avenue, Dallas, TX 75246, USA

Correspondence should be addressed to Jeffrey M. Schussler; jeffrey.schussler@baylorhealth.edu

Academic Editor: Kuan-Rau Chiou

Primary sarcomas of the great vessels (aorta, pulmonary artery, and inferior vena cava (IVC)) are exceedingly rare. We report a rare case of an undifferentiated intimal sarcoma of the IVC with extension to the right atrium, adrenal, and renal veins. The patient underwent extensive resection, reconstruction of the IVC, and subsequent adjuvant chemotherapy. Patient has tolerated chemotherapy and, at 17 months after resection, the patient remains free of tumor recurrence. Undifferentiated intimal sarcomas remain a rare entity with only five cases of venous undifferentiated intimal sarcomas reported in the literature, two of which occurred in the IVC. Intimal sarcomas tend to carry a poor prognosis with the limited literature available on treatment approaches. Our objective is to highlight this rare entity and possible treatment approach which we utilized. Primary sarcomas of IVC need to be included as part of a complete differential diagnosis in patients with atrial masses or recurrent pulmonary emboli.

1. Introduction

Primary sarcomas of the great vessels (aorta, pulmonary artery (PA), and inferior vena cava (IVC)) are seldom seen. IVC sarcomas have a female predominance and are typically present in the fifth decade [1]. These sarcomas are typically leiomyosarcoma or angiosarcoma which carry a better prognosis than undifferentiated sarcoma [1]. We highlight the case of a 52-year-old black female diagnosed with an undifferentiated intimal sarcoma, who then underwent extensive resection with reconstruction of IVC followed by chemotherapy over the past year and a half.

2. Case Presentation

A 52-year-old black female with past medical history of hypertension and atrial flutter presented to her primary care physician with a one-month history of shortness of breath, severe dyspnea on exertion, bilateral lower extremity edema, and fatigue. Her blood pressure was elevated at 187/119. Family history included prostate cancer in her father and was not

significant for clotting disorders. Home medications included amlodipine, aspirin, digoxin, and metoprolol.

A transthoracic echocardiogram (TTE) demonstrated an ejection fraction of 65%, and a 4.5 cm mass was visualized in the right atrium, extending into the IVC and restricting blood flow into the heart (Figures 1(a) and 1(b)). The mass was thought to be either clot or tumor. The patient was started on heparin drip and transferred for higher level of care.

On presentation, she did not appear in distress and was hemodynamically stable. Her lungs were clear to auscultation bilaterally. She had bilateral symmetric 2+ pitting edema of her lower extremities. An abdominal magnetic resonance imaging (MRI) demonstrated a 15.2 × 5.7 × 6.8 cm solid, heterogeneously enhancing tumor of the IVC with extension 4 cm distal to the right renal vein, 1.2 cm into the right renal vein, 1.0 cm into the left renal vein, and upper IVC with a 1.5 cm nodule within the inferior right atrium. The liver was enlarged but no mass extended into the liver or hepatoportal circulation (Figure 2). A cardiac MRI showed tumor within the upper IVC extending to the posterior aspect of the right atrium with a 2 cm thrombus adherent to the intracardiac

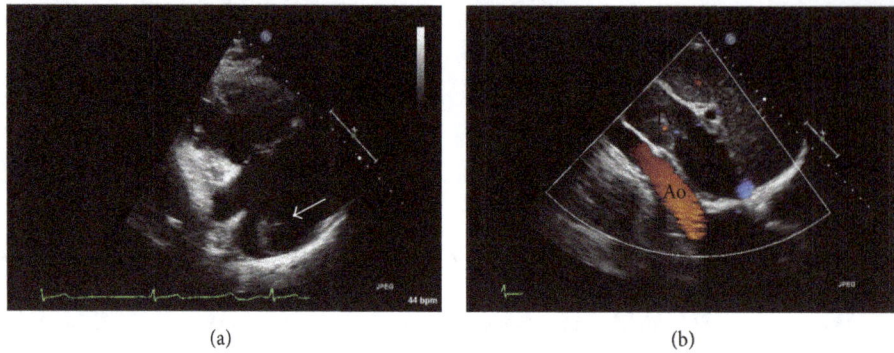

(a)   (b)

FIGURE 1: (a) Transthoracic echo showing right atrial mass (arrow). (b) Doppler flow showing IVC tumor restricting blood flow.

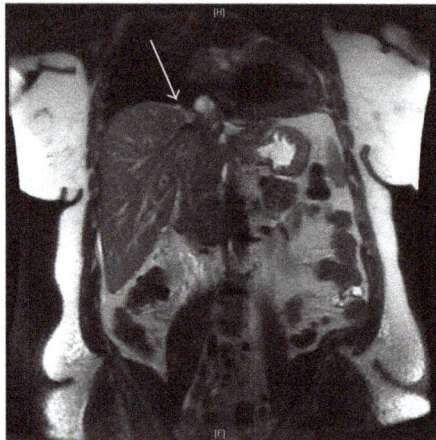

FIGURE 2: T1 MRI with sagittal view showing the tumor in the IVC with right atrial clot at the tip of the tumor (arrow).

portion of the tumor (Figure 2). A computed tomography (CT) of chest, abdomen, and pelvis along with an MRI of brain were negative for metastasis.

Due to extensive multiorgan involvement, a multidisciplinary team consisting of cardiothoracic, vascular, and transplant surgeons were involved for a combined cardiothoracic and hepatobiliary surgery. The patient underwent resection of IVC from the right atrium to the infrarenal IVC with reconstruction using a composite graft, right nephrectomy and adrenalectomy, left nephrectomy with autotransplantation in the right iliac fossa, total hepatectomy, and liver autotransplantation. The surgery lasted for about 7 hours with an estimated blood loss of 2 liters. The patient did not undergo sarcoma staging before surgery was performed.

Macroscopic examination of the IVC revealed a tan-gray tumor that measured 13.5 × 6.0 × 5.3 cm and completely filled the entire resected specimen. The tumor protruded through the cephalic end of the IVC and the ostium of right renal vein (Figure 3(a)). The cut surface of the tumor was tan-pink with focal areas of hemorrhage and necrosis.

Microscopically, the tumor was comprised of spindled cells in a fascicular growth pattern with cigar-shaped nuclei, intracytoplasmic vacuoles, and exhibited marked nuclear pleomorphism (Figure 3(b)). Mitotic figures were numerous

and necrosis was present. The tumor appeared to be arising from the intima of the vessel wall (Figure 3(c)) and focally infiltrated into the adjacent adventitial fibroadipose tissue with no extension to the serosal surface (Figure 3(d)). Immunohistochemistry had negative staining for epithelial differentiation (pancytokeratin AE1-3 and OSCAR), nerve sheath differentiation (S100), endothelial cell markers (CD31, CD34), and smooth muscle markers (smooth muscle actin, muscle specific actin, caldesmon, MYOD-1, and desmin). Tumor cells stained diffusely positive for Fli-1, an endothelial cell marker (Figure 3(e)). Ki-67 or the proliferative index measured 60%.

Given the histologic features and immunohistochemical staining pattern, this tumor was classified as a high grade undifferentiated intimal sarcoma of the IVC. While the margins after resection were free of tumor, the tumor protruded into the proximal and distal ends of the lumen of the IVC as well as into both renal veins.

Postoperatively, patient had an uneventful recovery and was discharged home 7 days after operation. A follow-up echo prior to chemotherapy initiation showed left ventricular hypertrophy with hyperdynamic ejection fraction of 70% but no evidence of residual tumor. She was started on doxorubicin and ifosfamide as the local and distant recurrence rate of a high-grade sarcoma is extremely high. She tolerated the first cycle; however, after the second cycle she developed encephalopathy attributed to ifosfamide. She was switched to a different regimen using gemcitabine and docetaxel, which has been previously utilized in soft tissue tumors. She received multiple cycles of this regimen over the past nine months, developing mild asymptomatic thrombocytopenia and anemia on the new regimen. Surveillance CT over the past year and a half shows that the patient remains free of tumor recurrence. At 19-month status after resection, she remains free of tumor recurrence.

3. Discussion

Sarcomas of the IVC have a female predominance and are typically present in the fifth decade [1]. These tumors are most often derived from the medial smooth muscle and are usually leiomyosarcomas, but intimal sarcomas, leiomyomas, synovial sarcoma, angiosarcoma, and rhabdomyosarcoma have

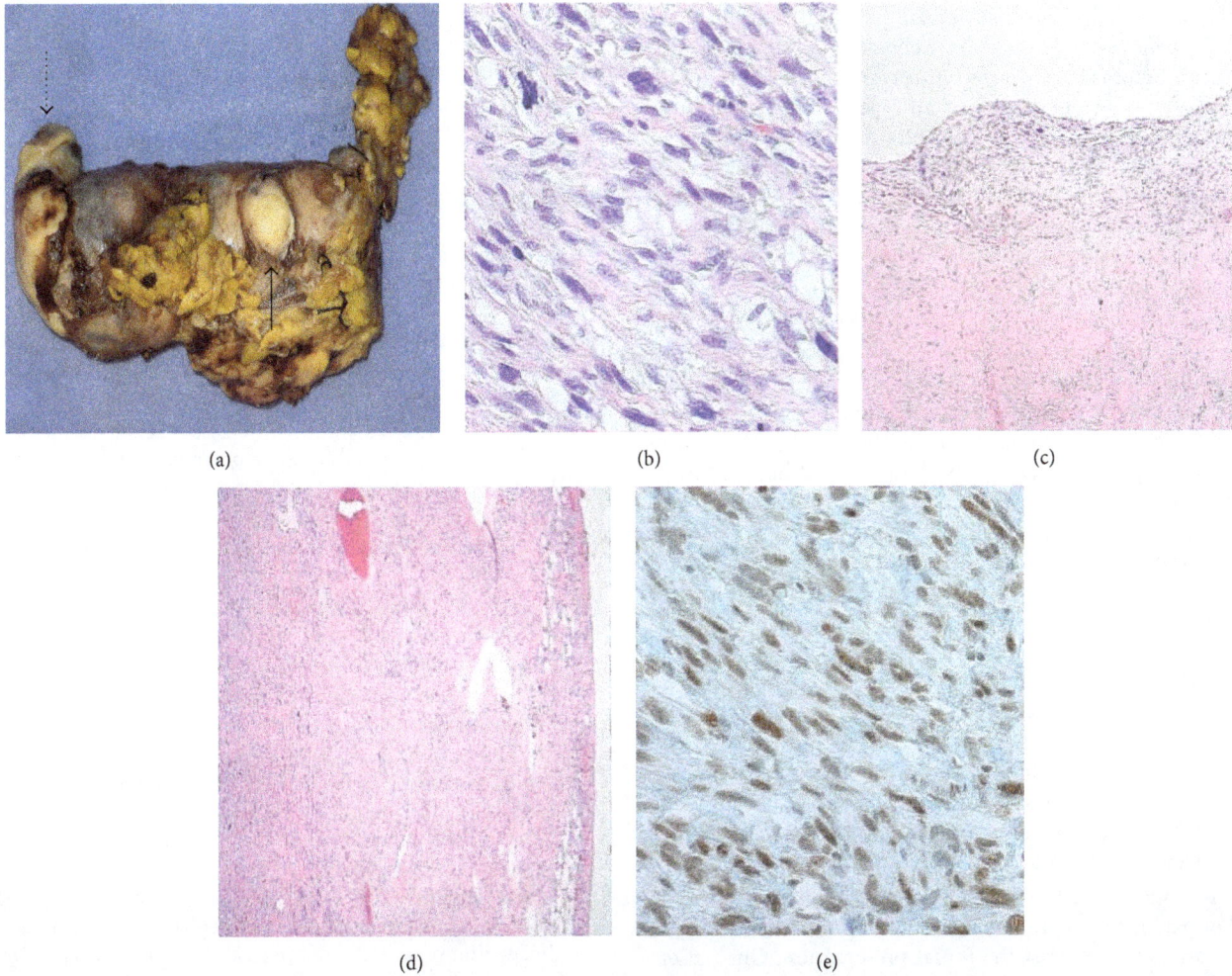

FIGURE 3: (a) The lumen of inferior vena cava distended by tumor. Dotted arrow specifies cranial end of specimen. Solid arrow indicates ostium of renal vein. (b) Spindled tumor cells in fascicles with nuclear pleomorphism and intracytoplasmic vacuoles (H&E 400x). (c) Neoplastic tumor cells lining the intimal surface of the inferior vena cava (H&E 40x). (d) Tumor invading into adjacent adventitial soft tissue (H&E 40x). (e) Tumor with positive staining for Fli-1 (400x).

been reported [1–4]. Nonmyogenic sarcomas, which are derived from the intima, are even more infrequent and are typically seen in the arterial system, particularly the PA [5, 6]. Intimal sarcomas have also been reported in the superior vena cava (SVC), IVC, and brachiocephalic vein [7, 8]. Typically leiomyosarcoma and angiosarcoma carry a better prognosis than undifferentiated intimal sarcoma with a mean 5-year survival of 33–53% [1].

There have been five cases of venous undifferentiated intimal sarcomas reported in the literature, two of which occurred in the IVC [7, 8]. A clinicopathologic study done by Burke and Virmani reviewed 16 cases of IVC sarcomas. 12 of the 16 patients were women and presented with symptoms of shortness of breath, pain, thrombosis, and IVC syndrome. Of the cases reviewed, 15 of the patients had leiomyosarcoma. Only one case of intimal sarcoma was reported and presented with symptoms of pulmonary embolus. The sarcoma was found to extend the renal and iliac veins. Thrombectomy was performed and the patient did relatively well postoperatively with no complications [1].

Primary sarcomas of IVC need to be included as part of a complete differential diagnosis in patients with atrial masses or recurrent pulmonary emboli. A presentation similar to that of our patient can be seen in patients with leiomyosarcoma, angiosarcoma, renal cell carcinoma with IVC extension, and right atrial thrombus. Clots are seen with tumors of the IVC, as these tumors result in turbulent flow and hemostasis. Only pathology can help differentiate between leiomyosarcoma, angiosarcoma, and intimal sarcoma.

Intimal sarcomas are comprised of epithelioid or haphazardly arranged spindled cells and express endothelial cell markers CD31 and Fli-1. In the case presented, the tumor was made of spindled cells with intracytoplasmic vacuoles and was arising from the intimal wall of the vena cava. The tumor expressed strong Fli-1 positivity, an endothelial marker. Despite not displaying reactivity for other endothelial markers, CD31 and CD34, the tumor was classified as an undifferentiated intimal sarcoma. The pathology results are important as they can affect the prognosis and treatment approach. Histology is important, but the size and grade of sarcoma, as well as adequacy of the resection, determine the need for therapy and outcome. Sebenik et al. suggested that intimal sarcomas are divided into two subtypes, the undifferentiated type and differentiated type [7]. The latter group represents intimal sarcoma of recognized type which may include myxofibrosarcoma, angiosarcoma, epithelioid hemangioendothelioma, and leiomyosarcoma [7]. Undifferentiated types often appear in an older patient population and have a shorter survival than differentiated subtypes [7].

Aggregate data shows poor prognosis for patients with intimal sarcoma, with an average survival of 27 months after chemotherapy and radiation [1]. Another poor prognostic indicator is location within the vessel lumen. Early surgical intervention and complete resection if possible are highly recommended and are the mainstay of therapy [9]. These surgeries are typically extensive in nature and if there is tumor, extension into the heart may require cardiopulmonary bypass with or without hypothermic circulatory arrest [9]. There are no current studies available that give specific guidelines for chemotherapy to treat intimal sarcomas of IVC. We treated our patient based on a meta-analysis done by Pervaiz et al. looking at efficacy of adjuvant chemotherapy for localized resectable soft-tissue sarcomas [10]. That meta-analysis confirmed marginal efficacy of chemotherapy in localized resectable soft-tissue sarcoma with respect to local recurrence, distant recurrence, overall recurrence, and overall survival [10]. The meta-analysis showed that addition of ifosfamide to doxorubicin has a higher antitumor activity on patients with advanced or metastatic soft-tissue sarcoma.

From a detailed literature review, there is record of two other patients who presented with an intimal sarcoma of the IVC and survived past the initial presentation. Our patient tolerated gemcitabine and docetaxel regimen relatively well and follow-up appointments have not documented any recurrences.

Consent

Informed consent was obtained from the patient or a surrogate that they consented to participate in a study in which the publication of case reports was permitted.

Disclosure

The institutional review board at Baylor University Medical Center at Dallas approved the study.

Conflict of Interests

The authors declare that there is no conflict of interests regarding the publication of this paper.

Authors' Contribution

All the authors have contributed substantively to (a) case reporting and discussion, (b) the drafting of the paper or critical revision for important intellectual content, and (c) the final approval of the version to be published.

Acknowledgments

Special thanks are due to Robert G. Mennel, M.D.; David L. Watkins, M.D.; and Metin Punar, M.D., for their assistance and contribution to this paper.

References

[1] A. P. Burke and R. Virmani, "Sarcomas of the great vessels. A clinicopathologic study," *Cancer*, vol. 71, no. 5, pp. 1761–1773, 1993.

[2] A. S. Griffin and J. M. Sterchi, "Primary leiomyosarcoma of the inferior vena cava: a case report and review of the literature," *Journal of Surgical Oncology*, vol. 34, no. 1, pp. 53–60, 1987.

[3] C. M. A. Bruyninckx and O. S. Derksen, "Leiomyosarcoma of the inferior vena cava. Case report and review of the literature," *Journal of Vascular Surgery*, vol. 3, no. 4, pp. 652–656, 1986.

[4] R. C. Wray Jr. and H. Dawkins, "Primary smooth muscle tumors of the inferior vena cava," *Annals of Surgery*, vol. 174, no. 6, pp. 1009–1018, 1971.

[5] H. Fujita, K. Kawata, T. Sawada et al., "Rhabdomyosarcoma in the inferior vena cava with secondary Budd-Chiari syndrome," *Internal Medicine*, vol. 32, no. 1, pp. 67–71, 1993.

[6] S. W. Weiss and J. R. Goldblum, *Enzinger and Weiss's Soft Tissue Tumors*, Mosby, Philadelphia, Pa, USA, 5th edition, 2007.

[7] M. Sebenik, A. Ricci Jr., B. DiPasquale et al., "Undifferentiated intimal sarcoma of large systemic blood vessels: report of 14 cases with immunohistochemical profile and review of the literature," *The American Journal of Surgical Pathology*, vol. 29, no. 9, pp. 1184–1193, 2005.

[8] E. R. C. Rytina, Y. K. Govil, K. Sabanathan, and R. Y. Ball, "Intimal sarcoma of the right brachiocephalic vein presenting as the superior vena caval syndrome," *Journal of Clinical Pathology*, vol. 49, no. 4, pp. 347–349, 1996.

[9] K. B. Wise, S. M. Said, C. J. Clark et al., "Resection of a giant primary synovial sarcoma of the inferior vena cava extending into the right atrium with caval reconstruction under cardiopulmonary bypass and circulatory arrest," *Perspectives in Vascular Surgery and Endovascular Therapy*, vol. 24, no. 2, pp. 95–101, 2012.

[10] N. Pervaiz, N. Colterjohn, F. Farrokhyar, R. Tozer, A. Figueredo, and M. Ghert, "A systematic meta-analysis of randomized controlled trials of adjuvant chemotherapy for localized resectable soft-tissue sarcoma," *Cancer*, vol. 113, no. 3, pp. 573–581, 2008.

10

Beneficial Effects of Isoproterenol and Quinidine in the Treatment of Ventricular Fibrillation in Brugada Syndrome

Melissa Dakkak, Khyati Baxi, and Ambar Patel

Departments of Cardiovascular Diseases and Internal Medicine, University of Florida Health, Jacksonville, FL 32209, USA

Correspondence should be addressed to Melissa Dakkak; melissa.dakkak@jax.ufl.edu

Academic Editor: Konstantinos P. Letsas

The use of an implantable cardiac defibrillator has been advocated as the only effective treatment for the management of ventricular fibrillation (VF) in patients with Brugada Syndrome (BrS). However, this device is only useful for terminating VF. Intermittent and/or recalcitrant VF for which lifesaving cardioversion occurs is a problematic situation in this patient population. The immediate use of appropriate antiarrhythmics in the acute setting has proven to be lifesaving. Quinidine has been well established as an effective antiarrhythmic in BrS, while isoproterenol (ISP) has had some recognition as well. The addition of drug therapy to prevent the induction of these arrhythmias has been shown to reduce the morbidity and mortality associated with BrS. It was proven to be especially effective in the presence of early repolarization, evidenced by the reduction or normalization of the early repolarization pattern on ECG. Thus, for the prophylactic management and long term suppression of VF in BrS, further prospective studies should be performed to determine the effectiveness of quinidine and ISP in this patient population.

1. Introduction

The use of an implantable cardiac defibrillator in patients with Brugada Syndrome (BrS) has been advocated as the first line therapy for managing recalcitrant ventricular fibrillation (VF). However, this device is only useful for terminating VF. Intermittent and/or refractory VF for which lifesaving cardioversion occurs is a problematic situation in this patient population. After an initial adverse arrhythmic event, such as cardiac arrest or syncope due to VF, approximately 60% of symptomatic patients will have a recurrent arrhythmic event within the next 4 years [1, 2]. Therefore, the addition of antiarrhythmic suppression therapy may reduce the morbidity and mortality associated with BrS. At this time, no pharmacologic intervention has been proven to be effective in reducing the risk of initial cardiac arrest from VF [3]. This case and literature review will focus on the effectiveness of isoproterenol (ISP) and quinidine in preventing VF in patients with BrS.

2. Case

A 25-year-old African American male with no significant past medical or family history of sudden cardiac arrest

(SCA) presented with VF. Electrocardiography (ECG) strip on arrival demonstrated VF (Figure 1). In the emergency department, the patient continued to have VF refractory to several antiarrhythmic agents, including amiodarone, esmolol, and lidocaine used alone or in combination. Physical examination while the patient was temporarily in sinus rhythm showed an obese afebrile male with no chest wall trauma and normal cardiac and pulmonary examination. Initial ECG demonstrated interventricular conduction delay with nonspecific ST-T wave changes as well as early repolarization pattern (ER) with QRS notching (Figure 2). Laboratory abnormalities included low magnesium (1.6 mg/dL) and potassium (3.3 mmol/L) levels, which were adequately replaced. The transthoracic echocardiogram showed a preserved left ventricular ejection fraction (EF) of 60–65% with normal wall motion, normal valvular function, and otherwise normal structure. The patient continued to have innumerable episodes of VF requiring a total of 63 shocks. Upon infusion of the beta-agonist ISP, an ECG performed during a temporary sinus rhythm showed a right bundle branch block morphology with a coved ST segment and negative T wave deflections in leads V1 and V2 (Figure 3). Urine drug screen was negative. The patient was continued on

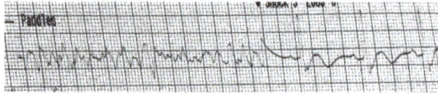

FIGURE 1: Electrocardiography strip demonstrating ventricular fibrillation with restoration of normal sinus rhythm after one cardioversion shock.

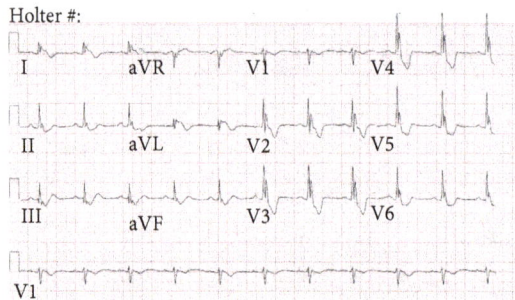

FIGURE 2: Baseline ECG on admission demonstrates interventricular conduction delay, QRS notching, and ST-T wave abnormalities.

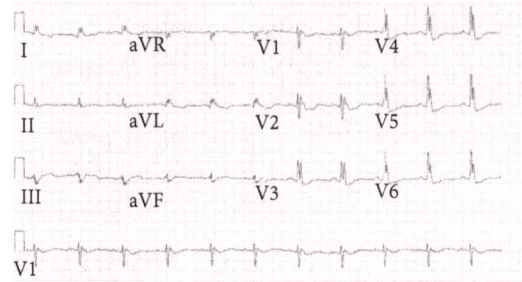

FIGURE 3: Baseline Electrocardiography during sinus rhythm showing coved-type ST segment in leads V1 and V2.

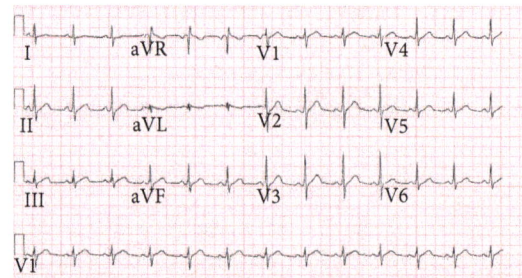

FIGURE 4: Electrocardiogram after Isoproterenol infusion and oral quinidine gluconate administration showing resolution of QRS notching and no J point elevation.

ISP at rate of 0.5 mcg/min. Once the patient status stabilized, ISP was weaned off and he was transitioned to oral quinidine gluconate 324 mg every 8 hours. No further arrhythmias occurred. The ECG on discharge showed near normalization of the ER pattern with resolution of the QRS notching and no J point elevation (Figure 4). The patient underwent further comprehensive testing including a coronary angiography, which demonstrated normal coronary arteries. Magnetic Resonance Imaging with and without gadolinium enhancement showed no myocardial scarring, inflammation, or infiltration, with a preserved EF of 62%. A diagnosis of Brugada syndrome (BrS) was established based on the characteristic ECG pattern in conjunction with documented VF. Prior to discharge, the patient received an implantable cardioverter defibrillator (ICD) for secondary prevention in conjunction with oral quinidine 324 mg every 8 hours for VF suppression. He has been free of arrhythmias for 7 months.

3. Discussion

BrS is diagnosed by characteristic ECG pattern in conjunction with at least one of the following: documented VF, self-terminating polymorphic VT, family history of sudden cardiac death, coved-type ECG pattern in family members, VF inducibility during electrophysiological study, syncope, or nocturnal agonal respirations [4, 5].

Criteria for Brugada Syndrome
ECG criteria

Type 1: elevation of the J point and coved-type ST segment elevation >2 mm followed by an inverted T wave that occurs spontaneously,

Type 2: saddle back-type ST segment elevation of >2 mm followed by either a positive T wave or biphasic T wave,

Type 3: either saddle back-type or coved-type ST segment elevation >1 mm.

Plus at least one of the following

(i) documented VF,

(ii) self-terminating polymorphic VT,

(iii) family history of sudden cardiac death,

(iv) coved-type ECG pattern in family members,

(v) VF inducibility during EP study,

(vi) syncope,

(vii) nocturnal agonal respirations.

There are 3 types of BrS based on ECG characteristics. Type 1 ECG pattern shows pronounced elevation of the J point and coved-type ST segment elevation ≥2 mm followed by an inverted T wave that occurs spontaneously. Type 2 ECG pattern consists of saddle back-type ST segment elevation of ≥2 mm followed by either a positive T wave or biphasic T wave. Lastly, type 3 ECG pattern shows either saddle back-type or coved-type ST segment elevation ≥1 mm (Figure 5). In contrary to type 1, type 2 and type 3 may not occur spontaneously and thus require a pharmacological challenge test [4, 6].

The prevalence of BrS appears to be low in the general population and occurs predominantly in young male adults less than 40 years of age. No precise data are available on the epidemiology of BrS. However, its prevalence is much higher in Asian and South Asian countries, reaching 0.5–1 per 1000.

V1

V2

Type 1:	Type 2:	Type 3:
coved-type	saddle back-type	saddle back-type
"ST segment	"ST segment	"ST segment
elevation"	elevation"	elevation"

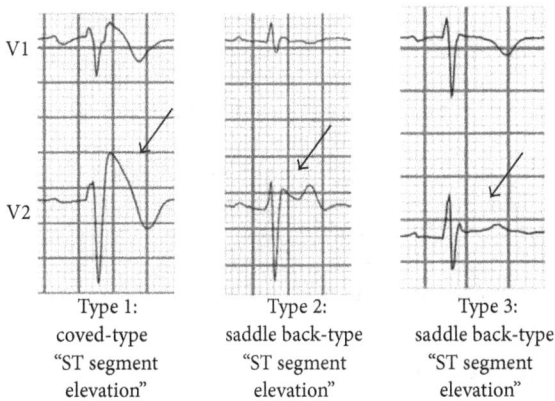

FIGURE 5: Three types of ECG pattern associated with BrS.

BrS is 8–10 times more prevalent in men than in women. Approximately 20% of BrS patients have been shown to have a mutation located in the SCN5A gene, which produces a complete loss of function of the cardiac sodium channel [4, 7].

Risk stratification is paramount in BrS since no medications have been proven to be effective in increasing the risk of ventricular arrhythmias. Patients who have experienced an episode of SCA are at the highest risk of arrhythmia recurrence. The presence of a spontaneous type I ECG associated with history of syncope defines the second highest risk group. Conversely, asymptomatic patients with spontaneous ECG characteristics, such as those with type 2 and 3 Brugada pattern, can be considered for an electrophysiology study for further risk stratification [8, 9]. Guidelines for genetic testing in patients with suspected BrS are not definitive [10]. As it stands, ICD implantation is advocated to be the first line therapy in SCA in BrS survivors [11].

Additionally, the combination of fractionated-QRS (f-QRS) with early repolarization (ER) abnormalities is useful for identifying high- and low-risk patients [12]. ER pattern on ECG is indicated by the presence of an elevation of the QRS-ST junction (J point) in at least two leads. The amplitude of J point elevation has to be at least 1 mm (0.1 mV) above the baseline level, either as QRS slurring depicted as a smooth transition from the QRS segment to the ST segment or notching represented by a positive J deflection inscribed on the S wave in the inferior lead (II, III, and aVF), lateral lead (I, aVL, and V4 to V6), or both [13]. An ER pattern is currently considered to be a benign electrocardiographic phenomenon affecting 2% to 5% of the general population and is most commonly observed in young men. However, recently, an ER pattern has been shown to be an additional risk marker for VF development, especially in inferolateral leads, in patients with BrS [14, 15]. The study performed by Tokioka et al. showed that the combination of f-QRS and inferolateral ER pattern was associated with the development of VF in these patients. Furthermore, repolarization abnormalities were independently associated with VF development. Moreover, VF and SCA episodes during follow-up and a history of VF episodes were more frequently observed in patients with an ER pattern than in those without an ER pattern ($p = 0.001$ and $p = 0.005$, resp.) [12].

The pathophysiology of BrS is complex but does impact the selection of antiarrhythmic medications to use for its management. The defective myocardial sodium channels reduce sodium inflow currents and consequentially reduce the duration of the normal action potential. Phase 0 of the action potential, which correlates with influx of sodium, is blunted and this results in reduction of calcium inflow and shortening of phase 2. The cells may therefore fail to conduct the action potential due to a shortened refractory period, which may give rise to localized reentry circuits and the potential of arrhythmias in the presence of ventricular premature beats. The effect is more pronounced when there are normal and abnormal sodium channels in the same tissue with heterogeneity of refractory periods [16]. Attacks of VF usually occur at the night during sleep during which there is an increase in vagal stimulation causing an increase in outward current and decrease in inward current, leading to a shortening of the action potential duration and excitation. Beta-adrenergic stimulation through the sympathetic nervous system induces the contrary, by increasing inward calcium current and attenuating the excess outward current and thus counterbalancing the changes in membrane potential [17].

Despite their anecdotal success and proven efficacy, ISP and Quinidine are Class IIa recommendations according to the HRS/EHRA/APHRS and Class IIa and Class IIb recommendations according to ACC/AHA, respectively, for the management of arrhythmic storms such as VF storm [18, 19].

Quinidine, a class IA antiarrhythmic, has been established as an effective drug in the management of BrS. It exerts its beneficial effects in BrS by inhibiting the outward current, thereby restoring electrical homogeneity. In addition, it prolongs ventricular refractoriness [20]. The study by Belhassen et al. demonstrated that quinidine had an 88% success rate in preventing VF induction in BrS patients with inducible VF. Furthermore, quinidine was effective in preventing spontaneous VF during follow-up ranging from 6 months to 18 years [20]. In a case series performed by Márquez et al., quinidine was effective in suppressing ventricular arrhythmias during a mean follow-up time of 4 years. Long-term use of quinidine was well tolerated at a low dose of <600 mg/d while maintaining an effectiveness of 85% [21]. The limiting factor for long-term compliance included noncardiac side effects such as abdominal cramping, diarrhea, cinchonism and anticholinergic effects and proarrhythmia in the setting of electrolyte abnormalities [22].

In contrast, ISP has not been as well studied as quinidine, though its efficacy has been documented. ISP is a beta-adrenergic agonist that increases intracellular calcium in order to stabilize and restore the dome in phase 2 of the action potential and reduce the electrical heterogeneity responsible for BrS. This stability reduces the susceptibility to VF triggered by premature beats. In addition to successfully terminating and suppressing the refractory ventricular fibrillation as in the above case, it has also been shown to normalize the electrocardiographic pattern and prevent ventricular fibrillation induction during electrophysiological study. ISP was effective in suppressing VF in a 36-year-old male with BrS and was also associated with the disappearance of the short-coupled premature ventricular beats, which trigger VF [23]. Its effect is also confirmed in a case series by Watanabe et al., in which ventricular arrhythmias were successfully abolished after the infusion of ISP in six patients with BrS. The suppressive effect continued for three days after the termination of the infusion. However, one patient had recurrent ventricular arrhythmias following the end of the isoproterenol infusion. The addition of quinidine was effective in terminating the arrhythmias. Thus, the direct effect of ISP on the myocardium to increase inward current is important for therapeutic effects in patients with BrS [17].

The infusion of ISP followed by the oral administration of quinidine used for the management of VF in BrS has been documented in very few case studies and small studies. A recent case report by Furniss confirmed its efficacy in terminating and preventing VF in a 3-year-old male with BrS who has been event-free for 1 year [16]. This was preceded by a case by Jongman et al, in which a 45-year-old male with BrS type 2 presented with numerous ICD shocks for VF [22]. A study performed in 2007 by Ohgo et al. demonstrated that ISP infusion was successful in terminating VF storm in the acute setting in patients with BrS. These patients were then successfully transitioned to oral antiarrhythmics including quinidine for chronic suppression of VT/VF [24]. Therefore, a prospective study to determine the long-term efficacy of ISP infusion followed by the administration of oral quinidine in remaining arrhythmia-free in BrS patients with an ICD would be of interest.

A multicenter study performed by Haïssaguerre et al. demonstrated the efficacy of ISP and quinidine to abolish and prevent recurrences of VF associated with early repolarization abnormality in the inferolateral leads. ISP was infused in 7 patients during repetitive episodes of VF at a rate of 1 to 5 μg/min, which eliminated all arrhythmias when the sinus heart rate was increased to above 120 beats/min. Any attempt to reduce the infusion and heart rate was associated with recurrence of VF in 3 of the patients. Isoproterenol was infused for a period ranging from 6 h to 5 days. In addition, quinidine (in 3) or hydroquinidine (in 6) was totally successful in 9 of 9 patients in decreasing the number of recurrent VF from a mean of 33 episodes to nil with follow-up of 25 ± 18 months on therapy. The study concluded that ISP and quinidine both reduced the ER pattern or restored a normal ECG, which also occurred in our patient. This demonstrates that ISP and quinidine are effective in preventing the recurrence of VF associated with ER abnormality. Thus, this study confirmed that the infusion of ISP can successfully manage electrical storms as a lifesaving therapy, while the oral administration of quinidine is effective chronically on a long-term basis [12].

4. Conclusion

In an otherwise young healthy male with no significant cardiac risk factors, hereditary channelopathies such as BrS should be higher in the differential. The immediate use of appropriate antiarrhythmics has proven to be lifesaving.

Quinidine has been well established as an effective antiarrhythmic in BrS, while ISP has had some recognition as well. Interestingly, the use of isoproterenol and quinidine has been successful in long-term prevention of VF in case reports and studies. It has been proven to be especially effective in the presence of ER pattern evident by the reduction or normalization of this pattern on ECG. Thus, further prospective studies should be performed to determine the effectiveness of quinidine and ISP therapy in early management and long-term suppression of VF in the BrS population.

Conflict of Interests

The authors declare that there is no conflict of interests regarding the publication of this paper.

Authors' Contribution

Melissa Dakkak and Khyati Baxi equally contributed to the paper.

References

[1] J. Brugada, R. Brugada, and P. Brugada, "Asymptomatic patients with a Brugada electrocardiogram: are they at risk?" *Journal of Cardiovascular Electrophysiology*, vol. 12, no. 1, pp. 7–8, 2001.

[2] J. Brugada, R. Brugada, C. Antzelevitch, J. Towbin, K. Nademanee, and P. Brugada, "Long-term follow-up of individuals with the electrocardiographic pattern of right bundle-branch block and ST-segment elevation in precordial leads V_1 to V_3," *Circulation*, vol. 105, no. 1, pp. 73–78, 2002.

[3] B. Belhassen, S. Viskin, and C. Antzelevitch, "The Brugada syndrome: is an implantable cardioverter defibrillator the only therapeutic option?" *Pacing and Clinical Electrophysiology*, vol. 25, no. 11, pp. 1634–1640, 2002.

[4] K. F. Kusano, "Brugada syndrome: recent understanding of pathophysiological mechanism and treatment," *Journal of Arrhythmia*, vol. 29, no. 2, pp. 77–82, 2013.

[5] A. A. M. Wilde, C. Antzelevitch, M. Borggrefe et al., "Proposed diagnostic criteria for the Brugada syndrome: consensus report," *Circulation*, vol. 106, no. 19, pp. 2514–2519, 2002.

[6] C. Antzelevitch, P. Brugada, M. Borggrefe et al., "Brugada syndrome: report of the second consensus conference," *Circulation*, vol. 111, no. 5, pp. 659–670, 2005.

[7] V. Probst, C. Veltmann, L. Eckardt et al., "Long-term prognosis of patients diagnosed with brugada syndrome: results from the finger brugada syndrome registry," *Circulation*, vol. 121, no. 5, pp. 635–643, 2010.

[8] S. G. Priori, C. Napolitano, M. Gasparini et al., "Natural history of Brugada syndrome: insights for risk stratification and management," *Circulation*, vol. 105, no. 11, pp. 1342–1347, 2002.

[9] D. P. Zipes, A. J. Camm, M. Borggrefe et al., "ACC/AHA/ESC 2006 guidelines for management of patients with ventricular arrhythmias and the prevention of sudden cardiac death—executive summary: a report of the American College of Cardiology/American Heart Association Task Force and the European Society of Cardiology Committee for Practice Guidelines," *Circulation*, vol. 114, no. 10, pp. 1088–1132, 2006.

[10] Y. Mizusawa and A. A. M. Wilde, "Brugada syndrome," *Circulation: Arrhythmia and Electrophysiology*, vol. 5, no. 3, pp. 606–616, 2012.

[11] E. S. Kaufman, "Genetic testing in brugada syndrome," *Journal of the American College of Cardiology*, vol. 60, no. 15, pp. 1419–1420, 2012.

[12] K. Tokioka, K. F. Kusano, H. Morita et al., "Electrocardiographic parameters and fatal arrhythmic events in patients with brugada syndrome: combination of depolarization and repolarization abnormalities," *Journal of the American College of Cardiology*, vol. 63, no. 20, pp. 2131–2138, 2014.

[13] M. Haïssaguerre, N. Derval, F. Sacher et al., "Sudden cardiac arrest associated with early repolarization," *The New England Journal of Medicine*, vol. 358, no. 19, pp. 2016–2023, 2008.

[14] A. Sarkozy, G.-B. Chierchia, G. Paparella et al., "Inferior and lateral electrocardiographic repolarization abnormalities in brugada syndrome," *Circulation: Arrhythmia and Electrophysiology*, vol. 2, no. 2, pp. 154–161, 2009.

[15] S. Kamakura, T. Ohe, K. Nakazawa et al., "Long-term prognosis of probands with Brugada-pattern ST-elevation in leads V1–V3," *Circulation: Arrhythmia and Electrophysiology*, vol. 2, no. 5, pp. 495–503, 2009.

[16] G. Furniss, "Isoprenaline and quinidine to calm Brugada VF storm," *BMJ Case Reports*, vol. 2012, Article ID bcr0420114156, 2012.

[17] A. Watanabe, K. Fukushima Kusano, H. Morita et al., "Low-dose isoproterenol for repetitive ventricular arrhythmia in patients with Brugada syndrome," *European Heart Journal*, vol. 27, no. 13, pp. 1579–1583, 2006.

[18] S. Priori, A. Wilde, M. Horie et al., "Executive summary: HRS/EHRA/APHRS expert consensus statement on the diagnosis and management of patients with inherited primary arrhythmia syndromes," *Europace*, vol. 15, no. 10, pp. 1389–1406, 2013.

[19] A. E. Epstein, J. P. DiMarco, K. A. Ellenbogen et al., "ACC/AHA/HRS 2008 guidelines for device-based therapy of cardiac rhythm abnormalities: a report of the American College of Cardiology/American Heart Association Task Force on Practice Guidelines (writing committee to revise the ACC/AHA/NASPE 2002 guideline update for implantation of cardiac pacemakers and antiarrhythmia devices): developed in collaboration with the American Association for Thoracic Surgery and Society of Thoracic Surgeons," *Circulation*, vol. 117, no. 21, pp. e350–e408, 2008.

[20] B. Belhassen, A. Glick, and S. Viskin, "Efficacy of quinidine in high-risk patients with Brugada syndrome," *Circulation*, vol. 110, no. 13, pp. 1731–1737, 2004.

[21] M. F. Márquez, A. Bonny, E. Hernández-Castillo et al., "Long-term efficacy of low doses of quinidine on malignant arrhythmias in Brugada syndrome with an implantable cardioverter-defibrillator: a case series and literature review," *Heart Rhythm*, vol. 9, no. 12, pp. 1995–2000, 2012.

[22] J. K. Jongman, N. Jepkes-Bruin, A. R. R. Misier et al., "Electrical storms in Brugada syndrome successfully treated with isoproterenol infusion and quinidine orally," *Netherlands Heart Journal*, vol. 15, no. 4, pp. 151–154, 2007.

[23] P. Maury, P. Couderc, M. Delay, S. Boveda, and J. Brugada, "Electrical storm in Brugada syndrome successfully treated using isoprenaline," *Europace*, vol. 6, no. 2, pp. 130–133, 2004.

[24] T. Ohgo, H. Okamura, T. Noda et al., "Acute and chronic management in patients with Brugada syndrome associated with electrical storm of ventricular fibrillation," *Heart Rhythm*, vol. 4, no. 6, pp. 695–700, 2007.

11

Transapical Implantation of a 2nd-Generation JenaValve Device in Patient with Extremely High Surgical Risk

Juan Mieres, Marcelo Menéndez, Carlos Fernández-Pereira, Miguel Rubio, and Alfredo E. Rodríguez

Cardiac Unit and Cardiovascular Surgery Department, Otamendi Hospital, Azcuènaga 870, C1115AAB Buenos Aires, Argentina

Correspondence should be addressed to Alfredo E. Rodríguez; arodriguez@centroceci.com.ar

Academic Editor: Henri Justino

Transcatheter Aortic Valve Replacement (TAVR) is performed in patients who are poor surgical candidates. Many patients have inadequate femoral access, and alternative access sites have been used such as the transapical approach discussed in this paper. We present an elderly and fragile patient not suitable for surgery for unacceptable high risk, including poor ventricular function, previous myocardial infarction with percutaneous coronary intervention, pericardial effusion, and previous cardiac surgery with replacement of mechanical mitral valve. Transapical aortic valve replacement with a second-generation self-expanding JenaValve is performed. The JenaValve is a second-generation transapical TAVR valve consisting of a porcine root valve mounted on a low-profile nitinol stent. The valve is fully retrievable and repositionable. We discuss transapical access, implantation technique, and feasibility of valve implantation in this extremely high surgical risk patient.

1. Introduction

Transcatheter Aortic Valve Replacement (TAVR) was introduced as a therapeutic option in treatment of severe aortic stenosis (AS) in elderly patients who are poor candidates for conventional surgical aortic valve replacement.

Since TAVR was first introduced [1], thousands of patients have been treated worldwide and their feasibility and safety have been demonstrated in randomized trials and large observational studies [2, 3]. Different prosthesis designs have been used, particularly two of them in the majority of the cases [4].

Femoral approach has been the most frequent access site, although vascular access site complications and cerebrovascular accident have been reported with this approach just as a significant increase in 30-day mortality [5].

For this reason other access sites are being used, such as transapical, carotid, subclavian, and transaortic, mainly when femoral approach is not feasible [6].

The purpose of this presentation is to report results achieved in a high risk patient with AS using transapical approach and implantation of second-generation JenaValve device [7, 8].

2. Case Presentation

83-year-old female presented hypertension, high cholesterol, and previous mechanical mitral valve replacement for severe mitral insufficiency in 1992.

Patient also has severe coronary artery disease treated with three bare metal stents (BMS) to left anterior descending artery (LAD) three years ago and non-ST elevation anterior myocardial infarction three months ago.

She was, at the time, symptomatic with multiple hospitalizations for heart failure and severe AS. In the last month, she had presented progressive dyspnea from functional classes II to IV NYHA associated with paroxysmal nocturnal dyspnea and orthopnea and lower extremities edema worsening in the 48 hours prior to hospital admission.

At physical examination she was lucid, normotensive, afebrile, and tachypneic with bilateral crackles to vertex and

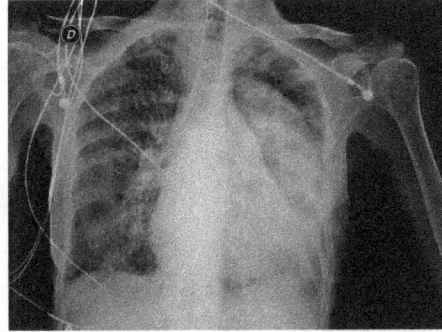

FIGURE 1: Chest X-ray showing pleural effusion.

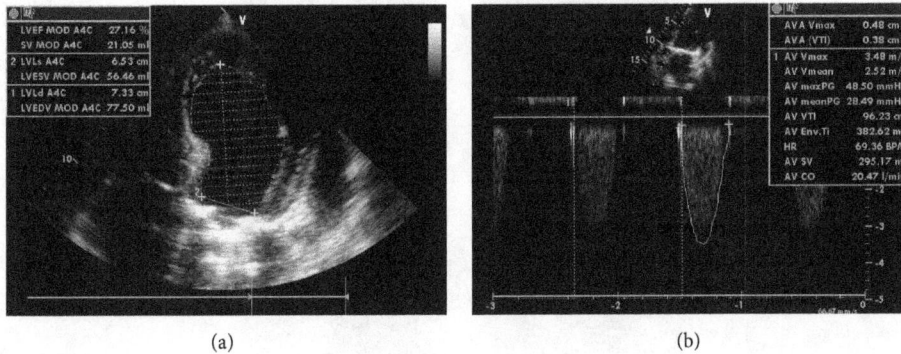

(a)　　　　　　　　　　　　　(b)

FIGURE 2: (a) Severe impairment of the left ventricular systolic function with pericardial effusion. (b) Severe aortic stenosis.

jugular engorgement 3/3 with hepatic jugular reflux; chest X-ray showed pleural effusion in left lung and signs of congestive heart failure (Figure 1).

EKG showed left anterior hemiblock, anterior myocardial infarction sequel, and negative T-waves in precordial and lateral leads.

Transthoracic echocardiogram presented akinesia of the apical segments and mid anterior septum and severe impairment in left ventricular systolic function and ejection fraction (EF) of 27% with mild to moderate pericardial effusion (Figure 2(a)).

There was a mechanical prosthesis in mitral position without signs of malfunction and we confirmed the presence of severe AS with aortic valve area of 0.5 cm^2 (Figure 2(b)).

Coronary angiography was performed, showing severe intrastent restenosis in mid portion of LAD and mild lesions on the other arteries. Taking into account the high surgical risk defined by our Heart Team, Euroscore II 23.1, and STS with a predicted morbidity or mortality of 50.2%, a conventional aortic valve replacement was ruled out and TAVR planned with transapical approach selected.

Reasons for this selection were the small size of both iliac arteries, <6 mm, and the presence of previous cardiac surgery with mitral valve prosthesis with a short distance between mitral and aortic rings.

First, as part of the strategy, a PCI to LAD with cutting balloon Boston Scientific (Marlborough, MA, USA) plus plain balloon angioplasty Ryujin Terumo (Somerset, NJ, USA) and balloon Quantum Maverick Boston Scientific (Marlborough, MA, USA) was performed without complications 72 hours previously to the percutaneous valve implantation.

Access site to the apical wall of left ventricle was previously guided by a 3D computer tomography angiogram, anterograde annulus entrance angle of 158°, and distance annulus to aortic arc of 68 mm (Figures 3(a), 3(b), and 3(c)). The patient had an annulus of 21.7 mm and a perimeter of 69.1 mm, so we selected a JenaValve size of 23.

A transapical access with a mini thoracotomy from fifth intercostal space was performed (Figure 4). We proceeded with transapical approach with initial insertion of a puncture needle using a Terumo (Somerset, NJ, USA) 0.35 J shape guiding wire to cross aortic valve through aortic arc; usually the aortic valve using this anterograde approach is crossed very easily independently of the degree of valvular stenosis. Afterwards a 6F sheath was implanted and a right coronary catheter Terumo (Somerset, NJ, USA) was crossing through the aortic valve, in direction of aortic arc and descendent aorta. At this point we change the wire guide and an extra shift Amplatz (Boston Scientific, Marlborough, MA, USA) 0,35 guide wire was deployed in descendent aorta to give extra backup support (Figure 5(a)).

Through the Amplatz guide an 18 Fr sheath crossing the left ventricular apex was deployed and aortic valvuloplasty with 22 mm Zelos PTA, Balloon Catheter (Ettlingen, Germany), was performed under temporary pacemaker

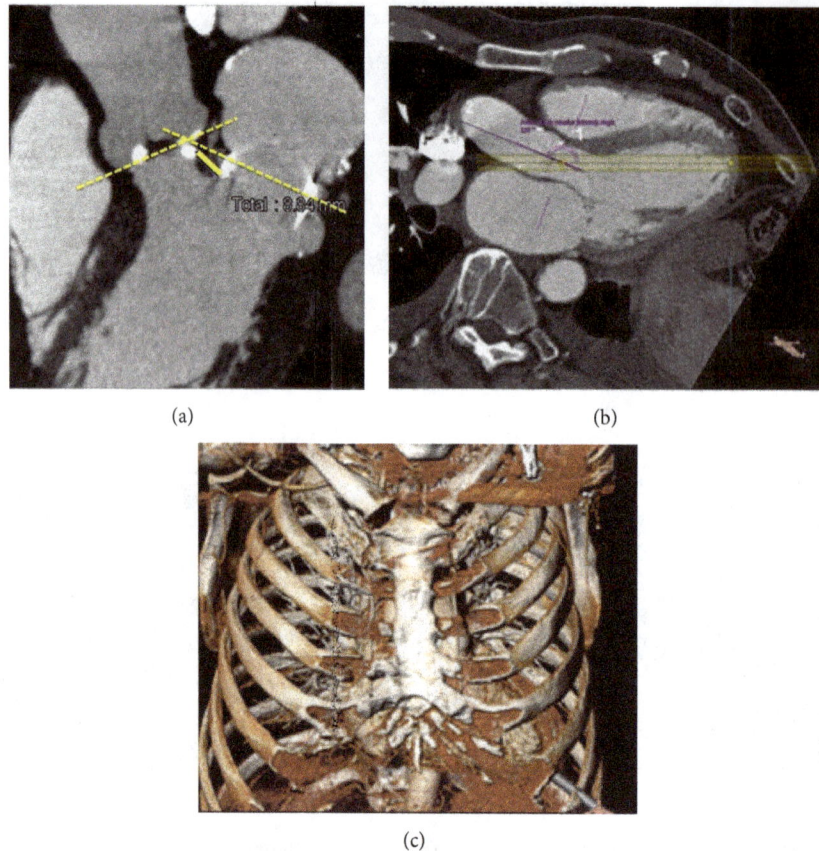

(a)

(b)

(c)

Figure 3: (a) 3D computer tomography images showing distance between aortic and mitral ring, (b) anterograde annulus entrance angles, and (c) place of transapical and 3D reconstruction of intercostal space site access.

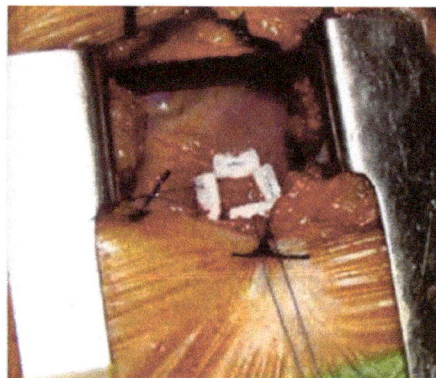

Figure 4: Transapical access with a mini thoracotomy.

(Figure 5(b)). Immediately after valvuloplasty, 18 Fr sheath was removed and in spite of poor left ventricular function and previous cardiac surgery, a 32-French size was successfully delivered and the JenaValve (Guerickestraße, München, Germany) device was implanted and a valve number 23 placed using a three-step deployment system (Figures 5(c) and 5(d)) under 3D fluoroscopy and transesophageal echo. After JenaValve implantation, the device was retrieved easily under simultaneous 150 pacing beats per minute.

Patient had no residual valve leak, with mild valve gradient and an aortic valve area of 1.42 cm^2 after implantation (Figure 6).

During the first 24 hours, patient presented low cardiac output and oliguria requiring dobutamine and intravenous furosemide.

With EKG showing no changes, temporary pacemaker was withdrawn 24 hours after valve implantation. Patient was discharged at day 6, asymptomatic, with 40 mg of furosemide,

(a)

(b)

(c)

(d)

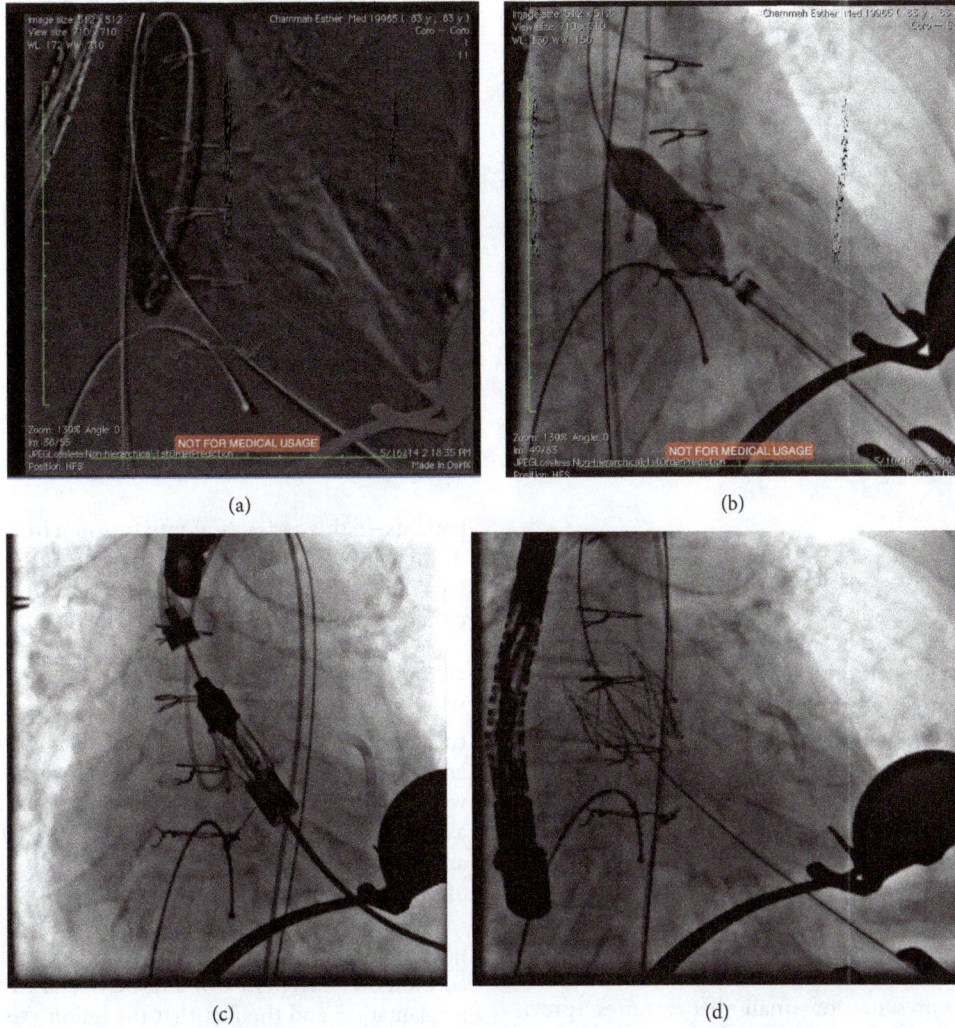

FIGURE 5: (a) Extra shift Amplatz 0,35 guide wire was deployed in descendent aorta to give extra backup support. (b) Aortic valvuloplasty with 22 mm balloon. ((c), (d)) A 32-French size delivery with its JenaValve device can be done, and a valve number 23 is implanted.

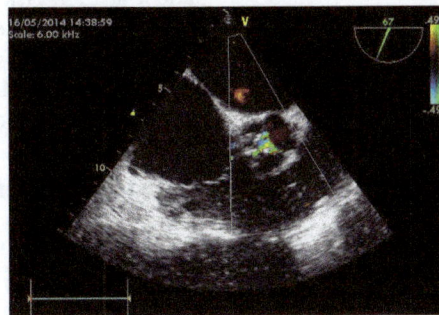

FIGURE 6: No residual valve leak, with mild valve gradient and an aortic valve area of 1.42 cm^2 after implantation.

75 mg clopidogrel, 100 mg aspirin, and 3.25 mg of bisoprolol daily.

At time of hospital discharge, transthoracic echocardiogram showed a significant improvement of left ventricular EF, 41% with an aortic valve area of 1.42 cm^2 (Figure 7).

Four months after implantation patient presented progressive chest pain with ischemic T-waves in lateral leads and was treated medically.

At one year follow-up, patient is alive, in functional classes I-II with an aortic valve area of 1.4 cm^2.

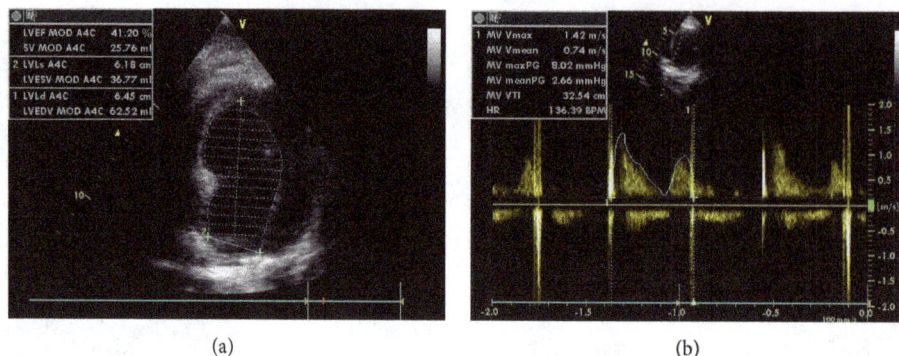

(a)   (b)

FIGURE 7: (a) Hospital discharge transthoracic ECHO showed a significant improvement of left ventricular EF, 41%, (b) 1.42 of aortic valve area and Vmax of 2.66.

3. Discussion

We are presenting a case of severe AS with a critical valve area of $0.5\,\text{cm}^2$ in a patient with high risk morbidity or mortality defined by Heart Team as "elderly female with previous cardiac surgery with mitral valve replacement, severe coronary artery disease, previous myocardial infarction, poor left ventricular EF, pleural and pericardial effusion and severe congestive heart failure." The case was successfully treated using a percutaneous transapical implantation of a second-generation JenaValve [9].

TAVR significantly improves survival and functional class in elderly patients with high surgical risk. Femoral approach is the most frequent access for valve implantation; however there are several circumstances where other access sites are chosen [10].

In this case, presence of small iliac arteries, previous mitral surgical valve implantation, and small distance between mitral and aortic rings almost contraindicated access needed for the other aortic valve device available in Argentina.

The use of CT angiogram previous to the procedure facilitates a better selection of the access site for transapical approach and selects the right coaxial approach of the left ventricle and aortic arch.

Pacing left ventricle during device retrieval allows a softer repossession of the 32 Fr JenaValve sheath without damage to the left ventricle wall in spite of previous valve replacement with pericardial effusion present in our patient.

Even though several large registries have shown that femoral access had lower incidence of morbidity or mortality risk compared to transapical access, the same registries also showed that patients with transapical approach also had significant poor baseline comorbidities associated with high procedural risk [11]. Furthermore, the same registries also showed that apical access was associated with lower incidence of vascular complications and perivalvular aortic leak, both complications linked with late follow-up mortality [12].

A multicenter registry in Europe with the JenaValve device reported high procedural success and very low incidence of cerebrovascular complications (1.1%) with residual moderate aortic regurgitation in only 0.6% of more than 150

patients. In this series, 6-month freedom from cardiovascular death was 90.6% [13]. The second-generation self-expanding JenaValve device is available to be used percutaneously in patients with AS and also with aortic insufficiency [14].

In our initial experience with this device [15] we reported 30-day results from the first 18 patients with a survival of 100% of them without vascular, cerebrovascular, or coronary complications. No patients had residual aortic insufficiency and none required permanent pacemaker. All procedures were performed together by all members of the Heart Team: a cardiac surgeon opened and closed the left ventricle and an interventional cardiologist performed the entire process of percutaneous valve implantation.

Finally, cutting and plain balloon angioplasty to mid portion LAD stenosis was selected as PCI strategy taking into account the short period of time between PCI and aortic valve implantation and the fact that the lesion was located at mid portion of LAD artery presenting an area with previous large anterior myocardial infarction.

In conclusion, we are reporting a case with clinical indication of percutaneous aortic valve replacement in a patient at high risk for femoral access, successfully treated with implantation of a second-generation JenaValve device. To our knowledge, only a few JenaValve patients have been reported in medical literature but none with the amount of comorbidities as our patient [16–19].

Conflict of Interests

The authors declare that there is no conflict of interests regarding the publication of this paper.

References

[1] A. Cribier, H. Eltchaninoff, A. Bash et al., "Percutaneous transcatheter implantation of an aortic valve prosthesis for calcific aortic stenosis: first human case description," Circulation, vol. 106, no. 24, pp. 3006–3008, 2002.

[2] M. B. Leon, C. R. Smith, M. Mack et al., "Transcatheter aortic-valve implantation for aortic stenosis in patients who cannot undergo surgery," The New England Journal of Medicine, vol. 363, no. 17, pp. 1597–1607, 2010.

[3] C. R. Smith, M. B. Leon, M. J. Mack et al., "Transcatheter versus surgical aortic-valve replacement in high-risk patients," *The New England Journal of Medicine*, vol. 364, no. 23, pp. 2187–2198, 2011.

[4] M. Abdel-Wahab, M. El-Mawardy, and G. Richardt, "Update on transcatheter aortic valve replacement," *Trends in Cardiovascular Medicine*, vol. 25, no. 2, pp. 154–161, 2015.

[5] H. Eggebrecht, A. Schmermund, T. Voigtländer, P. Kahlert, R. Erbel, and R. H. Mehta, "Risk of stroke after transcatheter aortic valve implantation (TAVI): a meta-analysis of 10,037 published patients," *EuroIntervention*, vol. 8, no. 1, pp. 129–138, 2012.

[6] V. H. Thourani, C. Li, C. Devireddy et al., "High-risk patients with inoperative aortic stenosis: use of transapical, transaortic, and transcarotid techniques," *Annals of Thoracic Surgery*, vol. 99, no. 3, pp. 817–823, 2015.

[7] H. R. Figulla and M. Ferrari, "Percutaneously implantable aortic valve: the JenaValve concept evolution," *Herz*, vol. 31, no. 7, pp. 685–687, 2006.

[8] J. Kempfert, A. J. Rastan, F.-W. Mohr, and T. Walther, "A new self-expanding transcatheter aortic valve for transapical implantation—first in man implantation of the JenaValve," *European Journal of Cardio-Thoracic Surgery*, vol. 40, no. 3, pp. 761–763, 2011.

[9] H. Treede, F.-W. Mohr, S. Baldus et al., "Transapical transcatheter aortic valve implantation using the JenavalVe system: acute and 30-day results of the multicentre CE-mark study," *European Journal of Cardio-Thoracic Surgery*, vol. 41, no. 6, pp. e131–e138, 2012.

[10] S. V. Lichtenstein, A. Cheung, J. Ye et al., "Transapical transcatheter aortic valve implantation in humans: initial clinical experience," *Circulation*, vol. 114, no. 6, pp. 591–596, 2006.

[11] A. Ghatak, C. Bavishi, R. N. Cardoso et al., "Complications and mortality in patients undergoing transcatheter aortic valve replacement with Edwards SAPIEN & SAPIEN XT valves: a meta-analysis of world-wide studies and registries comparing the transapical and transfemoral accesses," *Journal of Interventional Cardiology*, vol. 28, no. 3, pp. 266–278, 2015.

[12] E. Van Belle, F. Juthier, S. Susen et al., "Postprocedural aortic regurgitation in balloon-expandable and self-expandable transcatheter aortic valve replacement procedures: analysis of predictors and impact on long-term mortality: insights from the France2 registry," *Circulation*, vol. 129, no. 13, pp. 1415–1427, 2014.

[13] O. Wendler, U. Kappert, S. Ensminger et al., "The JUPITER registry: thirty-day primary endpoint results of a second generation transapical TAVI system," in *Proceedings of the EuroPCR Congress*, Abstracts Euro14A-OP289 PCR, Paris, France, May 2014.

[14] S. Bleiziffer, D. Mazzitelli, C. Nöbauer, T. Ried, and R. Lange, "Successful treatment of pure aortic insufficiency with transapical implantation of the jenavalve," *Thoracic and Cardiovascular Surgeon*, vol. 61, no. 5, pp. 428–430, 2013.

[15] J. Mieres, M. Menéndez, C. Fernández-Pereira et al., "Transapical approach of aortic valve implantation with JenaValve: initial experience from Cardiology Department of Otamendi Hospital," *Revista Argentina de Cardioangiología Intervencionista*, vol. 5, no. 4, pp. 268–274, 2014.

[16] V. T. Chao, P. T. Chiam, and S. Y. Tan, "Transcatheter aortic valve implantation with preexisting mechanical mitral prosthesis-use of CT angiography," *Journal of Invasive Cardiology*, vol. 22, no. 7, pp. 339–340, 2010.

[17] J. L. Soon, J. Ye, S. V. Lichtenstein, D. Wood, J. G. Webb, and A. Cheung, "Transapical transcatheter aortic valve implantation in the presence of a mitral prosthesis," *Journal of the American College of Cardiology*, vol. 58, no. 7, pp. 715–721, 2011.

[18] C. J. Beller, R. Bekeredjian, U. Krumsdorf et al., "Transcatheter aortic valve implantation after previous mechanical mitral valve replacement: expanding indications?" *Heart Surgery Forum*, vol. 14, no. 3, pp. E166–E170, 2011.

[19] K. E. O' Sullivan, I. Casserly, and J. Hurley, "Transapical JenaValve in a patient with mechanical mitral valve prosthesis," *Catheterization and Cardiovascular Interventions*, vol. 85, no. 5, pp. 916–919, 2015.

12

A Retained Bullet in Pericardial Sac: Penetrating Gunshot Injury of the Heart

Adnan Kaya,[1] **Emine Caliskan,**[2] **Mustafa Adem Tatlisu,**[3] **Mert Ilker Hayiroglu,**[3] **Ahmet Ilker Tekessin,**[3] **Yasin Cakilli,**[3] **Sahin Avsar,**[3] **Ahmet Oz,**[3] **and Osman Uzman**[3]

[1]*Cardiology, Suruc State Hospital, Sanliurfa, Turkey*
[2]*Radiology, Suruc State Hospital, Sanliurfa, Turkey*
[3]*Cardiology, Dr. Siyami Ersek Cardiovascular and Thoracic Surgery Hospital, Istanbul, Turkey*

Correspondence should be addressed to Adnan Kaya; adnankaya@ymail.com

Academic Editor: Assad Movahed

Penetrating cardiac trauma is rarely seen but when present there is a short time lag to keep the patients alive. Cardiac gunshot injuries are exceptional and it occurs mostly during interpersonal disagreements casualties or a mistakenly fired gun nowadays. Here we present a case of cardiac gunshot injury from the war of Kobani, Syria. The patient was mistakenly diagnosed to have a sole bullet in the left shoulder while he had a penetrating cardiac trauma with a bullet in the heart and pericardial effusion possibly giving rise to pericardial tamponade. Luckily the cardiac gunshot injury was noticed one day later and the patient was referred to a tertiary hospital. Intrapericardial bullet was conservatively followed up. The patient was discharged one week later after resection of the bullet in the shoulder.

1. Introduction

Penetrating cardiac trauma is rarely seen but when present there is a short time lag to keep the patients alive. Cardiac gunshot injuries are exceptional and they occur mostly during interpersonal disagreements casualties or a mistakenly fired gun nowadays. Most cases of the literature of cardiac gunshot injuries come from the data of World War II [1] and Lebanese civil war [2]. Nearly 81% of patients with cardiac gunshot injury lost their life [3]. When a cardiac gunshot injury is suspected computerized tomography, transthoracic echocardiography, and transesophageal echocardiography are suggested for evaluation of cardiac compromise, bullet trajectory, and the localization of the bullet [4]. Surgical intervention is gold standard when hemodynamic compromise like pericardial tamponade, hypovolemic shock due to bleeding is present. However, there is no treatment consensus of hemodynamic stable patient with cardiac gunshot injury and it varies from patient to patient.

Here we present a case of cardiac gunshot injury from the war of Kobani, Syria. The patient was mistakenly diagnosed to have a sole bullet in the left shoulder while he had a PCT with a bullet in the pericardial sac and pericardial effusion possibly giving rise to pericardial tamponade. One day later the bullet in the heart was noticed and luckily the pericardial effusion was shifted to the right pleura. With this case report we would like to point out cautious interrogation of gunshot wounds despite clinical stability at admission and follow-up.

2. Case Presentation

A 32-year-old male fighter was brought to our emergency department on the morning of 6th January, 2015, with several other wounded fighters from the war of Kobani, Syria. Because of the ongoing war, there have been many gunshot wounds, bomb blast wounds, and deaths admitted to our ED. Whenever a casualty arrived to the ED all the staff intensify for minimizing the time loss to save the patients. Fast triage for all the patients is required to determine which patients need to refer to tertiary hospitals and which patients to intervene on the scene. This patient arrived to our hospital after a suicide bomb attack with nine other

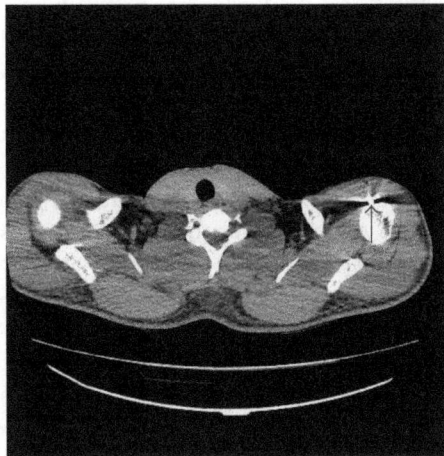

FIGURE 1: Transverse cut view of chest CT shows a bullet in the left shoulder at proximal humerus.

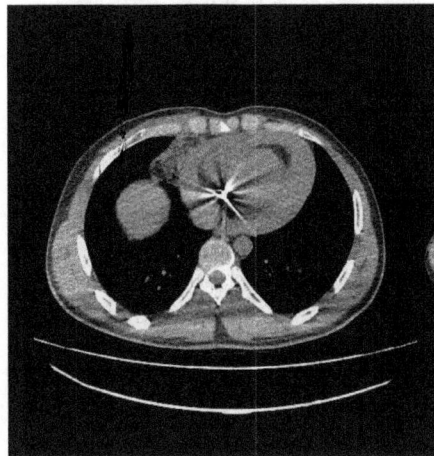

FIGURE 2: Transverse cut view of chest CT shows a bullet in the pericardial sac with pericardial effusion.

patients. Physical examination revealed a superficial wound on the left shoulder and another on the left side of thorax at the 6th intercostals space. There were no exit sides of these wounds which were thought to be bullet wounds. He was conscious with a Glasgow Coma Score of 15, a blood pressure of 110/55 mmHg, a body temperature of 36.3°C, respiratory rate of 22/minute, an oxygen saturation of 93% on room air, and a heart rate of 103 beats per minute. After first evaluation of the patient a thoracoabdominal computerized tomography (CT) was ordered. A bullet was seen in the left shoulder at proximal humerus (Figure 1). There was no fracture of the bone. Intravenous saline, antibiotic, and intramuscular tetanus vaccine were started and the patient was admitted to the general surgery ward for extraction of the bullet. There was moderate dyspnea of the patient which was attributed to anxiety and pain shock. The patient was mobilized during the evening. He had severe dyspnea which was resolved suddenly at 01.00 am and he slept till 06.30 without any symptoms.

The radiologist and the general surgeon of the hospital noticed a pericardial bullet in the patients CT while checking it. The CT shows a hyperdense material in the heart with up to 2 cm pericardial effusion. Transverse cut view of chest CT shows a bullet in the pericardial sac with pericardial effusion compressing the heart (Figure 2). Sagittal cut view of chest CT also revealed a bullet in the pericardial sac with pericardial effusion (Figure 3). There was no evident projectile trajectory.

Cardiology consultation was made. A bedside physical evaluation showed normal heart sounds without any murmurs. Electrocardiography showed sinus rhythm with a rate of 67 bpm and no abnormality. A bedside transthoracic echocardiography (TTE) showed a hyperechogenicity embedded near to the connection of interatrial and interventricular septum in apical 4-chamber view (Figure 4); however, a definite conclusion could not be made if the bullet is compromising the myocardium. There were no valvular insufficiency and no interventricular or interatrial connections. The pericardial effusion seen in CT was drained to the right pleura. The patient was stable. No pericardial effusion,

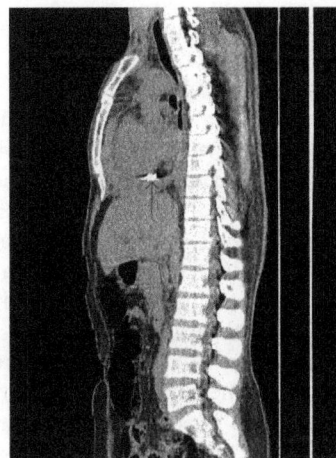

FIGURE 3: Sagittal cut view of chest CT shows a bullet in the pericardial sac with pericardial effusion.

no valvular insufficiency, and no rhythm abnormalities were observed.

The patient was referred to a tertiary cardiovascular institution for follow-up and definite treatment. After a detailed evaluation conservative follow-up was decided and the patient was observed one week in the coronary care unit. He was discharged on the 13th of January after resection of the bullet in the left shoulder. He showed up to his first month visit without any complaints. We do not have any news from him since then.

3. Discussion

The most important clinical presentation of cardiac gunshot injuries is those leading to the cardiac wound, pericardial tamponade, and intrathoracic bleeding. Valvular insufficiencies intracardiac shunts, and conduction defects could be seen in the early course of the trauma. Bacterial endocarditis [5], pericarditis [6], systemic or pulmonary embolization of

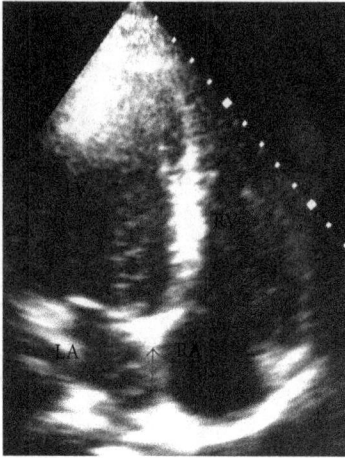

FIGURE 4: Modified apical 4-chamber view of TTE shows the bullet without pericardial effusion.

the missile or thrombi, and neurotic manifestations of various degrees could be late presentations.

The management of cardiac gunshot injuries depends on hemodynamic compromise of the patient. Surgical intervention and correction are an obligation when hemorrhagic shock due to blood loss and pericardial tamponade is present. Some patients may have no time to reach healthcare institution due to severe blood loss and tamponade. When a patient suffers from a cardiac gunshot injury with stable hemodynamic, a careful evaluation is warranted. A thorough physical examination with evaluation vital signs must be the first step. Then chest X-ray and chest CT must be ordered for the possible damage of the vital organs and for localization foreign material. TTE is performed to confirm pericardial effusion and localization of foreign material. Despite progress in surgical interventions and postoperative care the management of retained missiles in the heart and pericardium is still controversial [7–10].

Surgical care of gunshot wounds of the heart and the descending aorta and thoracic or abdominal aorta focuses on substantial and continuous blood loss [11]. Resuscitation management of these penetrating injuries involves massive volume replacement of colloid and crystalloid solutions as well as of blood [12]. Other organ injuries (liver, lungs, stomach, and small intestines) may worsen the situation and complicate the resuscitation. Early surgical intervention may be the only diagnostic and therapeutic procedure at hand, as rapid operative control of the hemorrhagic site is the most effective resuscitation manoeuvre [13]. Correction of damaged tissue must be performed as fast as possible. Projectile trajectory must be followed up for injured tissues. A successful surgical gunshot injury of 16-year-old boy was presented by Aydemir et al. [14]. In this case the projectile entered from right anterior thoracic cavity, passed through the right lung, right atrium, atrial septum, left ventricle, and left lung, and ended up between the eighth and ninth ribs. Early surgical intervention saved this patient's life.

In our case the first examination of the patient revealed a stable hemodynamic and two inlet wounds without exit.

A CT of chest was mistakenly reported as the patient has only one bullet in the left shoulder while he had one in the myocardium with pericardial effusion. Because of our increased workload with nine other casualties no one noticed the CT finding and the patient was interned to the ward for removal of the bullet in the shoulder. The patient's dyspnea is resolved by itself suddenly and he had a comfortable sleep. TTE was performed for the pericardial effusion and intracardiac bullet. TTE showed an embedded bullet to the connection of interatrial and interventricular septum. There was no valvular compromise and electrical instability. Pericardial effusion was drained to the right pleura and the patient was stable. Resection of the bullet of the shoulder was performed and the patient was discharged without any intervention after one-week follow-up in the ward of the tertiary hospital.

4. Conclusion

Cardiac gunshot injuries are very rare in daily routine of medical practice. Physical examination, chest X-ray, chest CT, and TTE are the key elements for rapid diagnosis and management. Here we present a case of cardiac gunshot injury and missed diagnosis because of increased workload. By this case we would like to draw attention to a careful evaluation of gunshot wounds whatever the clinical situation of the patient is.

Conflict of Interests

The authors certify that there is no conflict of interests with any financial organization regarding the material discussed in the paper.

Authors' Contribution

All authors have read and approved the paper.

References

[1] E. F. Bland and G. W. Beebe, "Missiles in the heart. A twenty-year follow-up report of World War II cases," *The New England Journal of Medicine*, vol. 274, no. 19, pp. 1039–1046, 1966.

[2] V. A. Jebara and B. Saade, "Penetrating wounds to the heart: a wartime experience," *The Annals of Thoracic Surgery*, vol. 47, no. 2, pp. 250–253, 1989.

[3] N. C. Campbell, S. R. Thomson, D. J. J. Muckart, C. M. Meumann, I. Van Middelkoop, and J. B. C. Botha, "Review of 1198 cases of penetrating cardiac trauma," *British Journal of Surgery*, vol. 84, no. 12, pp. 1737–1740, 1997.

[4] C. E. M. Brathwaite, R. L. Weiss, W. A. Baldino, N. Hoganson, and S. E. Ross, "Multichamber gunshot wounds of the heart: the utility of transesophageal echocardiography," *Chest*, vol. 101, no. 1, pp. 287–288, 1992.

[5] H. R. Decker, "Foreign bodies in the heart and pericardium: should they be removed?" *The Journal of Thoracic Surgery*, vol. 32, pp. 62–79, 1939.

[6] J. M. Fritz, M. M. Newman, R. W. Jampolis, and W. E. Adams, "Fate of cardiac foreign bodies," *Surgery*, vol. 25, no. 6, pp. 869–879, 1949.

[7] L. F. Parmley, T. W. Mattingly, and W. C. Manion, "Penetrating wounds of the heart and aorta," *Circulation*, vol. 17, no. 5, pp. 953–973, 1958.

[8] A. Hassett, J. Moran, D. C. Sabiston, and J. Kisslo, "Utility of echocardiography in the management of patients with penetrating missile wounds of the heart," *Journal of the American College of Cardiology*, vol. 7, no. 5, pp. 1151–1156, 1986.

[9] R. J. Robison, J. W. Brown, R. Caldwell, K. S. Stone, and H. King, "Management of asymptomatic intracardiac missiles using echocardiography," *The Journal of Trauma*, vol. 28, no. 9, pp. 1402–1403, 1988.

[10] P. N. Symbas, S. E. Vlasis-Hale, A. L. Picone, and C. R. Hatcher Jr., "Missiles in the heart," *The Annals of Thoracic Surgery*, vol. 48, no. 2, pp. 192–194, 1989.

[11] K. K. Nagy, R. R. Roberts, R. F. Smith et al., "Trans-mediastinal gunshot wounds: are 'stable' patients really stable?" *World Journal of Surgery*, vol. 26, no. 10, pp. 1247–1250, 2002.

[12] M. F. Rotondo, C. W. Schwab, M. D. McGonigal et al., "'Damage control': an approach for improved survival in exsanguinating penetrating abdominal injury," *Journal of Trauma*, vol. 35, no. 3, pp. 375–383, 1993.

[13] M. M. Carrick, C. A. Morrison, D. J. Alexis et al., "Thoracoabdominal shotgun wounds: an evaluation of factors associated with the need for surgical intervention," *The American Journal of Surgery*, vol. 198, no. 1, pp. 64–69, 2009.

[14] N. A. Aydemir, I. Bakir, F. Altin, S. Sahin, and M. S. Bilal, "A magic bullet through the heart," *Circulation*, vol. 115, no. 20, pp. e467–e468, 2007.

13

Reversibility of High-Grade Atrioventricular Block with Revascularization in Coronary Artery Disease without Infarction: A Literature Review

Rhanderson Cardoso, Carlos E. Alfonso, and James O. Coffey

Miller School of Medicine, University of Miami, Miami, FL 33136, USA

Correspondence should be addressed to James O. Coffey; jamesodellcoffey@gmail.com

Academic Editor: Konstantinos P. Letsas

Complete atrioventricular (AV) block is known to be reversible in some cases of acute inferior wall myocardial infarction (MI). The reversibility of high-grade AV block in non-MI coronary artery disease (CAD), however, is rarely described in the literature. Herein we perform a literature review to assess what is known about the reversibility of high-grade AV block after right coronary artery revascularization in CAD patients who present without an acute MI. To illustrate this phenomenon we describe a case of 2:1 AV block associated with unstable angina, in which revascularization resulted in immediate and durable restoration of 1:1 AV conduction, thereby obviating the need for permanent pacemaker implantation. The literature review suggests two possible explanations: a vagally mediated response or a mechanism dependent on conduction system ischemia. Due to the limited understanding of AV block reversibility following revascularization in non-acute MI presentations, it remains difficult to reliably predict which patients presenting with high-grade AV block in the absence of MI may have the potential to avoid permanent pacemaker implantation via coronary revascularization. We thus offer this review as a potential starting point for the approach to such patients.

1. Introduction

Permanent pacing is the routine treatment for irreversible third-degree and advanced second-degree atrioventricular (AV) block [1, 2]. Although necessary and effective in most patients with such conditions, the implantation of a permanent pacemaker is costly [3, 4] and is associated with significant potential acute complications, including but not limited to infection [5], bleeding [6], hematoma [2], hemothorax [7], lead dislodgement [8], and atrial [9, 10] or ventricular [9, 11] rupture. Moreover, pacemaker leads over time are subject to fracture, insulation break, or recall, which may require lead extraction, a potentially high-risk procedure [12, 13]. It is therefore desirable from both societal [14] and individual [15] patient points of view to thoroughly rule out all reversible causes of bradyarrhythmia before commitment to a permanent device [2]. Reversible causes of high-grade AV block include hypothyroidism [16], hyperthyroidism [17], lymphoma [18], herbal medications [19], chemotherapeutic

agents [20], Lyme disease [21], viral myocarditis [22], apical ballooning syndrome [23], and negative chronotropic agents [24].

Acute myocardial infarction (MI), particularly with injury to the inferior wall, is also a well-described cause of reversible AV block [25–27]. Potential reversibility of high-grade AV block in coronary artery disease (CAD) patients without an acute MI, in contrast, is a relatively unexplored concept. Herein, we present a literature review prompted by a case of unexpected postrevascularization reversal of symptomatic AV block.

2. Illustrative Case Description

An 85-year-old man with a history of ischemic cardiomyopathy and baseline ejection fraction of 40% following an inferior wall MI in 1996 presented with approximately one week of lightheadedness and chest pain at rest. Previously, his symptoms of chronic stable angina were well controlled

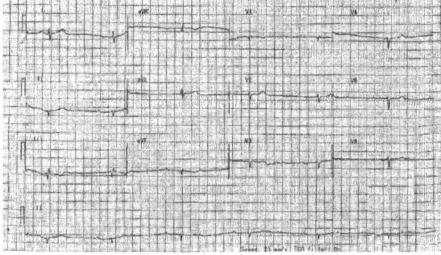

FIGURE 1: Two : one atrioventricular block in a patient with unstable angina prior to revascularization.

with isosorbide mononitrate. An electrocardiogram was performed, revealing 2 : 1 AV block with a ventricular rate of 37 beats per minute (Figure 1). The patient had no prior history of conduction system abnormality. Common causes of reversible AV block were excluded, and the patient was admitted in anticipation of permanent pacemaker implantation. Cardiac biomarkers were negative. Cardiac monitoring continued to show 2 : 1 and occasionally higher-grade AV block.

Given the history of ischemic cardiomyopathy and symptoms consistent with unstable angina, a decision was made to proceed with left heart catheterization before pacemaker implantation. Coronary angiography revealed a dominant right coronary artery (RCA) with 80% ostial stenosis (Figure 2(a)). A drug-eluting stent was successfully deployed to the ostial RCA lesion with an outstanding angiographic result (Figure 2(b)). Upon revascularization, the patient immediately reverted to 1 : 1 AV conduction (Figure 3) and has remained in normal sinus rhythm with mild first-degree AV block since then. The lightheadedness and fatigue have entirely resolved. Permanent pacemaker implantation was avoided.

3. Theoretical Mechanisms of AV Block Reversibility in Coronary Artery Disease

The noteworthy finding in this case is the complete resolution of symptomatic high-grade AV block upon revascularization of the RCA. Review of the literature reveals two possible mechanisms for the presence of clinically significant AV block in patients without MI who experience restoration of normal AV conduction following coronary revascularization. These mechanisms are vagally mediated heart block and ischemia-driven conduction delay.

3.1. Vagal Hypothesis. Vagally mediated bradyarrhythmia is well documented in patients with myocardial ischemia or injury. Ischemic-mediated mechanical stretch and chemical substances stimulate receptors located in the inferior and posterior left ventricular walls [28]. These receptors lead to activation of nonmyelinated afferent C-fibers from the vagus nerve, which in turn result in increased vagal tone and bradyarrhythmia [28, 29]. This mechanism is known as the Bezold-Jarisch reflex. One case report discusses a patient with non-ST elevation MI who developed complete heart block in the setting of a 90% stenosis of the RCA acute marginal

branch. The AV block resolved after balloon angioplasty of this lesion. Because the acute marginal branch does not supply the AV node, the mechanism for third-degree AV block was attributed to the Bezold-Jarisch reflex triggered by inferior wall ischemia [29].

Patients with CAD are especially susceptible to vagal stimulation, as demonstrated by the frequency of carotid sinus hypersensitivity in this population, as well as by the correlation of carotid hypersensitivity with the severity of CAD [30–32]. Jick and Linenthal, for example, reported a case of 2 : 1 AV block in an 85-year-old man with two previous myocardial infarctions and ischemic cardiomyopathy. In a time before percutaneous coronary intervention was available, they observed complete reversal of the 2 : 1 AV block to 1 : 1 AV conduction with atropine administration, as well as progression to complete heart block with carotid sinus massage, phenomena consistent with a vagal etiology of the conduction system disease [33]. Furthermore, coronary revascularization has been shown to attenuate postexercise heart rate decay in patients with RCA lesions, which suggests decreased vagal activity following reperfusion in inferior wall ischemia [34].

Although these descriptions confirm biologic plausibility, whether the decreased cardiac sensitivity to vagal stimuli after revascularization can fully reverse 2 : 1 AV block and avoid further episodes of high-grade AV block is difficult to prove and appears to be a rare phenomenon. Moreover, if the heart block was solely mediated by increased vagal tone, one would expect to see episodes of intermittent AV block during times of high vagal tone, despite revascularization.

3.2. Ischemia Hypothesis. AV conduction defects that resolve with revascularization may occur as a direct result of ischemia, a circumstance more consistent with complete postrevascularization restoration of 1 : 1 AV conduction, such as that observed in the case above. The AV node blood supply is provided by the AV nodal branch, which most commonly arises from the RCA [35], although it can rarely be a branch of the circumflex artery in patients with left coronary artery dominance [36–38]. Meanwhile, infranodal conduction system structures are supplied almost entirely by the septal perforator branches of the LAD artery, with variable dual supply provided by either the RCA or left circumflex artery [38–41]. Decreased flow to the septal branches or RCA is therefore associated with a variety of conduction disturbances [42, 43]. Importantly, the presence of high-grade AV block is associated with a 4-fold and 3-fold increased risk of in-hospital mortality for anterior and inferior wall acute infarctions, respectively [44]. Further, the presence of third-degree AV block in inferior MI has also been associated with an increased incidence of sustained hypotension and ventricular tachyarrhythmia [45].

In acute inferior wall MI, where the RCA is often the culprit, high-grade AV block has been described in up to 17% of cases [26]. Most of these cases are transient and resolve either spontaneously or with revascularization, whereas approximately 9% will ultimately require a permanent pacemaker, implicating permanent damage to AV conduction tissue prior to or due to lack of revascularization

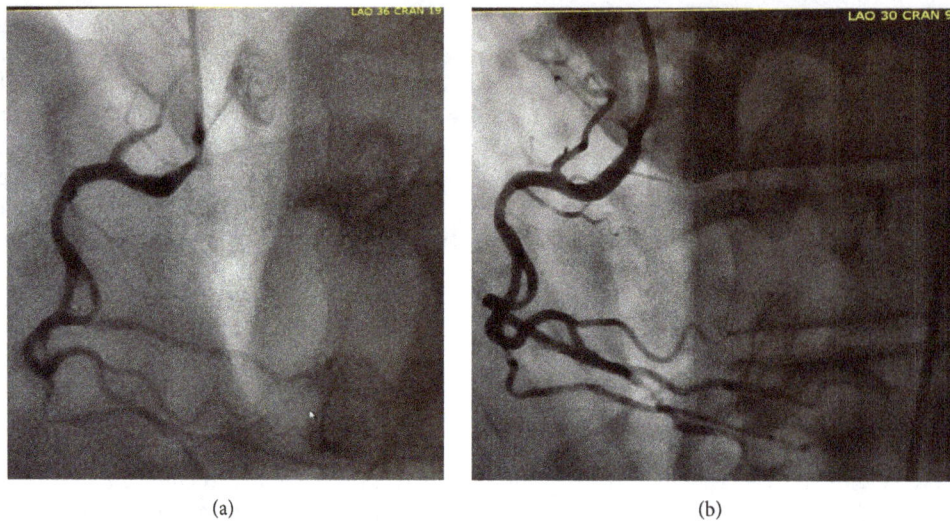

(a)   (b)

FIGURE 2: (a) Angiography revealed an 80% ostial stenosis in the right coronary artery; (b) right coronary artery after successful deployment of drug-eluting stent to ostial lesion.

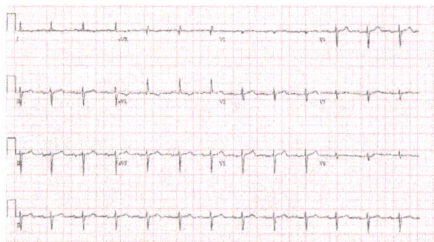

FIGURE 3: Resolution of 2:1 AV block after revascularization; residual 1st-degree AV block (PR 220 ms).

[46, 47]. The 2008 ACC/AHA/HRS Guidelines for Device-Based Therapy acknowledge that, in cases of third-degree AV block complicating inferior wall MI, permanent pacing should be reserved for patients in whom the block does not resolve with revascularization [1]. The possibility of transient AV block secondary to myocardial ischemia in patients without MI is not discussed in current practice guidelines [1].

3.3. AV Block Reversibility in Non-Myocardial Infarction Presentations. In patients with CAD presenting without acute MI, the reversibility of high-grade AV block and the avoidance of pacemaker implantation via revascularization are infrequently described in the literature. In a single-center retrospective study evaluating the reversibility of AV block in patients with CAD, Hwang et al. assessed 188 patients with high-grade AV block for the presence of concomitant CAD. Fifty-eight (30.8%) individuals were found to have CAD, distributed as follows: stable angina, 41; acute MI, 15; and unstable angina, 2. As expected, AV block was reversible with revascularization in 13 of the 15 patients presenting with acute MI. The culprit lesion was located in the RCA in 14 of the 15 acute MI patients. Conversely, only 1 of the 43 patients (2.3%) with stable angina and none of the 2 patients with unstable angina reverted to 1:1 AV conduction after revascularization,

despite the fact that roughly 60% (26/43) of these patients also had significant RCA lesions [48].

Yesil et al. studied 53 pacemaker patients with complete heart block and significant CAD, defined by the presence of a coronary lesion with greater than 70% stenosis. In this study, patients with acute coronary syndrome were excluded. After a mean follow-up of 36 ± 6 months, third-degree AV block persisted in 13/16 (81%) patients treated medically and in 27/37 (73%) of the revascularized patients. Despite most of the lesions being in the RCA, the difference was not significant, leading the authors to conclude that, in the absence of acute MI, coronary revascularization has minimal impact on regaining normal AV function in patients with concomitant third-degree AV block and CAD [49].

The remaining published assessments of AV block in CAD patients without MI are smaller case series. Omeroglu et al., for example, reported a series of 8 patients who presented with new-onset complete AV block and severe CAD requiring coronary artery bypass grafting. Revascularization was performed on the same admission, but none of the patients had resolution of complete AV block in a follow-up of 10 ± 1.07 days [50]. Narin et al. reported two cases of complete heart block in patients with unstable angina that required CABG. When AV block in one of the patients remained on postoperative day 15, he received a permanent pacemaker. The other patient, however, reverted to 1:1 AV conduction immediately after surgical revascularization, and the absence of significant AV block remained at a follow-up of 27.7 months [51]. Such an outcome, we believe, is likely analogous to the fortuitous clinical course experienced by the patient we describe above.

4. Conclusion

In summary, while new-onset high-grade AV block in the setting of CAD is less likely to be reversible in patients without acute MI, there are patients in whom revascularization leads to immediate and durable resolution of 1:1 AV conduction. Examples of this phenomenon include the case illustration above as well as anecdotal cases in the literature. This clinical course is fairly unusual and the mechanism responsible is uncertain. Possible mechanisms include vagal mediation and, more likely, ischemia. The majority of published data suggest that high-grade AV block is usually not reversible with revascularization in patients who have CAD and do not present with an acute MI. The rare case such as the one we describe above is a fortunate but currently unpredictable exception to the rule that such patients will require pacemaker implantation. Nevertheless, in light of the potential negative impacts of permanent pacemakers, it may be prudent to observe postrevascularization conduction before committing patients to device implantation.

Conflict of Interests

The authors declare that there is no conflict of interests regarding the publication of this paper.

Authors' Contribution

All authors participated in concept/design, literature review, drafting of the paper, critical revision of the paper, and final approval of the paper submitted.

References

[1] A. E. Epstein, J. P. DiMarco, K. A. Ellenbogen et al., "ACC/AHA/HRS 2008 guidelines for device-based therapy of cardiac rhythm abnormalities: a report of the American College of Cardiology/American Heart Association Task Force on Practice Guidelines: developed in collaboration with the American Association for Thoracic Surgery and Society of Thoracic Surgeons," *Circulation*, vol. 117, pp. e350–e408, 2008.

[2] M. Brignole, A. Auricchio, G. Baron-Esquivias et al., "2013 ESC guidelines on cardiac pacing and cardiac resynchronization therapy: the Task Force on cardiac pacing and resynchronization therapy of the European Society of Cardiology (ESC)," *Europace*, vol. 15, pp. 1070–1118, 2013.

[3] E. Castelnuovo, K. Stein, M. Pitt, R. Garside, and E. Payne, "The effectiveness and cost-effectiveness of dual-chamber pacemakers compared with single-chamber pacemakers for bradycardia due to atrioventricular block or sick sinus syndrome: systematic review and economic evaluation," *Health Technology Assessment*, vol. 9, pp. 1–246, 2005.

[4] F. Osman, S. Krishnamoorthy, A. Nadir, P. Mullin, A. Morley-Davies, and J. Creamer, "Safety and cost-effectiveness of same day permanent pacemaker implantation," *The American Journal of Cardiology*, vol. 106, no. 3, pp. 383–385, 2010.

[5] J. B. Johansen, O. D. Jørgensen, M. Møller, P. Arnsbo, P. T. Mortensen, and J. C. Nielsen, "Infection after pacemaker implantation: infection rates and risk factors associated with infection in a population-based cohort study of 46299 consecutive patients," *European Heart Journal*, vol. 32, no. 8, pp. 991–998, 2011.

[6] C. Tompkins, A. Cheng, D. Dalal et al., "Dual antiplatelet therapy and heparin 'bridging' significantly increase the risk of bleeding complications after pacemaker or implantable cardioverter-defibrillator device implantation," *Journal of the American College of Cardiology*, vol. 55, no. 21, pp. 2376–2382, 2010.

[7] G. B. Forleo, J. Zeitani, T. Perretta et al., "Acute left hemothorax as a late complication of an active-fixation pacemaker lead," *Annals of Thoracic Surgery*, vol. 95, no. 3, pp. 1081–1084, 2013.

[8] A. Bashir, N. Noroozian, W. Bradlow, and H. Marshall, "Malposition of pacing lead into the left ventricle: a rare complication of pacemaker insertion," *BMJ Case Reports*, 2014.

[9] J. Piekarz, J. Lelakowski, A. Rydlewska, and J. Majewski, "Heart perforation in patients with permanent cardiac pacing—pilot personal observations," *Archives of Medical Science*, vol. 8, no. 1, pp. 70–74, 2012.

[10] A. J. Trigano and T. Caus, "Lead explantation late after atrial perforation," *Pacing and Clinical Electrophysiology*, vol. 19, no. 8, pp. 1268–1269, 1996.

[11] F. Migliore, A. Zorzi, E. Bertaglia et al., "Incidence, management, and prevention of right ventricular perforation by pacemaker and implantable cardioverter defibrillator leads," *PACE*, vol. 37, no. 12, pp. 1602–1609, 2014.

[12] E. Buch, N. G. Boyle, and P. H. Belott, "Pacemaker and defibrillator lead extraction," *Circulation*, vol. 123, no. 11, pp. e378–e380, 2011.

[13] B. L. Wilkoff, C. J. Love, C. L. Byrd et al., "Transvenous lead extraction: Heart Rhythm Society expert consensus on facilities, training, indications, and patient management: this document was endorsed by the American Heart Association (AHA)," *Heart Rhythm*, vol. 6, no. 7, pp. 1085–1104, 2009.

[14] A. A. Choby and A. M. Clark, "What costs matter? Rethinking social costs of new device technologies," *Europace*, vol. 15, no. 11, pp. 1538–1539, 2013.

[15] M. A. Wood and K. A. Ellenbogen, "Cardiology patient pages. Cardiac pacemakers from the patient's perspective," *Circulation*, vol. 105, no. 18, pp. 2136–2138, 2002.

[16] J. B. Singh, O. E. Starobin, R. L. Guerrant, and E. K. Manders, "Reversible atrioventricular block in myxedema," *Chest*, vol. 63, no. 4, pp. 582–585, 1973.

[17] R. H. Miller, F. H. Corcoran, and W. P. Baker, "Second and third degree atrioventricular block with Graves' disease: a case report and review of the literature," *Pacing and Clinical Electrophysiology*, vol. 3, no. 6, pp. 702–711, 1980.

[18] R. K. Crisel, B. P. Knight, and S. S. Kim, "Reversible, complete atrioventricular block caused by primary cardiac lymphoma in a nonimmunocompromised patient," *Journal of Cardiovascular Electrophysiology*, vol. 23, no. 12, pp. 1386–1389, 2012.

[19] S. Guha, B. Dawn, G. Dutta, T. Chakraborty, and S. Pain, "Bradycardia, reversible panconduction defeat and syncope following self-medication with a homeopathic medicine," *Cardiology*, vol. 91, no. 4, pp. 268–271, 1999.

[20] C.-H. Huang, W.-J. Chen, C.-C. Wu, Y.-C. Chen, and Y.-T. Lee, "Complete atrioventricular block after arsenic trioxide treatment in an acute promyelocytic leukemic patient," *Pacing and Clinical Electrophysiology*, vol. 22, no. 6, pp. 965–967, 1999.

[21] I. S. Bhattacharya, M. Dweck, and M. Francis, "Lyme carditis: a reversible cause of complete atrioventricular block," *Journal of the Royal College of Physicians of Edinburgh*, vol. 40, no. 2, pp. 121–122, 2010.

[22] T. H. Yu, G. F. Guo, M. C. Chen, and C. H. Yang, "Reversible infra-Hisian atrioventricular block in acute myocarditis," *Chang Gung Medical Journal*, vol. 24, no. 10, pp. 651–656, 2001.

[23] H. M. Nef, H. Möllmann, J. Sperzel et al., "Temporary third-degree atrioventricular block in a case of apical ballooning syndrome," *International Journal of Cardiology*, vol. 113, no. 2, pp. E33–E35, 2006.

[24] D. Osmonov, I. Erdinler, K. S. Ozcan et al., "Management of patients with drug-induced atrioventricular block," *Pacing and Clinical Electrophysiology*, vol. 35, no. 7, pp. 804–810, 2012.

[25] M. C. Gupta, M. M. Singh, P. K. Wahal, M. P. Mehrotra, and S. K. Gupta, "Complete heart block complicating acute myocardial infarction," *Angiology*, vol. 29, no. 10, pp. 749–757, 1978.

[26] A. C. Tans, K. I. Lie, and D. Durrer, "Clinical setting and prognostic significance of high degree atrioventricular block in acute inferior myocardial infarction: a study of 144 patients," *American Heart Journal*, vol. 99, no. 1, pp. 4–8, 1980.

[27] P. Nicod, E. Gilpin, H. Dittrich, R. Polikar, H. Henning, and J. Ross Jr., "Long-term outcome in patients with inferior myocardial infarction and complete atrioventricular block," *Journal of the American College of Cardiology*, vol. 12, no. 3, pp. 589–594, 1988.

[28] J. A. Chiladakis, N. Patsouras, and A. S. Manolis, "The Bezold-Jarisch reflex in acute inferior myocardial infarction: clinical and sympathovagal spectral correlates," *Clinical Cardiology*, vol. 26, no. 7, pp. 323–328, 2003.

[29] O. Bolorunduro, R. N. Khouzam, and D. Dishmon, "Resolution of complete heart block after revascularization of acute marginal branch of the right coronary artery," *Turk Kardiyoloji Dernegi Arsivi*, vol. 42, no. 7, pp. 667–670, 2014.

[30] C. P. Tsioufis, I. E. Kallikazaros, K. P. Toutouzas, C. I. Stefanadis, and P. K. Toutouzas, "Exaggerated carotid sinus massage responses are related to severe coronary artery disease in patients being evaluated for chest pain," *Clinical Cardiology*, vol. 25, no. 4, pp. 161–166, 2002.

[31] I. Kallikazaros, C. Stratos, C. Tsioufis et al., "Carotid sinus hypersensitivity in patients undergoing coronary arteriography: relation with the severity of carotid atherosclerosis and the extent of coronary artery disease," *Journal of Cardiovascular Electrophysiology*, vol. 8, no. 11, pp. 1218–1228, 1997.

[32] K. A. Brown, J. D. Maloney, H. C. Smith, G. O. Haritzler, and D. M. Ilstrup, "Carotid sinus reflex in patients undergoing coronary angiography: relationship of degree and location of coronary artery disease to response to carotid sinus massage," *Circulation*, vol. 62, no. 4, pp. 697–703, 1980.

[33] H. Jick and A. J. Linenthal, "Reversible Wenckebach type atrioventricular block associated with severe coronary artery disease," *Circulation*, vol. 20, no. 2, pp. 262–266, 1959.

[34] N. Tahara, H. Takaki, A. Taguchi et al., "Pronounced HR variability after exercise in inferior ischemia: evidence that the cardioinhibitory vagal reflex is invoked by exercise-induced inferior ischemia," *The American Journal of Physiology—Heart and Circulatory Physiology*, vol. 288, no. 3, pp. H1179–H1185, 2005.

[35] S. H. El-Maasarany, E. E. B. Elazab, S. Jensen, and M. Y. Henein, "A-V nodal artery anatomy and relations to the posterior septal space and its contents," *International Journal of Cardiology*, vol. 141, no. 1, pp. 92–98, 2010.

[36] J.-L. Lin, S. K. S. Huang, L.-P. Lai et al., "Distal end of the atrioventricular nodal artery predicts the risk of atrioventricular block during slow pathway catheter ablation of atrioventricular nodal re-entrant tachycardia," *Heart*, vol. 83, no. 5, pp. 543–550, 2000.

[37] M. C. Hutchinson, "A study of the artrial arteries in man," *Journal of Anatomy*, vol. 125, pp. 39–54, 1978.

[38] P. J. Zimetbaum and M. E. Josephson, "Use of the electrocardiogram in acute myocardial infarction," *The New England Journal of Medicine*, vol. 348, no. 10, pp. 933–940, 2003.

[39] D. Harpaz, S. Behar, S. Gottlieb, V. Boyko, Y. Kishon, and M. Eldar, "Complete atrioventricular block complicating acute myocardial infarction in the thrombolytic era," *Journal of the American College of Cardiology*, vol. 34, no. 6, pp. 1721–1728, 1999.

[40] R. M. Norris, "Heart block in posterior and anterior myocardial infarction," *British Heart Journal*, vol. 31, no. 3, pp. 352–356, 1969.

[41] L. G. van der Hauwaert, R. Stroobandt, and L. Verhaeghe, "Arterial blood supply of the atrioventricular node and main bundle," *British Heart Journal*, vol. 34, no. 10, pp. 1045–1051, 1972.

[42] S. Wei, L. Zhong, S. Chen, and X. Li, "The status of coronary artery lesions in patients with conduction disturbance," *Journal of Cardiovascular Medicine*, vol. 12, no. 10, pp. 709–713, 2011.

[43] M. Yesil, E. Arikan, N. Postaci, S. Bayata, and R. Yilmaz, "Locations of coronary artery lesions in patients with severe conduction disturbance," *International Heart Journal*, vol. 49, no. 5, pp. 525–531, 2008.

[44] K. McDonald, J. J. O'Sullivan, R. M. Conroy, K. Robinson, and R. Mulcahy, "Heart block as a predictor of in-hospital death in both acute inferior and acute anterior myocardial infarction," *Quarterly Journal of Medicine*, vol. 74, no. 275, pp. 277–282, 1990.

[45] P. Clemmensen, E. R. Bates, R. M. Califf et al., "Complete atrioventricular block complicating inferior wall acute myocardial infarction treated with reperfusion therapy. TAMI Study Group," *American Journal of Cardiology*, vol. 67, no. 4, pp. 225–230, 1991.

[46] C. Giglioli, M. Margheri, S. Valente et al., "Timing, setting and incidence of cardiovascular complications in patients with acute myocardial infarction submitted to primary percutaneous coronary intervention," *Canadian Journal of Cardiology*, vol. 22, no. 12, pp. 1047–1052, 2006.

[47] U. J. O. Gang, A. Hvelplund, S. Pedersen et al., "High-degree atrioventricular block complicating ST-segment elevation myocardial infarction in the era of primary percutaneous coronary intervention," *Europace*, vol. 14, no. 11, pp. 1639–1645, 2012.

[48] I.-C. Hwang, W.-W. Seo, I.-Y. Oh, E.-K. Choi, and S. Oh, "Reversibility of atrioventricular block according to coronary artery disease: results of a retrospective study," *Korean Circulation Journal*, vol. 42, no. 12, pp. 816–822, 2012.

[49] M. Yesil, S. Bayata, E. Arikan, R. Yilmaz, and N. Postaci, "Should we revascularize before implanting a pacemaker?" *Clinical Cardiology*, vol. 31, no. 10, pp. 498–501, 2008.

[50] S. N. Omeroglu, H. Ardal, H. B. Erdogan et al., "Can revascularization restore sinus rhythm in patients with acute onset

atrioventricular block?" *Journal of Cardiac Surgery*, vol. 20, no. 2, pp. 136–141, 2005.

[51] C. Narin, A. Ozkara, A. Soylu et al., "The effect of coronary revascularization on new-onset complete atrioventricular block due to acute coronary syndrome," *Heart Surgery Forum*, vol. 12, no. 1, pp. E30–E34, 2009.

14

Biatrial Cardiac Metastases in a Patient with Uterine Cervix Malignant Melanoma

Caglayan Geredeli,[1] **Melih Cem Boruban,**[2] **Necdet Poyraz,**[3]
Mehmet Artac,[2] **Alpay Aribas,**[4] **and Lokman Koral**[2]

[1]*Department of Medical Oncology, Konya Training and Research Hospital, 42090 Konya, Turkey*
[2]*Department of Medical Oncology, Meram Medical Faculty, Necmettin Erbakan University, 42080 Konya, Turkey*
[3]*Department of Radiology, Meram Medical Faculty, Necmettin Erbakan University, 42080 Konya, Turkey*
[4]*Department of Cardiology, Meram Medical Faculty, Necmettin Erbakan University, 42080 Konya, Turkey*

Correspondence should be addressed to Caglayan Geredeli; caglayange@hotmail.com

Academic Editor: Monvadi Barbara Srichai

Primary malignant melanomas of uterine cervix are quite rarely seen neoplasms, and long-life prognosis of patients with this disease is poor. Immunohistochemical methods and exclusion of other primary melanoma sites are used to confirm the diagnosis. As with other melanomas, cervix malignant melanomas may also cause cardiac metastases. Cardiac metastases are among rarely seen but more commonly encountered cases, compared to primary cardiac tumors. Here, we present a case of biatrial cardiac metastases in a 73-year-old patient with uterine cervix malignant melanomas. The patient underwent echocardiography, cardiac magnetic resonance imaging, and computed tomography. Our report shows the importance of advanced diagnostic techniques, such as cardiac magnetic resonance, not only for the detection of cardiac masses, but for a better anatomic definition and tissue characterization. Although the cases of malignant melanomas leading to multiple cardiac metastasis were reported in literature, the metastatic concurrence of malignant melanomas in both right and left atriums is quite rarely encountered as metastatic malignant melanomas. Also, another intriguing point in our case is that the primary lesion of our case was stemmed from uterine cervix, but not skin.

1. Introduction

Malignant melanomas, common neoplasms of the mucous membranes and skin, constitute almost 2% of all newly diagnosed cancers [1]. Although malignant melanomas can occur in several mucosal sites, genital area in women is an extremely unusual involvement site. Among women, 3 to 7% of all cases are observed within genital tract, and the most witnessed sites are vulva and vagina. Primary malignant melanomas of uterine cervix are extremely rare neoplasms for which only 80 cases have been reported [2, 3].

Malignant melanomas are among the tumors with the highest rates of cardiac metastasis. However, cardiac metastases are diagnosed in about 1% of patients with malignant melanomas because nearly one-tenth of these patients present with cardiac symptoms [4]. The identification of cardiac metastases arising from melanomas usually demonstrates that systemic metastases are the reason of suffering in patients. In our report, we present a rare case with biatrial cardiac metastasis caused by uterine cervix malignant melanomas.

2. Case Presentation

A 73-year-old Caucasian woman had been admitted to the gynaecology and obstetrics department of our hospital with the complaint of vaginal bleeding. On the gynaecologic examination, a mass in size of nearly 5 cm was determined in uterine cervix. Magnetic resonance imaging (MRI) was performed, and a mass in size of 5.5×7.5 cm involving contrast material was detected in cervix area. The mass expanding into uteral parenchyma was seen to cause pressure on

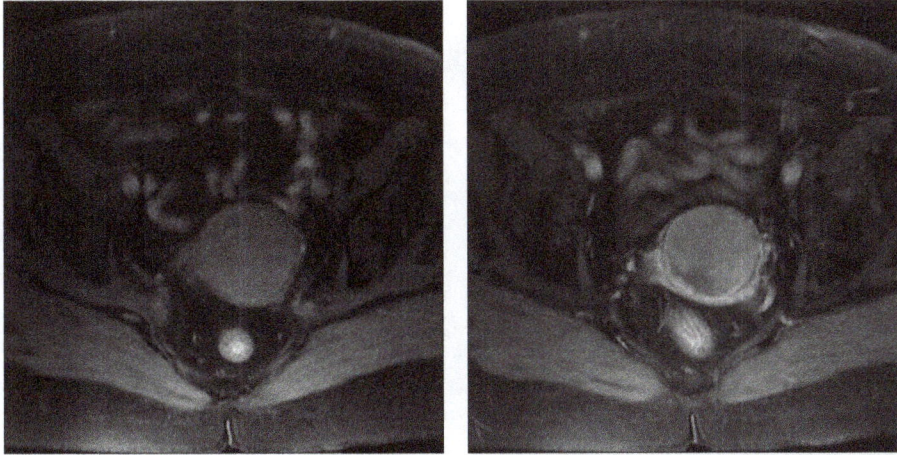

FIGURE 1: Pelvic MRI demonstrates a mass of malignant melanoma in size of 5.5 × 7.5 cm in uterine cervix area.

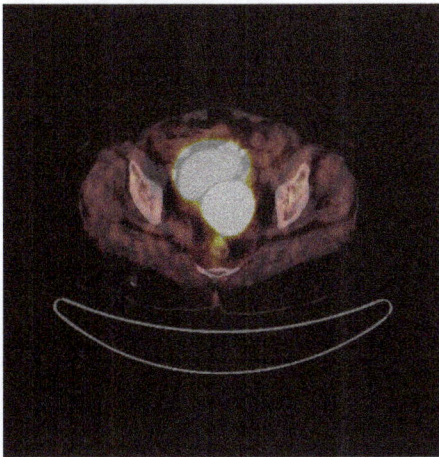

FIGURE 2: PET-CT demonstrates a mass of malignant melanoma in size of 65 × 63 × 98 mm with the uptake of fluoro-2-deoxy-D-glucose (FDG) (suv MAX 27.37) in uterine cervix area.

endometrium. Myometrium and uterine serosa were within normal limits (Figure 1). Positron emission tomography and computed tomography (PET-CT) revealed a mass of 65 × 63 × 98 mm with the uptake of fluoro-2-deoxy-D-glucose (FDG) (suv MAX 27.37) (Figure 2). The patient was surgically treated with type III hysterectomy + bilateral salpingooophorectomy + pelvic and para-aortic lymph node dissection + partial omentectomy. On pathologic examination, a mass of 4 × 3 × 1.8 cm immunohistochemically stained with HMB-45 and S-100 was detected and reported as malignant melanoma. No malignant melanoma metastases were witnessed in all of 38 resected lymph nodes. Within the postop period, the patient was referred to and followed up in the medical oncology department for the adjuvant therapy. Her initial blood pressure was 110/70 mm Hg, pulse rate 70 beats/min, respiratory rate 20/min, and body temperature 36.1°C. The general medical examination showed no pathology of respiratory, cardiovascular, or gastrointestinal systems. On the dermatologic investigation, no cutaneous lesion was observed in all parts of her skin. The treatment of adjuvant interferon alpha-2b (10 million IU/m^2, three days a week) was commenced in the patient in whom no metastases were determined in any other parts of the body via PET-CT. On the thoracic CT performed four months after the initial treatment, two masses were seen, one in size of 36 × 37 mm in right atrium and the other in size of 26 × 20 mm in the left atrium (Figure 3). Via the transesophageal echocardiography, the images of two mobile masses were seen in each atrium, one attached to free wall in size of 29 × 21 mm in right atrium and the other attached to interatrial septum in size of 20 × 17 mm in the left atrium (Figure 4). Also, biatrial dilatation and ejection fraction were found as 55%. The images seen on CT and echocardiography were confirmed by performing cardiac MRI and commented as metastasis. Cardiac MRI demonstrates two masses with biatrial cardiac metastases of malignant melanomas in uterine cervix; one is 37 mm and the other is 20 mm in right and left atriums (Figure 5). Upon the evaluation as cardiac metastasis of uterine cervix malignant melanoma, systemic chemotherapy was administered, and the patient died three months after the initiation of systemic chemotherapy.

3. Discussion

Primary malignant melanomas of uterine cervix are difficultly diagnosed due to the lack of symptoms but may rarely lead to vaginal bleeding, as in our case. Meticulous examinations and detailed clinical investigations should be performed in order to diagnose correctly and early such an ailment with rare clues [5].

Malignant melanomas are known to show an aggressive biological behavior and a great tendency to cardiac metastases [6]. Most of such metastases occur after multifocal hematologic dissemination and may occur anywhere in the heart. Melanotic metastases can invade the walls of four cardiac chambers, and the right atrium is the most frequently involved site. Cardiac metastases typically involve the pericardium and myocardium while the endocardial layer is rarely involved. Additionally, metastatic melanomas of

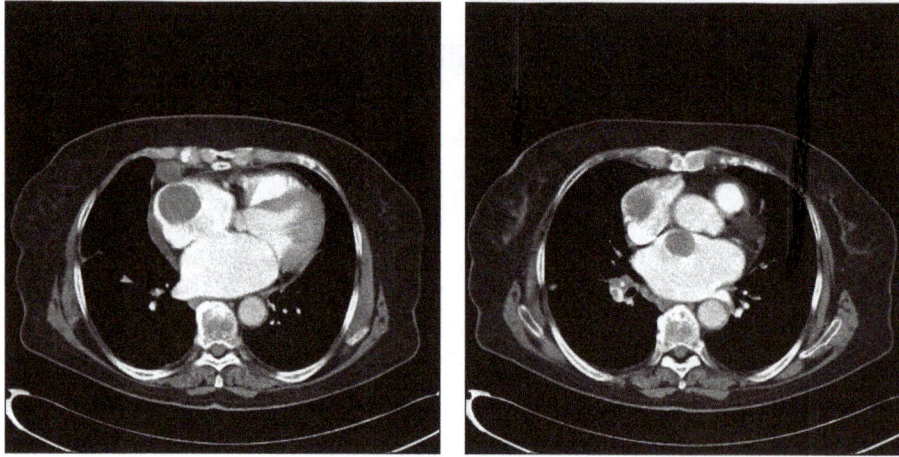

FIGURE 3: Thoracic CT demonstrates two masses with biatrial cardiac metastases of malignant melanomas in uterine cervix: one is 36 × 37 mm and the other is 26 × 20 mm in right and left atriums.

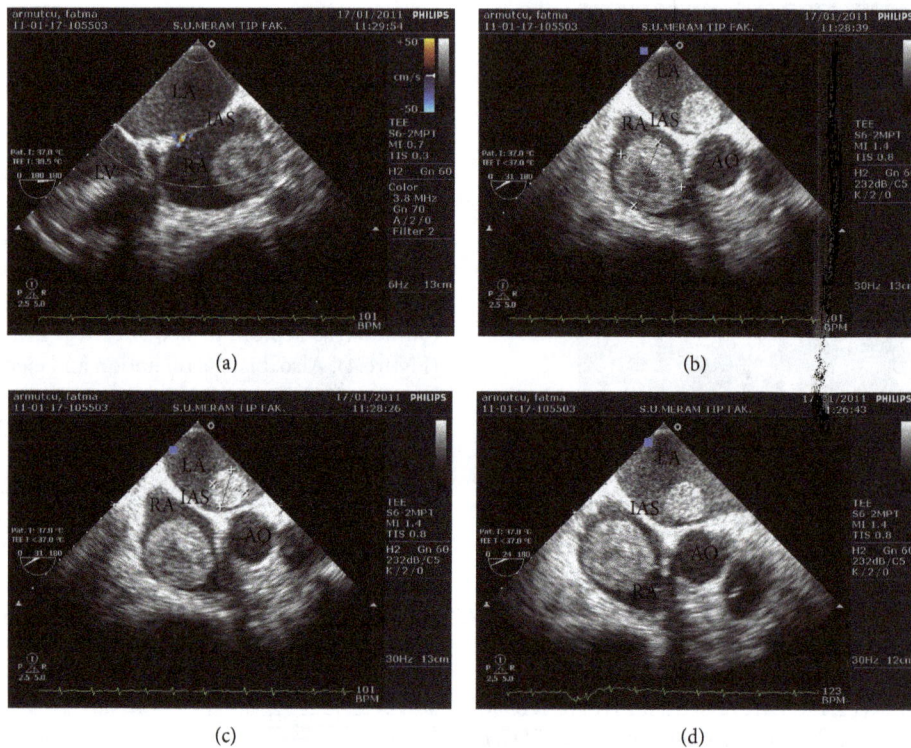

(a)

(b)

(c)

(d)

FIGURE 4: Transesophageal echocardiography demonstrates two mobile masses with biatrial cardiac metastases of malignant melanomas in uterine cervix, one attached to free wall (29 × 21 mm) in right atrium and the other attached to interatrial septum (20 × 17 mm) in the left.

the pericardium and myocardium are usually multifocal lesions [7–9].

While cardiac metastases are the rarely seen initial manifestations, cardiac involvement usually occurs during the late stages of the disease. Therefore, the initial definitive antemortem diagnosis of metastatic melanomas of the heart is rare. Suspicious symptoms include otherwise-unexplained fever, heart murmurs, dysrhythmia, pericardial effusion, or heart failure [10–12].

CT or MRI may be beneficial in providing information, and PET is a noninvasive imaging technique used to detect occult or distant metastases at a relatively early stage and to clarify abnormal radiologic findings [10–12]. Cardiac metastases are seen as hypodense mass leading to filling defect after the injection of contrast material on CT images. A hypodense mass leading to filling defect in right atrium after contrast material injection is seen on our CT images as well (Figure 2). In the cardiac metastasis of malignant melanomas, hyperintense involvements are usually seen on T1-weighted cardiac MR images, heterogeneous hypointense involvements on T2-weighted images, and intense contrast material involvement after the injection of contrast material injection [13, 14]. In

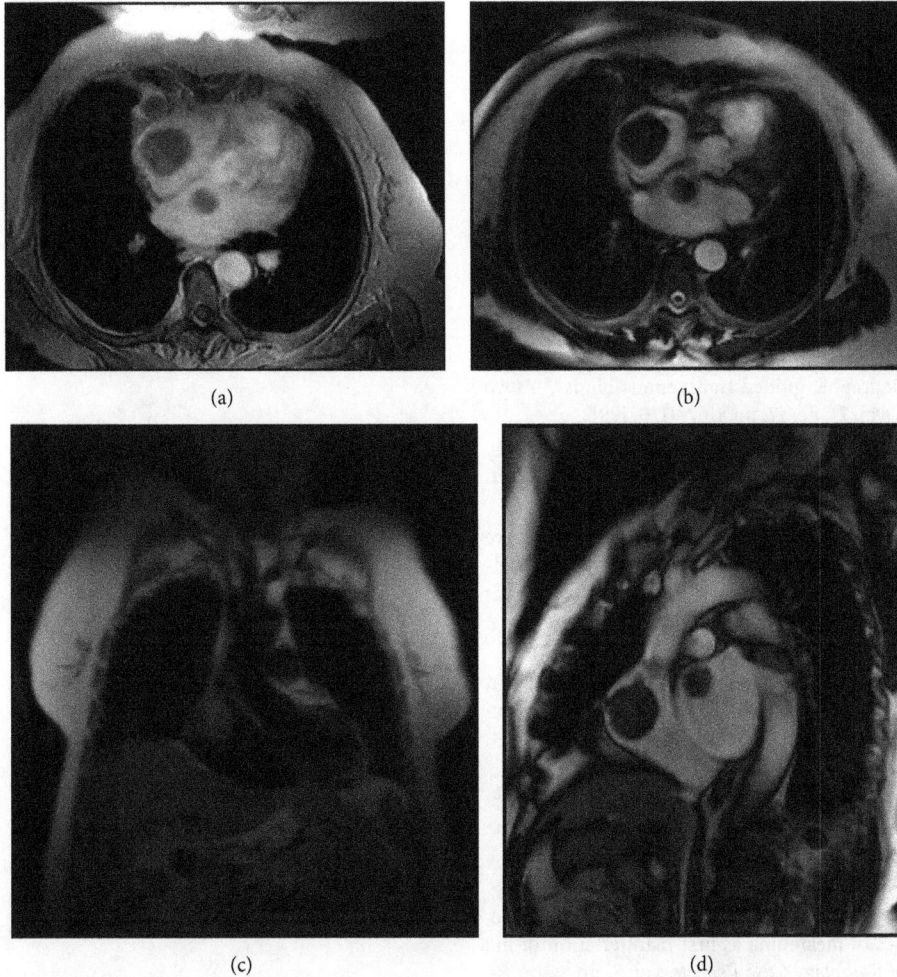

(a)

(b)

(c)

(d)

FIGURE 5: Cardiac MRI demonstrates two masses with biatrial cardiac metastases of malignant melanomas in uterine cervix: one is 37 mm and the other is 20 mm in right and left atriums.

our cardiac MR images, heterogeneous hypointensity is seen on T2-weighted images, as well. An anatomic location of a tumor and the extent of invasion determine the feasibility of surgical intervention, which should optimally be performed during the early stages of the disease. Completely resecting an intracardiac melanoma prevents potential morbidities associated with progressive intracardiac growth, such as superior vena cava syndrome, right ventricular outflow and inflow obstruction, dysrhythmia, cardiac tamponade, and heart failure [10–12].

The medical therapy of patients with metastatic melanomas consists of the palliation of symptoms and systemic therapy with cytotoxic drugs, biotherapy, or immunotherapy. Long-term survival in these patients is associated with a complete response to systemic treatment. Although the cases of malignant melanomas leading to multiple cardiac metastasis were reported in literature [7], the metastatic concurrence of malignant melanomas in both right and left atriums is quite rarely encountered as metastatic malignant melanomas. Also, another intriguing point in our case is that the primary lesion of our case was stemmed from uterine cervix, but not skin.

Conflict of Interests

The authors declare that there is no conflict of interests regarding the publication of this paper.

References

[1] J. Tomicic and H. J. Wanebo, "Mucosal melanomas," *Surgical Clinics of North America*, vol. 83, no. 2, pp. 237–252, 2003.

[2] C. C. McLaughlin, X.-C. Wu, A. Jemal, H. J. Martin, L. M. Roche, and V. W. Chen, "Incidence of noncutaneous melanomas in the U.S.," *Cancer*, vol. 103, no. 5, pp. 1000–1007, 2005.

[3] W. Kedzia, S. Sajdak, H. Kedzia, and M. Spaczyński, "Primary melanoma of the uterine cervix in a 19 year old woman—case report," *Ginekologia polska*, vol. 68, no. 8, pp. 386–389, 1997.

[4] E. Y. Lee, J.-O. Choi, H. N. Park et al., "Malignant melanoma of unknown primary origin presenting as cardiac metastasis," *Korean Circulation Journal*, vol. 42, no. 4, pp. 278–280, 2012.

[5] J. Baruah, K. K. Roy, S. Kumar, and L. Kumar, "A rare case of primary malignant melanoma of cervix," *Archives of Gynecology and Obstetrics*, vol. 280, no. 3, pp. 453–456, 2009.

[6] N. Ozyuncu, M. Sahin, T. Altin, R. Karaoguz, M. Guldal, and O. Akyurek, "Cardiac metastasis of malignant melanoma: a rare cause of complete atrioventricular block," *Europace*, vol. 8, no. 7, pp. 545–548, 2006.

[7] D. N. Chrissos, P. N. Stougiannos, D. Z. Mytas, A. A. Katsaros, G. K. Andrikopoulos, and I. E. Kallikazaros, "Multiple cardiac metastases from a malignant melanoma," *European Journal of Echocardiography*, vol. 9, no. 3, pp. 391–392, 2008.

[8] P. Savoia, M. T. Fierro, A. Zaccagna, and M. G. Bernengo, "Metastatic melanoma of the heart," *Journal of Surgical Oncology*, vol. 75, no. 3, pp. 203–207, 2000.

[9] J. F. Malouf, R. C. Thompson, W. J. Maples, and J. T. Wolfe, "Diagnosis of right atrial metastatic melanoma by transesophageal echocardiographic-guided transvenous biopsy," *Mayo Clinic Proceedings*, vol. 71, no. 12, pp. 1167–1170, 1996.

[10] B. Onan, I. S. Onan, and B. Polat, "Surgical resection of solitary metastasis of malignant melanoma to the right atrium," *Texas Heart Institute Journal*, vol. 37, no. 5, pp. 598–601, 2010.

[11] I. Basarici, I. Demir, H. Yilmaz, and R. E. Altekin, "Obstructive metastatic malignant melanoma of the heart: imminent pulmonary arterial occlusion caused by right ventricular metastasis with unknown origin of the primary tumor," *Heart and Lung*, vol. 35, no. 5, pp. 351–354, 2006.

[12] L. Kontozis, M. Soteriou, D. Papamichael et al., "Isolated right atrial metastasis of malignant melanoma mimicking a myxoma," *Hellenic Journal of Cardiology*, vol. 52, no. 3, pp. 281–284, 2011.

[13] B. C. Allen, T. L. Mohammed, C. D. Tan, D. V. Miller, E. E. Williamson, and J. S. Kirsch, "Metastatic melanoma to the heart," *Current Problems in Diagnostic Radiology*, vol. 41, no. 5, pp. 159–164, 2012.

[14] A. Villa, E. Eshja, S. Dallavalle, E. M. Bassi, and A. Turco, "Cardiac metastases of melanoma as first manifestation of the disease," *Journal of Radiology Case Reports*, vol. 8, no. 4, pp. 8–15, 2014.

15

Hypereosinophilic Syndrome:
A Case of Fatal Löffler Endocarditis

Mario Enrique Baltazares-Lipp,[1] **Juan Ignacio Soto-González,**[1]
Carlos Manuel Aboitiz-Rivera,[1] **Héctor A. Carmona-Ruíz,**[1] **Benito Sarabia Ortega,**[1]
and Ruben Blachman-Braun[2]

[1]*Departamento de Hemodinamia y Ecocardiografía, Instituto Nacional de Enfermedades Respiratorias "Ismael Cosío Villegas",
14080 Mexico City, Mexico*
[2]*Facultad de Ciencias de la Salud, Universidad Anáhuac México Norte, 52786 Estado de México, Mexico*

Correspondence should be addressed to Mario Enrique Baltazares-Lipp; sclc1961@yahoo.com.mx

Academic Editor: Ertuğurul Ercan

Hypereosinophilic syndrome (HES) is a rare disorder with unknown global prevalence, barely reported in Hispanic population, and characterized by persistent eosinophilia in association with organ dysfunctions directly attributable to eosinophilic infiltration. Cardiac involvement may be present in 50 to 60% of the patients. This is known as Löffler endocarditis. We present a case of a 36-year-old Hispanic man with signs of heart failure. Laboratory studies showed eosinophilia ($23{,}100/\mu L$). Thoracic computer tomography showed bilateral pleural effusion and a large left ventricular mass. Transthoracic echocardiography showed left ventricle apical obliteration and a restrictive pattern. Pulmonary angiography demonstrated a thrombus in the lingular and middle lobe. Despite treatment, the patient deceased seven days after admission. Autopsy confirmed the diagnosis of Löffler endocarditis.

1. Introduction

Hypereosinophilic syndrome (HES) is a rare disorder with unknown global prevalence, barely reported in Hispanic population [1]. HES is traditionally defined as persistent eosinophilia with more than 1500 cells per microliter for at least six months, which remains unexplained despite a comprehensive evaluation, in association with organ dysfunctions directly attributable to eosinophilic infiltration [2, 3]. In 1936, Löffler described the first cases of HES with cardiac involvement (Löffler endocarditis) [4].

Cardiac involvement is secondary to the myocardium and endocardium damage due to the eosinophils infiltration and degranulation, which release toxic proteins, thus creating tissue inflammation and later fibrosis. Löffler endocarditis is present in 50 to 60% of HES cases; this is usually characterized by endocardial thickening, atrial dilatation, a restrictive pattern in Doppler echocardiography, and ventricular obliteration by an echogenic material, suggestive of fibrosis or thrombosis frequently located in the apical region of the left

and right ventricles. HES can present a slow or a rapid (acute) progression, this last one especially when the heart or central nervous system is involved. The prognosis is poor, and death is usually due to congestive heart failure, often with associated renal, hepatic, or respiratory dysfunction [5–7].

In this paper, we present one of the few reported cases of Löffler endocarditis in Hispanic population in addition to a clinical, radiological, tomographic, echocardiographic, and pathological correlation with literature review of this rare entity.

2. Case Presentation

A 36-year-old Hispanic male admitted with persistent symptoms of congestive heart failure that began 12 days before admission and persists despite standard medical treatment. During physical examination, he presents atypical chest pain, progressive dyspnea, orthopnea, palpitation, productive cough, and fever. Physical examination revealed normal

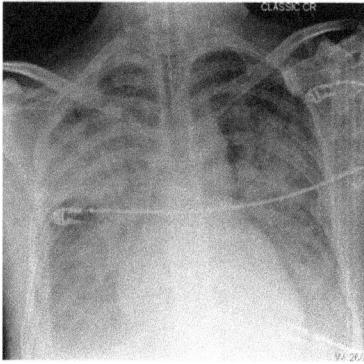

FIGURE 1: Anteroposterior chest radiography, which shows diffuse pulmonary congestion with bilateral pleural effusion.

blood pressure (110/70 mmHg), tachycardia, tachypnea, elevated jugular vein pressure, and congestive hepatomegaly, in functional class III according to the New York Heart Association (NYHA). Cardiac auscultation revealed a third heart sound as well as mitral and tricuspid holosystolic murmurs; crackles were heard in both lungs and edema was observed in both legs.

Chest radiography demonstrated pulmonary congestion with bilateral pleural effusion and cardiomegaly (Figure 1). Laboratory test revealed a marked leukocytosis ($23,100/\mu L$) with hypereosinophilia (59%, $13,360/\mu L$). Computed tomography of the chest showed bilateral pleural effusion and a large left ventricular mass (Figure 2). The transthoracic echocardiogram showed moderate tricuspid and mild mitral regurgitation with normal left ventricular dimensions and systolic function; left ventricular filling was reduced because of endocardial thickening together with a large homogeneous mass at the apex that occupied 50 to 65% of the left ventricular cavity (Figure 3). Echocardiographic Doppler detected restrictive-type diastolic filling an E/A ratio greater than 2. The echocardiography also revealed another mass in the right ventricle. A coronary angiography was performed and found no significant coronary artery disease; pulmonary angiography demonstrated a thrombus in the lingular and middle lobe.

An endomyocardial biopsy was performed; however, pathologic examination of the obtained specimens revealed mainly thrombus with some necrotic tissue. Despite the biopsy results, a diagnosis of endomyocardial fibrosis secondary to HES was made, on the basis of the imaging, clinical, and laboratory findings, and other secondary causes of hypereosinophilia were ruled out. Despite the team effort and adequate treatment, patient deteriorates to NYHA class IV and died seven days after admission. Then, autopsy was done which confirms the diagnosis of Löffler endocarditis (Figure 4).

3. Discussion

Although the real epidemiology of HES is unknown, it is estimated that 90% of patients are men; the majority of the cases occur between 20 and 50 years of age, with a peak in

the fourth decade of life [3]. The clinical manifestations of HES are markedly heterogeneous with a wild clinical spectrum from a completely asymptomatic to a life-threatening condition; this pathology can involve many organs and systems such as skin, lungs, nervous system, gastrointestinal tract, kidneys, and heart; therefore the diagnosis could be a challenge [3, 4]. The major morbidity and mortality in HES patients are cardiovascular complication, which is found in 40 to 50% of the cases [3].

Löffler endocarditis presents with extensive infiltration of the ventricular endocardium by eosinophils, with degranulation and arteriolar necrosis with subsequent endomyocardial fibrosis. The inflammatory changes result in thrombus formation, in this case occupying both ventricular cavities, with impairment of diastolic filling and a resultant restrictive cardiomyopathy [8, 9]. The clinical presentation was consistent with heart failure with NYHA functional class III that rapidly progressed to functional class IV, despite the treatment. HES is a potentially fatal disease, with a survival rate of less than 50% after 10-year follow-up. There are several predictors of early mortality that includes intraventricular conduction delay, duration of symptoms prior to presentation, NYHA functional classes III and IV, and the presence of an embolic event. Our patient had two of these early mortality predictors (NYHA functional class IV and pulmonary embolism) and rapid deterioration; finally he deceased [10, 11].

Echocardiographic and radiological studies could be a useful tool in determining cardiac anatomy and function; however, Löffler endocarditis requires a pathological diagnosis; therefore endocardial biopsy remains the gold standard. Nevertheless, in some cases the cardiac biopsy could be a risky procedure; therefore the clinician should assess the inherent risk of this intervention in each particular clinical setting. In addition, it is indispensable to rule out Löffler endocarditis when diagnosis of pulmonary disorders associated with hypereosinophilia is considered. Additionally, it is important to discard the main differential diagnosis of HES when assessing the possibility of Löffler endocarditis, which includes hypereosinophilia secondary to hypersensitivity reactions and parasite infections [4].

In this case, despite the endomyocardial biopsy result, the patient had peripheral hypereosinophilia and typical echocardiographic findings of restrictive cardiomyopathy; therefore the diagnosis of Löffler endocarditis was established and then was confirmed during autopsy. Pathological finding in Löffler endocarditis includes fibrous thickening of the endocardium, leading to apical obliteration, thrombus formation, and restrictive cardiomyopathy, which clinically manifest as heart failure, thromboembolic event, and atrial fibrillation [5–7].

HES treatment primary goals are to reduce eosinophil level in peripheral blood and tissue, preventing end-organ damage and avoiding adverse thrombotic events. Heart failure in Löffler endocarditis is mainly due to diastolic rather than systolic dysfunction; therefore treatment includes intravenous diuretics to decrease cardiac preload [4]. In addition, for the treatment of symptomatic patients, such as this case, the first-line drug of choice is corticosteroids followed by cytotoxic agents such as hydroxyurea or

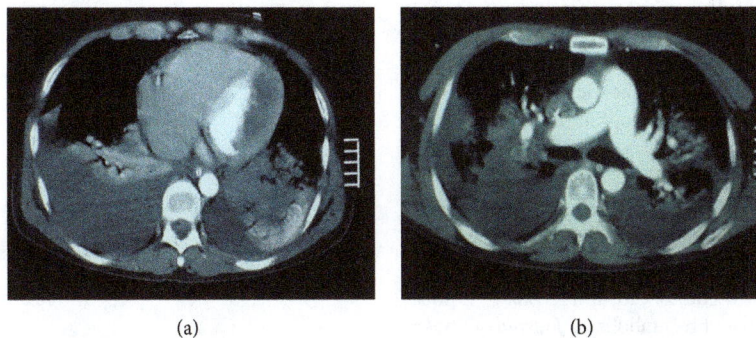

(a)   (b)

FIGURE 2: Chest computer tomography with contrast showing (a) a thrombus in the left ventricle and (b) bilateral pleural effusion and dilated main pulmonary artery and its branches.

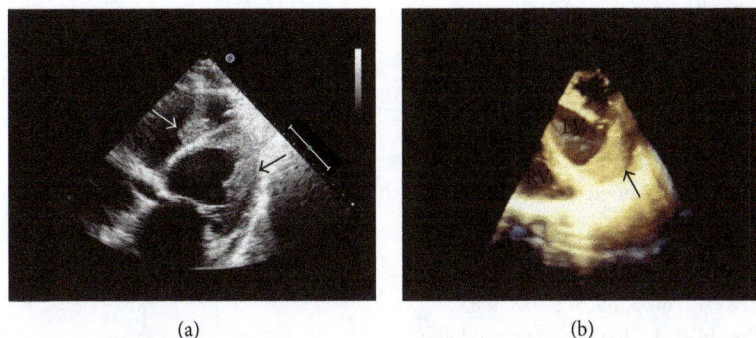

(a)   (b)

FIGURE 3: (a) Transthoracic echocardiogram in a modified apical four-chamber view, showing the left ventricular apex with obliteration and the lateral wall thickened by an image suggestive of a thrombus (black arrow) in the right ventricle and image suggestive of a smaller thrombus attached to the septum (white arrow). (b) Transesophageal echocardiogram with a 3D reconstruction, showing a thrombus in the left ventricle (black arrow). LV = left ventricle; RV = right ventricle.

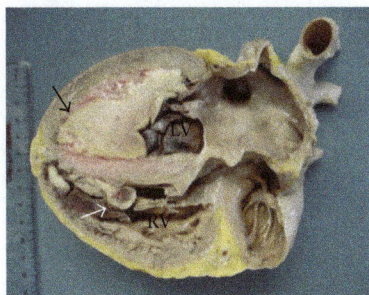

FIGURE 4: Patients heart, showing a thrombus located in the left ventricle (black arrow), with an endothelium cover, and myocardial infiltration. Additionally, a right ventricular thrombus (white arrow) attached to the septum and covered by endothelium. In addition, there is right ventricular thickness of the free wall. LV = left ventricle; RV = right ventricle.

immunomodulatory agents such as interferon-alpha. Gluco-corticoid treatment resulted in clinical and biopsy-proven improvement of eosinophilic and myocardial damage as well as normalization of peripheral hypereosinophilia [12, 13]. Other recent therapeutics includes tyrosinase inhibitors and new types of monoclonal antibodies (Imatinib) [4, 14]. The patient received glucocorticoid treatment without favorable response; his heart failure continued to worsen and led to his death within one week.

4. Conclusion

Löffler endocarditis is a rare entity probably underdiagnosed and underreported worldwide and, in Hispanic popula-tions, this pathology represents a diagnosis challenge for the attending physician. Therefore, when HES is suspect, an echocardiographic study should be indicated with the intention of determining if there is a restrictive pattern, and if this pattern is present, a biopsy is indicated. When there is a high clinical suspicion of HES and image studies that support the possibility of Löffler endocarditis and early mortality predictors are present, we consider that treatment should be initiated immediately even in the absence of a definitive pathological diagnosis.

Conflict of Interests

Authors declare no conflict of interests.

References

[1] E. González Torrecilla, M. Rey Pérez, C. Maraví Petri, L. Alvarez Lacruz, and M. Córdoba Polo, "Diagnostic usefulness of 2-dimensional echocardiography in eosinophilic endomyocardial disease (Loeffler disease)," *Revista Espanola de Cardiologia*, vol. 42, no. 2, pp. 126–130, 1989.

[2] M. J. Chusid, D. C. Dale, B. C. West, and S. M. Wolff, "The hypereosinophilic syndrome: analysis of fourteen cases with review of the literature," *Medicine*, vol. 54, no. 1, pp. 1–27, 1975.

[3] S. Wang, A. Wang, B. Guo, S. Zhu, Z. Chi, and X. Zhao, "Löffler endocarditis with multiple cerebral embolism," *Journal of Stroke and Cerebrovascular Diseases*, vol. 23, no. 6, pp. 1709–1712, 2014.

[4] Q. Zhuang, Z. Y. Zheng, W. Mao et al., "Right ventricular apical obstruction in a patient with hypereosinophilia: Löffler endocarditis," *Heart & Lung*, vol. 44, no. 2, pp. 165–169, 2015.

[5] E. P. M. Corssmit, M. D. Trip, and J. D. Durrer, "Loffler's endomyocarditis in the idiopathic hypereosinophilic syndrome," *Cardiology*, vol. 91, no. 4, pp. 272–276, 1999.

[6] J. Benezet-Mazuecos, A. de la Fuente, P. Marcos-Alberca, and J. Farre, "Loeffler endocarditis: what have we learned?" *American Journal of Hematology*, vol. 82, no. 10, pp. 861–862, 2007.

[7] J. S. Gottdiener, B. J. Maron, R. T. Schooley, J. B. Harley, W. C. Roberts, and A. S. Fauci, "Two-dimensional echocardiographic assessment of the idiopathic hypereosinophilic syndrome. Anatomic basis of mitral regurgitation and peripheral embolization," *Circulation*, vol. 67, no. 3, pp. 572–578, 1983.

[8] C. Lofiego, M. Ferlito, G. Rocchi et al., "Ventricular remodeling in Loeffler endocarditis: implications for therapeutic decision making," *European Journal of Heart Failure*, vol. 7, no. 6, pp. 1023–1026, 2005.

[9] G. C. Salanitri, "Endomyocardial fibrosis and intracardiac thrombus occurring in idiopathic hypereosinophilic syndrome," *American Journal of Roentgenology*, vol. 184, no. 5, pp. 1432–1433, 2005.

[10] P. N. Gupta, M. S. Valiathan, K. G. Balakrishnan, C. C. Kartha, and M. K. Ghosh, "Clinical course of endomyocardial fibrosis," *Heart*, vol. 62, no. 6, pp. 450–454, 1989.

[11] B. H. Chao, K. Cline-Parhamovich, J. D. Grizzard, and T. J. Smith, "Fatal Loeffler's endocarditis due to hypereosinophilic syndrome," *American Journal of Hematology*, vol. 82, no. 10, pp. 920–923, 2007.

[12] A. D. Klion, "Approach to the therapy of hypereosinophilic syndromes," *Immunology and Allergy Clinics of North America*, vol. 27, no. 3, pp. 551–560, 2007.

[13] H. J. Yoon, H. Kim, H. S. Park et al., "Loeffler's endocarditis due to idiopathic hypereosinophilic syndrome," *Journal of Cardiovascular Ultrasound*, vol. 16, no. 4, pp. 136–139, 2008.

[14] J. Gotlib, "World Health Organization-defined eosinophilic disorders: 2014 update on diagnosis, risk stratification, and management," *American Journal of Hematology*, vol. 89, no. 3, pp. 325–337, 2014.

16

Rare Cause of Wide QRS Tachycardia

Nikolay Yu. Mironov,[1] **Natalia A. Mironova,**[1] **Marina A. Saidova,**[2]
Olga V. Stukalova,[3] **and Sergey P. Golitsyn**[1]

[1]*Department of Clinical Electrophysiology, Russian Cardiology Research Center, Russia*
[2]*Department of Sonography, Russian Cardiology Research Center, Russia*
[3]*Department of Tomography, Russian Cardiology Research Center, Russia*

Correspondence should be addressed to Nikolay Yu. Mironov; hukmup@gmail.com

Academic Editor: Hiroaki Kitaoka

Cardiac involvement is a well-known feature of neuromuscular diseases. Most commonly cardiac manifestations occur later in the course of the disease. Occasionally severe cardiac disease, including conduction disturbances, life-threatening arrhythmias, and cardiomyopathy, with its impact on prognosis, may be dissociated from peripheral myopathy. We report a case of bundle branch reentrant ventricular tachycardia as primary manifestation of myotonic dystrophy and discuss associated diagnostic and treatment challenges.

1. Introduction

Myotonic dystrophy (MD) is a rare genetic progressive neuromuscular disease. The prevalence of MD in general population is 1 : 8000 [1]. MD affects skeletal muscle resulting in increased muscular tonus (myotonia) and progressive muscular weakness. Multiple organs are also involved. Disease is associated with significant morbidity and mortality. Respiratory failure and cardiovascular pathology were the most prevalent causes of death, accounting for about 40% and 30% of fatalities, respectively. Cardiac mortality occurs because of progressive left ventricular dysfunction, ischaemic heart disease, or pulmonary embolism or as a result of sudden death [2]. Commonly cardiac involvement develops later in the course of disease in patients with previously established diagnosis and prominent neuromuscular symptoms. Occasionally, cardiac involvement may be the first sign of MD [3]. We report a case of bundle branch reentrant VT as primary manifestation of MD and discuss diagnostic and treatment challenges.

2. Case Presentation

A 45-year-old male with no previous cardiac disease and unremarkable familial history was admitted due to recurrent hour-lasting episodes of chest pain that was caused by wide QRS tachycardia that required DC cardioversion.

Upon admission patient was oriented, in no acute distress, well developed, and well nourished (body mass index 30 kg/m^2). He denied smoking, alcohol abuse, and illicit drug use. Physical examination revealed hyperhidrosis. Patient's axillar temperature was 36.4°C (97.5°F), blood pressure was 110/80 mmHg on both arms, pulse was 86 bpm with a regular rhythm, and respiratory rate was 18 breaths/min. Chest and abdomen investigation was unremarkable. Extremities were warm and well perfused, with normal range of motion and no edema. Slight binocular ptosis and moderate peripheral muscle weakness were noted. Patient had no severe cognitive defects.

Clinical blood, thyroid, and coagulogic profiles were normal. Biochemistry panel revealed hyperlipidemia (total cholesterol 6.5 mmol/L [253 mg/dL], LDL-cholesterol 3.8 mmol/L [148.3 mg/dL]), and modestly elevated creatine kinase 347 U/L. Troponin test was negative. HbA1c level was 6.1%. BNP level was less than 10 pg/mL.

ECG at rest displayed sinus rhythm (95 bpm), PQ (200 ms), QRS (120 ms), and single premature ventricular complexes (Figure 1). 24-hour ECG monitoring registered 524 single premature ventricular beats with no significant sustained arrhythmias and pauses. Echocardiography revealed

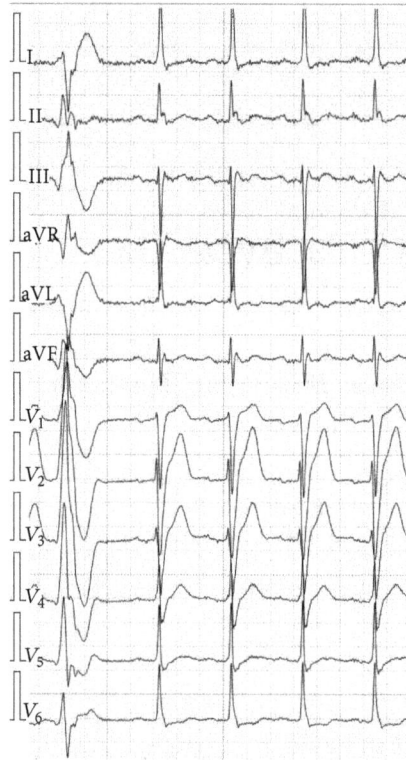

FIGURE 1: ECG at rest. Sinus rhythm 94 bpm, single premature ventricular complexes. Signs of left ventricular hypertrophy and atrioventricular (PQ 220 ms) and interventricular conduction abnormalities (QRS 120 ms). Recorded at 25 mm/sec, 10 mm/mV.

asymmetric nonobstructive hypertrophy of ventricular septum (up to 16 mm in basal segment) with preserved LVEF, no wall motion abnormalities, and enlarged LA (4.4 cm; volume 90 mL).

Cardiac MRI demonstrated areas of subendocardial late gadolinium enhancement in septal, inferior, and lateral walls of LV, indicating focal fibrosis (Figure 2). Although subendocardial accumulation is typical for ischemic lesions, coronary angiography revealed intact arteries.

Electrophysiologic study showed delayed conduction in His-Purkinje system (HPS). HV interval duration was 74 ms (Figure 3(a)). Right ventricle pacing repeatedly induced bundle branch reentrant VT with a rate of 250 bpm and RBBB morphology with anterograde conduction over RBB and retrograde conduction over LBB (Figure 3(b)). All episodes of VT very successfully terminated by burst pacing. Considering structural heart disease and HPS involvement the decision was to refrain from radiofrequency ablation (RFA) and to implant 2-chamber ICD.

Brain MRI prior to implantation showed multiple vascular lesions in white matter and anterior temporal lobe hyperintensities on T2-weighted and FLAIR images (Figure 4).

Patient was discharged on Bisoprolol 7.5 mg OD and referred to neurological center for further investigation where diagnosis of myotonic dystrophy (MD) was confirmed by electromyography. Genetic test revealed multiple CTG repeats in DMPK gene.

A 10-month follow-up was remarkable for significant progression of neuromuscular symptoms. However there were no signs of heart disease progression on ECG and echocardiography. ICD telemetry showed 4 appropriate shocks delivered to one episode of fast VT and multiple long-lasting episodes of Afib with mean ventricular rate of 86 bpm that were asymptomatic and diagnosed only at ICD interrogation. Considering hypertrophic cardiomyopathy anticoagulant therapy by rivaroxaban 20 mg OD was initiated.

We desired to refrain from RFA procedure again. ICD was reprogrammed to more aggressive antitachycardial pacing by addition of 4 extra burst pacing packs of shorter cycle length. In subsequent 8-month follow-up there were 3 sustained fast VT detections. All of them were terminated by burst pacing and were asymptomatic.

3. Discussion

Myotonic dystrophy type (MD) is the most common muscular dystrophy in adults. There are 2 forms of disease: MD type 1 (caused by expansion of a CTG trinucleotide repeat in the $3'$-untranslated region of the dystrophia myotonica protein kinase gene [DMPK gene]) and MD type 2 (caused by an expanded CCTG tetranucleotide repeat expansion located in intron 1 of the zinc finger protein 9 gene [ZNF9]). Exact proportions in prevalence of MD type 1 and MD type 2 are unknown [1].

Cardiac involvement is frequent in both forms of MD but commonly affects patients with prominent neuromuscular symptoms [3, 4]. Cardiac disease is characterized by progressive conduction system abnormalities, supraventricular and

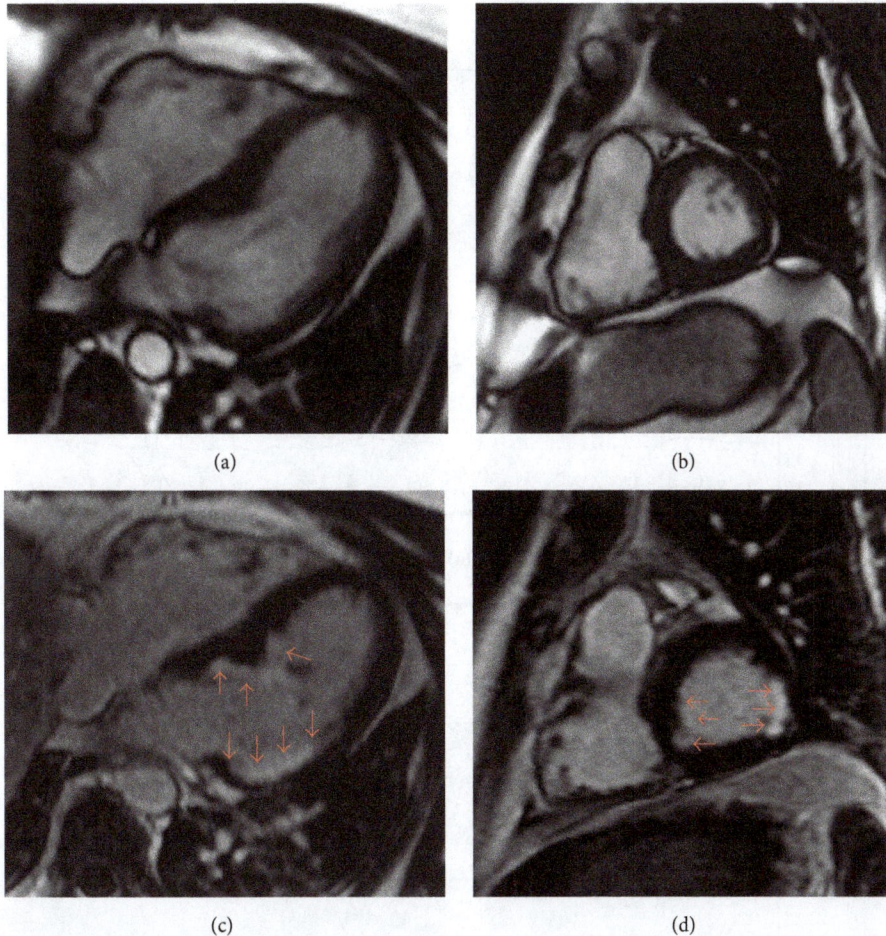

FIGURE 2: Cardiac magnetic resonance. Cine images in four-chamber long-axis view (a) and short-axis view (b). Late gadolinium enhancement (LGE) images in four-chamber long-axis view (c) and in short-axis view (d). Arrows point to regions of increased signal intensity, indicating focal fibrosis, visible as subendocardial enhancement.

ventricular arrhythmias, sudden death, and, less frequently, myocardial dysfunction (hypertrophic and, rarely, dilative cardiomyopathy) and ischaemic heart disease [5]. Conduction abnormalities that are of progressive course and potentially malignant may be found at any level of cardiac conduction system but commonly are located in HPS [4, 6]. In a study of 408 patients Groh et al. found that severe ECG abnormalities (rhythm other than sinus, PR interval of 240 ms or more, QRS duration of 120 ms or more, or second-degree or third-degree atrioventricular block) predict sudden death in type 1 MD [4]. ESC guidelines recommend pacemaker implantation if patient with MD develops any symptoms that may be caused by conduction system defect even if he has minor conduction abnormalities and does not meet classic pacemaker indications [7]. Tachyarrhythmias are also prevalent in MD patients. Most common arrhythmia is AFib. It is observed in up to 25% of patients in both sustained and non-sustained forms [4, 6, 8]. Since there are no data on risk of thromboembolic complications in that subset of patients, it is reasonable to use CHA_2DS_2-VASc score to define indications to anticoagulants. Malignant ventricular arrhythmias including monomorphic and polymorphic VT and spontaneous VF

are also described. Delayed impulse conduction along HPS represents ideal substrate for bundle branch reentrant VT [9]. ICD is indicated in all patients with MD with sustained ventricular arrhythmias due to high risk of sudden death [4, 10]. RFA of RBB or LBB may be successfully applied in patients with bundle branch reentrant VT [1, 6].

Brain involvement is common, resulting in cognitive dysfunction, behavioral changes, apathy, and excessive daytime somnolence [1]. It should be noted that almost exclusively white matter lesions are found in MRI scans of patients with MD [11]. The origin of glious lesions in grey matter of both temporal lobes in our patient remained unknown.

In our case upon admission patient had only moderate neuromuscular symptoms but severe life-threatening ventricular arrhythmias that required ICD implantation. Furthermore, his familial history was unremarkable. Verification of uncommon cardiac lesions led to extensive diagnostic approach with suspicion of neuromuscular disease and subsequent referral to neurologic center, where the exact diagnosis of MD was made.

Taking into consideration small number of episodes of bundle branch reentrant VT, cardiac conduction system

(a)

(b)

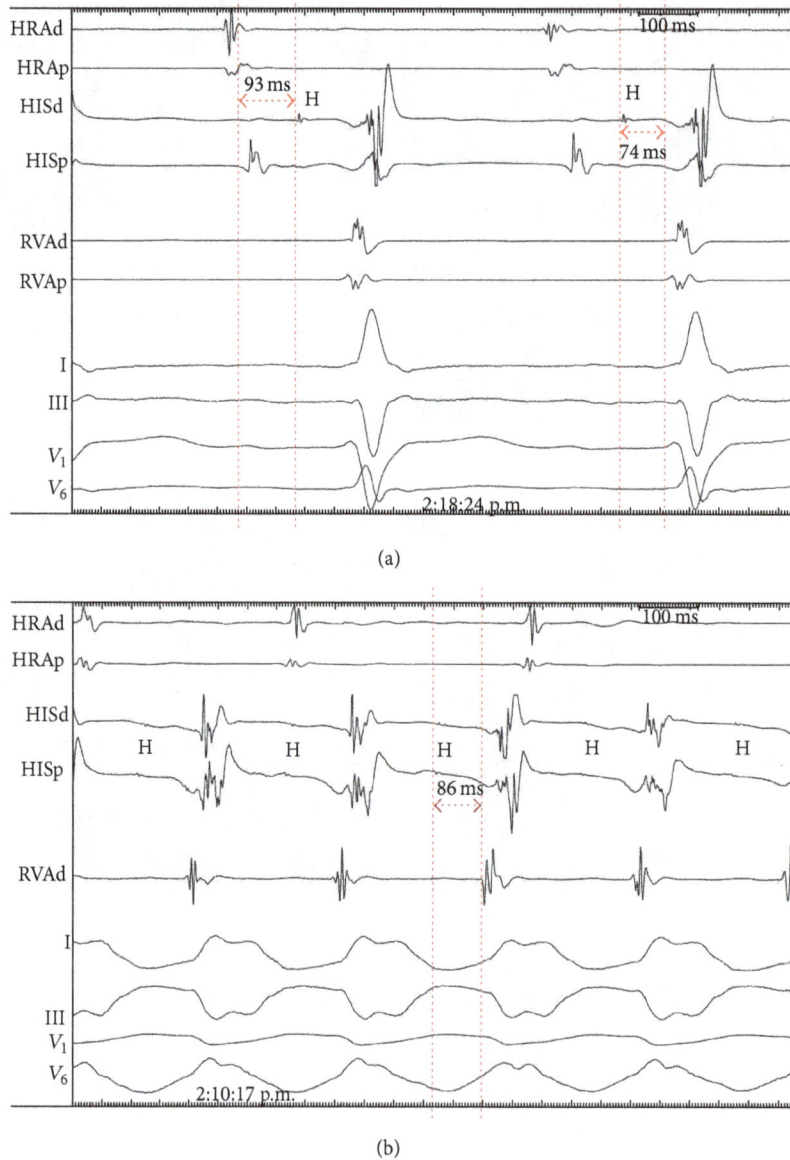

FIGURE 3: Results of electrophysiological investigation: (a) sinus rhythm; His bundle electrogram shows normal AH interval (93 ms) and delayed conduction in His-Purkinje system (HV interval 74 ms); (b) Bundle branch reentrant ventricular tachycardia: VA dissociation points to localization of reentrant circle within ventricles; typical bundle branch reentrant tachycardia features are (1) His bundle potential (H) precedes QRS in every beat and (2) HV interval in LBBB-shaped tachycardia (86 ms) is longer than HV interval on sinus rhythm. Tachycardia uses RBB as anterograde limb and LBB as retrograde limb of reentrant circuit; HRA, high right atrium; RVA, right ventricle apex; HIS, His bundle electrogram.

defects, and increased risk of LV dysfunction progression on permanent pacing, we desired to refrain from RFA, which is frequently referred to as method of choice in management of bundle branch reentrant VT. Thorough optimization of ICD antitachycardiac pacing parameters helped to terminate recurrent paroxysms. We did not initiate amiodarone therapy that time based on data that antiarrhythmic drugs rarely prevent bundle branch reentrant VT [9] and because of the risks of neurotoxicity that may be higher in patients with pre-existent neurological disorders. We continued a close follow-up and if patient will have multiple episodes of bundle branch reentrant VT, either antiarrhythmic drug therapy might be

initiated or he might be readmitted for RFA procedure. It should be noted that there was no significant cardiac disease progression in 18-month follow-up which could be frequently observed in patients with LBBB after bundle branch reentrant VT ablation [12].

Despite hyperlipidemia and high cardiometabolic risk, decision to refrain from statin prescription was made, powered by transient creatine kinase elevations and observations that patients with muscular metabolic abnormalities are more prone to statin-induced myopathy [13].

In the case described patient developed AFib significantly later than VT in the course of the disease. From the onset of

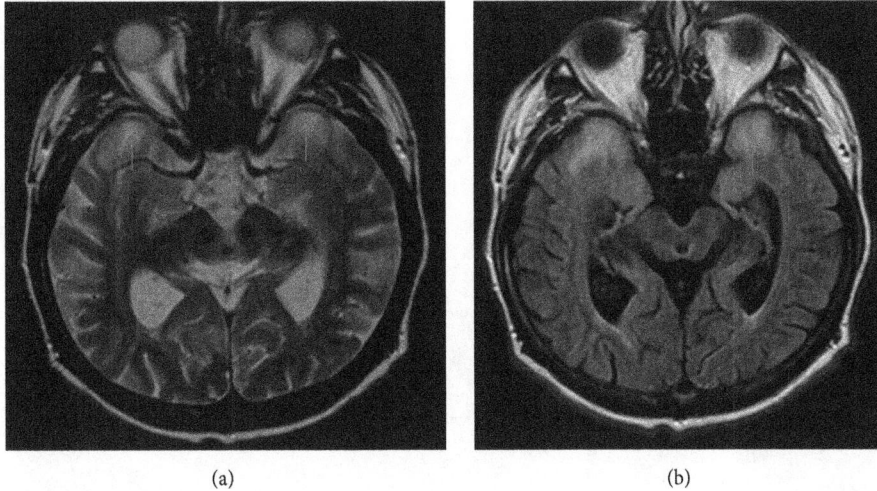

FIGURE 4: Brain MRI. Anterior temporal lobe hyperintensities on T2-weighted (a) and FLAIR (b) images.

the first paroxysm there is clear trend in AFib progression to permanent form. Although AFib was generally asymptomatic, it was clinically significant and required anticoagulation taking into consideration the presence of significant LV septal hypertrophy and high risk of cardioembolic events in patients with hypertrophic cardiomyopathy and AFib [14, 15]. Noteworthy, in this case $CHADS_2$ and CHA_2DS_2-VASc scales were useless as the patient's score was zero.

4. Conclusion

Our case illustrates that cardiac arrhythmias in patients with MD may be more severe than neuromuscular symptoms, and their management could be challenging. Stepwise approach should be applied. Thorough consideration of pros and contras of any therapeutic modality is mandatory because these patients may not benefit from routine treatment strategies.

Conflict of Interests

The authors declare that there is no conflict of interests regarding the publication of this paper.

Acknowledgment

The authors would like to thank Drs. Sergey Sokolov, Nikolay Shlevkov, and Yury Mareev for their contribution to diagnostic work-up and follow-up of patient.

References

[1] B. T. Darras and D. A. Chad, "Myotonic dystrophy: etiology, clinical features, and diagnosis," May 2015, http://www.uptodate.com/contents/myotonic-dystrophy-etiology-clinical-features-and-diagnosis.

[2] J. Mathieu, P. Allard, L. Potvin, C. Prévost, and P. Begin, "A 10-year study of mortality in a cohort of patients with myotonic dystrophy," *Neurology*, vol. 52, no. 8, pp. 1658–1662, 1999.

[3] V. A. Sansone, E. Brigonzi, B. Schoser et al., "The frequency and severity of cardiac involvement in myotonic dystrophy type 2 (DM2): long-term outcomes," *International Journal of Cardiology*, vol. 168, no. 2, pp. 1147–1153, 2013.

[4] W. J. Groh, M. R. Groh, C. Saha et al., "Electrocardiographic abnormalities and sudden death in myotonic dystrophy type 1," *The New England Journal of Medicine*, vol. 358, no. 25, pp. 2688–2697, 2008.

[5] M. F. Phillips and P. S. Harper, "Cardiac disease in myotonic dystrophy," *Cardiovascular Research*, vol. 33, no. 1, pp. 13–22, 1997.

[6] G. Pelargonio, A. Dello Russo, T. Sanna, G. De Martino, and F. Bellocci, "Myotonic dystrophy and the heart," *Heart*, vol. 88, no. 6, pp. 665–670, 2002.

[7] M. Brignole, A. Auricchio, G. Baron-Esquivias et al., "2013 ESC Guidelines on cardiac pacing and cardiac resynchronization therapyThe Task Force on cardiac pacing and resynchronization therapy of the European Society of Cardiology (ESC). Developed in collaboration with the European Heart Rhythm Association (EHRA)," *Europace*, vol. 15, no. 8, pp. 1070–1118, 2013.

[8] B. Udd and R. Krahe, "The myotonic dystrophies: molecular, clinical, and therapeutic challenges," *The Lancet Neurology*, vol. 11, no. 10, pp. 891–905, 2012.

[9] J. L. Merino, J. R. Carmona, I. Fernández-Lozano, R. Peinado, N. Basterra, and J. A. Sobrino, "Mechanisms of sustained ventricular tachycardia in myotonic dystrophy: implications for catheter ablation," *Circulation*, vol. 98, no. 6, pp. 541–546, 1998.

[10] D. Bhakta, C. Shen, J. Kron, A. E. Epstein, R. M. Pascuzzi, and W. J. Groh, "Pacemaker and implantable cardioverter-defibrillator use in a US myotonic dystrophy type 1 population," *Journal of Cardiovascular Electrophysiology*, vol. 22, no. 12, pp. 1369–1375, 2011.

[11] M.-L. Caillet-Boudin, F.-J. Fernandez-Gomez, H. Tran, C.-M. Dhaenens, L. Buee, and N. Sergeant, "Brain pathology in myotonic dystrophy: when tauopathy meets spliceopathy and RNAopathy," *Frontiers in Molecular Neuroscience*, vol. 6, article 57, 2014.

[12] C. Reithmann, B. Herkommer, A. Huemmer, F. Von Hoch, and M. Fiek, "The risk of delayed atrioventricular and intraventricular conduction block following ablation of bundle branch

reentry," *Clinical Research in Cardiology*, vol. 102, no. 2, pp. 145–153, 2013.

[13] G. D. Vladutiu, Z. Simmons, P. J. Isackson et al., "Genetic risk factors associated with lipid-lowering drug-induced myopathies," *Muscle and Nerve*, vol. 34, no. 2, pp. 153–162, 2006.

[14] B. J. Gersh, B. J. Maron, R. O. Bonow et al., "2011 ACCF/AHA guideline for the diagnosis and treatment of hypertrophic cardiomyopathy," *Circulation*, vol. 124, no. 24, pp. e783–e831, 2011.

[15] I. Olivotto, F. Cecchi, S. A. Casey, A. Dolara, J. H. Traverse, and B. J. Maron, "Impact of atrial fibrillation on the clinical course of hypertrophic cardiomyopathy," *Circulation*, vol. 104, no. 21, pp. 2517–2524, 2001.

17

Mitral Subvalvular Aneurysm in a Patient with Chagas Disease and Recurrent Episodes of Ventricular Tachycardia

Tereza Augusta Grillo,[1,2] **Guilherme Rafael S. Athayde,**[3,4] **Ana Flávia L. Belfort,**[5]
Reynaldo C. Miranda,[1,4] **Andrea Z. Beaton,**[6] **and Bruno R. Nascimento**[2,3,5,7]

[1]*Electrophysiology Department, Hospital Universitário São José-INCOR Minas, 30140-073 Belo Horizonte, MG, Brazil*
[2]*Interventional Cardiology Department, Hospital Universitário São José-INCOR Minas, 30140-073 Belo Horizonte, MG, Brazil*
[3]*Division of Cardiology and Cardiovascular Surgery, Hospital das Clínicas, Universidade Federal de Minas Gerais,*
 30130-100 Belo Horizonte, MG, Brazil
[4]*Electrophysiology Department, Universidade Federal de Minas Gerais, 30130-100 Belo Horizonte, MG, Brazil*
[5]*School of Medicine, Universidade Federal de Minas Gerais, 30130-100 Belo Horizonte, MG, Brazil*
[6]*Children's National Health System, Washington, DC 20010, USA*
[7]*Interventional Cardiology Department, Hospital das Clínicas, Universidade Federal de Minas Gerais,*
 30130-100 Belo Horizonte, MG, Brazil

Correspondence should be addressed to Bruno R. Nascimento; ramosnas@gmail.com

Academic Editor: Kjell Nikus

Subvalvular left ventricular aneurysm is a rare disease of obscure origin suggesting unique causes such as congenital, traumatic, and inflammatory or infectious diseases. Its mortality is closely related to heart failure, mitral insufficiency, thromboembolic phenomena, and cardiac arrhythmias. Although association with coronary artery disease is not described, the compression of epicardial vessels by the aneurysm may lead to ischemic manifestations. We report here a case of mitral subvalvular left ventricular aneurysm of probable chagasic origin, in a patient with normal left ventricular function evolving with repeated episodes of monomorphic ventricular tachycardia, despite noninducible electrophysiological testing and the use of optimal medical treatment, including amiodarone. The indication for implantable cardioverter-defibrillator in patients with Chagas cardiomyopathy and segmental wall motion abnormalities but without global systolic dysfunction remains unclear in literature, even in the presence of complex ventricular arrhythmias. A brief review of the literature on morphological features, diagnosis, prognosis, and treatment will be also discussed.

1. Introduction

Mitral subvalvular left ventricular (LV) aneurysm is a rare abnormality of unclear, likely varied, etiology. Suggested origins include congenital defects, traumatic injuries, and the sequel of inflammatory or infectious diseases [1, 2]. Similarly, the clinical manifestations, which include heart failure, mitral regurgitation, thromboembolic phenomena, and cardiac arrhythmias, are incompletely described in literature. Sudden death is among the rare reported presentations of subvalvular LV aneurysms (both submitral and subaortic), believed to be caused by direct coronary artery compression by the aneurysm. Here, we present a case of mitral subvalvular

LV aneurysm in a patient with positive Chagas serology and normal global systolic function evolving with repeated episodes of monomorphic ventricular tachycardia (MVT), refractory to oral amiodarone, despite no inducible complex arrhythmias in electrophysiological (EP) testing.

2. Case Report

A 42-year-old Brazilian woman presented in 2010 to the local emergency department (ED) with new-onset sustained palpitations, hemodynamically stable and denying chest pain, or dizziness. Her past medical history was negative for hospitalizations, trauma, major illness, or surgery. She took no

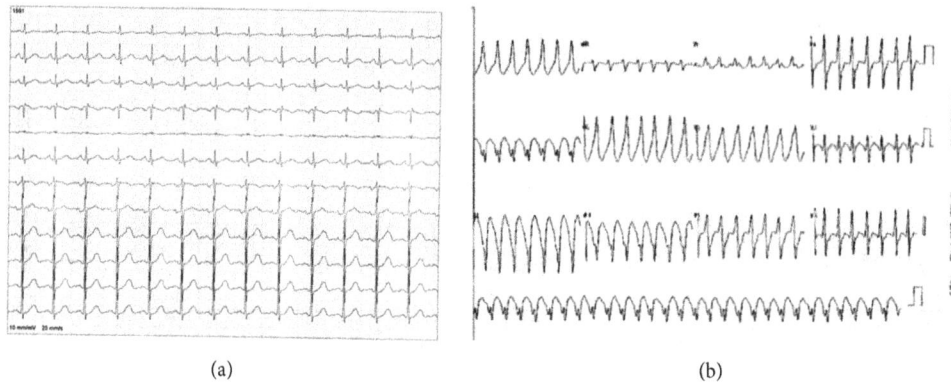

(a)   (b)

FIGURE 1: (a) Baseline electrocardiogram, showing no atrioventricular or intraventricular conduction abnormalities, nor fragmenting of the QRS complex. (b) Electrocardiogram performed in the emergency department showing monomorphic ventricular tachycardia with Rr' pattern in V1, late R/S transition, and left axis deviation.

medications and had no known drug allergies. Electrocardiogram (ECG) revealed MVT, HR = 280 bpm, with Rr' pattern in V1, late R/S transition, and left axis deviation, suggesting probable origin in the basal posterior inferior segment of the LV (Figure 1). The patient received high-dose intravenous (IV) amiodarone (300 mg), which ultimately converted the MVT to normal sinus rhythm (NSR). The baseline ECG (Figure 1) had neither atrioventricular or intraventricular conduction abnormalities, nor other abnormalities such as pathologic Q waves, low voltage, or QRS fragmentation. She was discharged on oral amiodarone 600 mg/day. In 2011 the drug was discontinued and the patient was switched to Atenolol 50 mg once daily. The patient was being managed by the primary care physician and had not received cardiology referral.

The patient remained asymptomatic in NSR until April 2012, when once more she was admitted to the ED with palpitations, weakness, dizziness, and presyncopal symptoms. On physical examination the patient was diaphoretic, hypotensive (BP 100/60 mmHg), and tachycardic (HR = 250 bpm). Again, ECG was consistent with MVT with the same pattern as the index event, which again converted to NSR with IV amiodarone.

Chest radiography was normal. Transthoracic echocardiography (TTE) revealed a subvalvular LV aneurysm (basal portion of the inferolateral wall) with preserved LV systolic function (LVEF = 65%), as confirmed later by ventriculography (Figure 2, Supplementary File in Supplementary Material available online at http://dx.doi.org/10.1155/2015/213104). Treadmill stress test was negative for inducible ischemia. Invasive coronary angiography was also normal (Supplementary File). Laboratory tests were positive for Chagas disease (hemagglutination inhibition and indirect immunofluorescence). Electrophysiology testing failed to induce sustained ventricular tachycardia after extensive endocardial and epicardial mapping: the programmed ventricular stimulation protocol was conducted in two basic cycles (450 and 600 ms) at the right ventricular apex and outflow tract with up to three extra stimuli and finalized when the ventricular refractory period or a minimum coupling of 200 ms was reached. As no sustained ventricular tachycardia was induced, the protocol was then repeated after infusion of Isoproterenol. No evidence of epicardial circuit was found. The noninducibility was taken as a reassurance of benign prognosis (high negative predictive value). At that point, electroanatomic mapping (EAM) was not available in our institution. She did not meet criteria for implantable cardioverter-defibrillator (ICD)—in the attending heart-team's point of view—and was discharged from the hospital after one week on oral amiodarone (800 mg/day, to be progressively reduced).

Despite good compliance with oral amiodarone, the patient once again presented to our hospital in August 2013, this time with hemodynamically unstable MVT. She was successfully converted to NSR with synchronized cardioversion. Her echocardiogram remained unchanged, and no other abnormalities were observed besides the mitral subvalvular LV aneurysm. The patient was then referred to cardiology, where the decision was made to go forward with ICD implantation. The patient remains stable and asymptomatic on oral Propafenone, with preserved LV function. She has not had recurrence of her MVT and has never required any type of therapy by her ICD after 2 years of device implantation.

3. Discussion

The present case illustrates a common dilemma on whether a patient with Chagas cardiomyopathy without global systolic dysfunction but with segmental wall-motion abnormalities should maintain drug therapy or have ICD implanted after an episode of sustained ventricular tachycardia without hemodynamic compromise. It also remarks the pattern of symptoms and short-term evolution of subvalvular LV aneurysm evolving with repeated episodes of MVT in which the final approach was ICD implantation.

Chagas disease affects approximately 20 million people in Latin America. Cardiac involvement is the most serious manifestation and accounts for more than 21,000 deaths every year. The majority of these deaths result from heart failure or sudden cardiac death secondary to malignant ventricular arrhythmias [3].

Our case was also complicated by the presence of a mitral subvalvular LV aneurysm, a rare cardiac abnormality

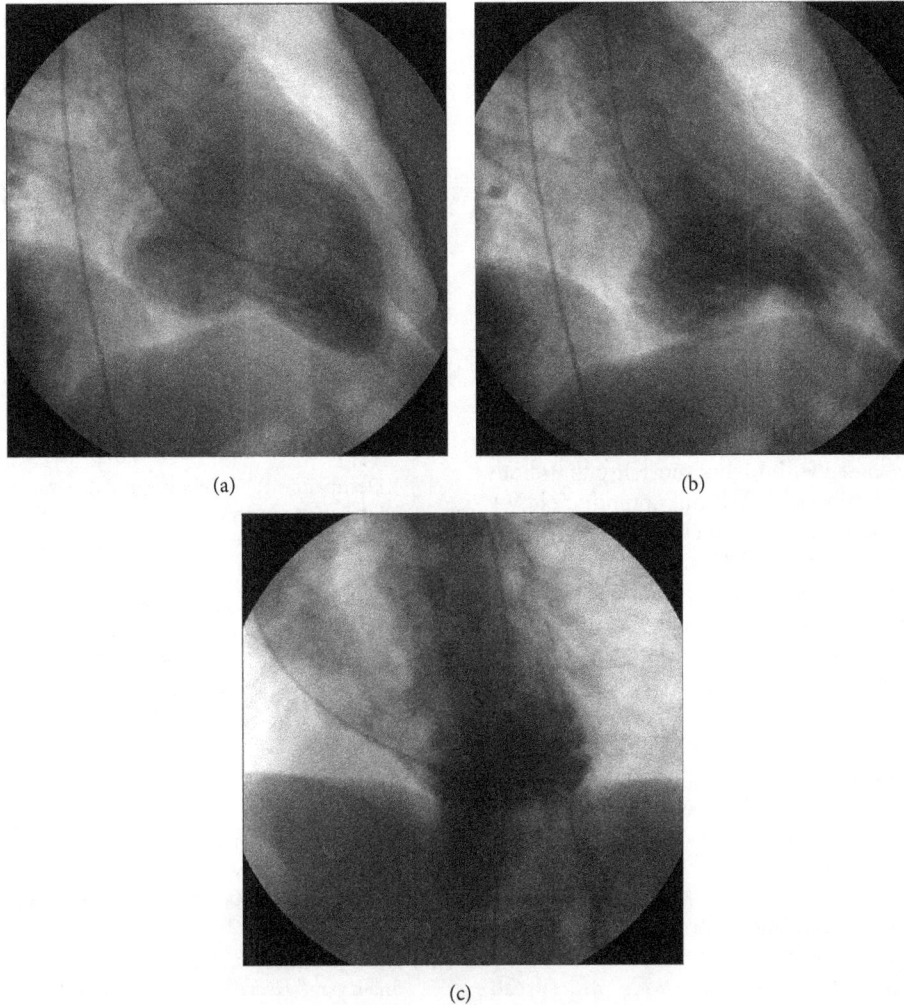

FIGURE 2: Left ventriculography, showing the mitral subvalvular aneurysm: (a) right anterior oblique, end-diastole; (b) right anterior oblique, end-systole; (c) left anterior oblique, end-systole.

first described in 1962 by Abrahams et al., thought to be caused by a congenital defect in the posterior portion of the mitral annulus and also by trauma, inflammatory, and infectious diseases, and may produce symptoms through diastolic overload [2, 4, 5], which has also been suggested as an additional focus of arrhythmogenic substratum in patients with Chagas disease [2, 4]. The mechanism of these arrhythmias is not always clear, but in some cases, compression of the circumflex artery has been observed [1, 5]. In the current case, the role of the subvalvular aneurysm is unclear, though we presume it could have contributed to the refractoriness of her ventricular arrhythmia. Indeed, while rare—Deshpande et al. reported 16 cases (0.7%) of subvalvular aneurysms from 2,285 consecutive autopsies in 10 years [1]—subvalvular aneurysms have been previously reported in patients with Chagas disease, sometimes associated with complex arrhythmias [2, 5]. In these cases, the probable arrhythmogenic substrate may also include reentry in a scar derived from necrosis and fibrosis caused by chronic inflammation of the myocardium. The reentrant circuits can originate from subendocardial, subepicardial, and intramyocardial injuries. For the latter,

intramural circuits may be kept by subepicardial fibers [6].

The effectiveness of ICD for primary prevention of ventricular fibrillation (VF) and sustained VT for patients with LVEF <35%, as well as for secondary prevention of VT/VF, is well established [7] but primarily derived from data on ischemic heart disease. More recently the ACCF/AHA/HRS joint working group advocated for inclusion of other high-risk profile diseases, including Chagas cardiomyopathy, as class IIa indications for ICD implantation. This recommendation is made without regard to ventricular function, given the high risk of ventricular tachyarrhythmias in patients with Chagas [3]. Moreover, for this case, these newer 2013 recommendations also put forward a IIa-C recommendation for ICD in patients with sustained VT, regardless of hemodynamic significance [7]. Thus, our patient met two class II-a, level of evidence C recommendations.

However, this case still presented a challenge in management, as the patient presented initially with signs of good prognosis: no significant abnormalities (conduction abnormalities, pathologic Q waves, and low-voltage) in baseline ECG, preserved LV systolic function with no significant structural cardiac disease, noninducible VT on electrophysiologic study, and a good response to class III antiarrhythmic medication. The positive Chagas serology was only known after the second episode. Indeed, even if the Chagas serology had been known, there is some debate if ICD implantation prevents mortality in this population. Though the total proportion of patients with Chagas disease was low, a retrospective case review of patients with ventricular tachycardia and normal LV function showed increased all-cause mortality in patients treated with ICD plus antiarrhythmic drugs versus amiodarone alone [8]. Specifically looking at a population with Chagas disease, Leite et al. showed that, in a group of 150 patients with symptomatic VT and moderate LV dysfunction, inducible hemodynamically unstable VT was associated with higher mortality than both inducible hemodynamically stable VT and noninducible VT [9]. Contrasting this, data from patients that received ICD for secondary prevention show that Chagas disease doubles the risk of appropriate therapies and appropriate therapies or death [10]. The sample, however, included mostly patients with severe LV dysfunction, with functional impairment. In a Latin American registry that included 89 chagasic patients with ICD (91% for secondary prevention), 66% of the individuals with LV dysfunction received therapy, while only 18% of those with markers of good prognosis, such as our patient, required any therapy. Moreover, compared to our case the population was older (59 ± 10 years), 72% were male, the mean LVEF was lower (40±11%), and most of the patients were symptomatic [11].

Some doubts remain regarding substrate ablation in Chagas heart disease. It is known that the disease leads to slowly progressive but incessant myocarditis, with widespread destruction of myocytes, diffuse fibrosis, mononuclear cell infiltration of the myocardium, and scarring of the conduction system [12, 13]. Thus, although the recurrence rate of malignant ventricular arrhythmias seems to decrease with the advent of EAM to establish the scar extension and limits [4, 6], it is not uncommon for patients with good LV function and favorable ablations to return 5 years afterwards presenting LV dysfunction and recurrence of new sustained ventricular tachycardias [6]. Recurrence rates are as high as 50% in some series [14], and current guidelines recommend ablation (class I) only for incessant MVT or recurrent MVT after ICD implantation [14]. In our case, it was not considered at first due to the noninducibility during endocardial and epicardial stimulation protocols. After recurrences, EAM could have been useful [4], but it was not available in our institution and in most of the tertiary hospitals in Brazil, since the Public Health System does not reimburse it. However, irrespective of availability, EAM should not defer ICD implantation [6]. There is no robust data to support surgical ventriculectomy in chagasic aneurysms [14], although there are some reports of successful suppression of ventricular arrhythmias after surgical repair of subvalvular aneurysms [15].

Given this case, we recommend routine testing for Chagas in patients presenting with VT of unclear etiology who reside in or have traveled to endemic areas. And we await more specific recommendations for indication of ICD in the context of primary prevention of sudden death in patients with Chagas disease that will be answered by the on-going CHAGASICS trial [16]. Though the data is still minimal, in the future we would consider the presence of a subvalvular aneurysm in a patient with Chagas disease an additional risk factor for malignant ventricular arrhythmias—even in the absence of global LV dysfunction—and consider this increased risk in our decision-making regarding ICD placement.

Conflict of Interests

The authors have no conflict of interests to disclose.

References

[1] J. Deshpande, P. Vaideeswar, and A. Sivaraman, "Subvalvular left ventricular aneurysms," *Cardiovascular Pathology*, vol. 9, no. 5, pp. 267–271, 2000.

[2] N. García Hernández, B. Espinosa Caleti, and X. Palacios Macedo, "Mitral subvalvular aneurysm of probable chagasic etiology," *Archivos del Instituto de Cardiología de Mexico*, vol. 65, no. 3, pp. 265–269, 1995.

[3] M. C. P. Nunes, W. Dones, C. A. Morillo, J. J. Encina, and A. L. Ribeiro, "Chagas disease: an overview of clinical and epidemiological aspects," *Journal of the American College of Cardiology*, vol. 62, no. 9, pp. 767–776, 2013.

[4] B. P. Valdigem, F. B. F. C. G. Pereira, N. J. Carneiro Da Silva et al., "Ablation of ventricular tachycardia in chronic chagasic cardiomyopathy with giant basal aneurysm carto sound, CT, and MRI merge," *Circulation: Arrhythmia and Electrophysiology*, vol. 4, no. 1, pp. 112–114, 2011.

[5] A. V. Deshpande, S. V. Vaidya, and A. Kumar, "Submitral aneurysm," *Heart*, vol. 90, article 988, 2004.

[6] M. Scanavacca, "Epicardial ablation for ventricular tachycardia in chronic Chagas heart disease," *Arquivos Brasileiros de Cardiologia*, vol. 102, no. 6, pp. 524–528, 2014.

[7] A. E. Epstein, J. P. DiMarco, K. A. Ellenbogen et al., "2012 ACCF/AHA/HRS focused update incorporated into the ACCF/AHA/HRS 2008 guidelines for device-based therapy of cardiac rhythm abnormalities: a report of the American College of Cardiology Foundation/American Heart Association task force on practice guidelines and the Heart Rhythm Society," *Journal of the American College of Cardiology*, vol. 61, pp. e6–e75, 2012.

[8] S. J. Connolly, A. P. Hallstrom, R. Cappato et al., "Meta-analysis of the implantable cardioverter defibrillator secondary prevention trials. AVID, CASH and CIDS studies. Antiarrhythmics vs implantable defibrillator study. Cardiac arrest study Hamburg. Implantable defibrillator study," *European Heart Journal*, vol. 21, no. 24, pp. 2071–2078, 2000.

[9] L. R. Leite, G. Fenelon, A. Simoes Jr., G. G. Silva, P. A. Friedman, and A. A. V. de Paola, "Clinical usefulness of electrophysiologic testing in patients with ventricular tachycardia and chronic chagasic cardiomyopathy treated with amiodarone or sotalol," *Journal of Cardiovascular Electrophysiology*, vol. 14, no. 6, pp. 567–573, 2003.

[10] M. P. Barbosa, M. O. da Costa Rocha, A. B. de Oliveira, F. Lombardi, and AL. Ribeiro, "Efficacy and safety of implantable cardioverter-defibrillators in patients with Chagas disease," *Europace*, vol. 15, no. 7, pp. 957–962, 2013.

[11] C. A. Muratore, L. A. Batista Sa, P. A. Chiale et al., "Implantable cardioverter defibrillators and Chagas' disease: results of the ICD registry Latin America," *Europace*, vol. 11, no. 2, pp. 164–168, 2009.

[12] A. Rassi Jr., A. Rassi, and J. A. Marin-Neto, "Chagas disease," *The Lancet*, vol. 375, no. 9723, pp. 1388–1402, 2010.

[13] A. L. Ribeiro, M. P. Nunes, M. M. Teixeira, and M. O. C. Rocha, "Diagnosis and management of Chagas disease and cardiomyopathy," *Nature Reviews Cardiology*, vol. 9, no. 10, pp. 576–589, 2012.

[14] J. P. Andrade, J. A. Marin Neto, A. A. Paola et al., "I Latin American guidelines for the diagnosis and treatment of Chagas cardiomyopathy," *Arquivos Brasileiros de Cardiologia*, vol. 97, no. 6, pp. 1–48, 2011.

[15] R. Geukens, F. Van de Werf, H. Ector, G. Stalpaert, and H. De Geest, "Ventricular tachycardia as a complication of annular subvalvular ventricular aneurysm in a Caucasian woman," *European Heart Journal*, vol. 8, no. 4, pp. 431–434, 1987.

[16] M. Martinelli, A. Rassi Jr., J. A. Marin-Neto et al., "CHronic use of amiodarone aGAinSt implantable cardioverter-defibrillator therapy for primary prevention of death in patients with Chagas cardiomyopathy Study: rationale and design of a randomized clinical trial," *American Heart Journal*, vol. 166, no. 6, pp. 976–982.e4, 2013.

18

A Complicated Case of Triple Valve Infective Endocarditis in an IV Drug User with a Bicuspid Aortic Valve Requiring Three Separate Salvage Operations: A Case Report and Literature Review

Shahzad Khan, Athanasios Smyrlis, Dmitry Yaranov, David Oelberg, and Eric Jimenez

Danbury Hospital, Western Connecticut Health Network, 187 Willow Springs, New Milford, CT 06776, USA

Correspondence should be addressed to Shahzad Khan; shahzadwkhan@gmail.com

Academic Editor: Yoshiro Naito

Infective endocarditis (IE) is an infection of the endocardium that involves valves and adjacent mural endocardium or a septal defect. Local complications include severe valvular insufficiency, which may lead to intractable congestive heart failure and myocardial abscesses. If left untreated, IE is generally fatal. Diagnosing IE can be straightforward in patients with the typical oslerian manifestations such as bacteremia, evidence of active valvulitis, peripheral emboli, and immunologic vascular phenomena. In the acute course, however, the classic peripheral stigmata may be few or absent, particularly among intravenous drug abuse (IVDA) patients in whom IE is often due to a *S. aureus* infection of right-sided heart valves. We present a complicated case of a very aggressive native aortic valve *MSSA (methicillin sensitive Staphylococcus aureus)* IE in a young adult male with a past medical history of bicuspid aortic valve and IV drug abuse. His clinical course was complicated by aortic valve destruction and development of third-degree AV block, as well as an aorto-left atrial fistula requiring emergent operation for AV replacement and patch repair. The patient required two reoperations for recurrent endocarditis and its complications.

1. Background

Infective endocarditis (IE) is an infection of the endocardium that could involve or affect the valves and adjacent structures of the heart. IE can be caused by a wide variety of microorganisms fungal or bacteria (*Streptococcus viridans, Streptococcus gallolyticus, Staphylococcus aureus, HACEK* group). Although not common, it can be a fatal pathological condition if not identified and treated especially in those that are older and have congenital or valvular heart defects or other comorbidities that delay or impede the healing process. Different reports indicate that, in the United States, there may be up 15,000 new cases of IE reported every year [1].

High risk patient groups for developing IE include those with a history of IV drug use, congenital heart disease, increased age, prosthetic heart valves, and end stage renal disease on hemodialysis [2].

5% to 15% of hospital admissions of IV drug users (IDU) are attributed to IE [2]. Female gender and HIV have been identified as risk factors among IDU. Intravenous drug use increased chances of getting IE similar to those found in the prosthetic heart valve population, around 1% per year [3].

Bicuspid aortic valve is the most common congenital malformation. It affects 1-2% of the general population and has a 3:1 predilection of males to females and is a well-described risk factor for IE [4]. Lamas and Eykyn demonstrated that 7–25% of the IE population had a past medical history of a congenital bicuspid aortic valve. They also found that these patients are more likely to have a worse prognosis such as developing heart failure, valvular destruction, and/or perivalvular/myocardial abscess [5]. Abscess formation in the aortic annulus can be complicated by complete heart block or bundle branch block in up to 45% of cases.

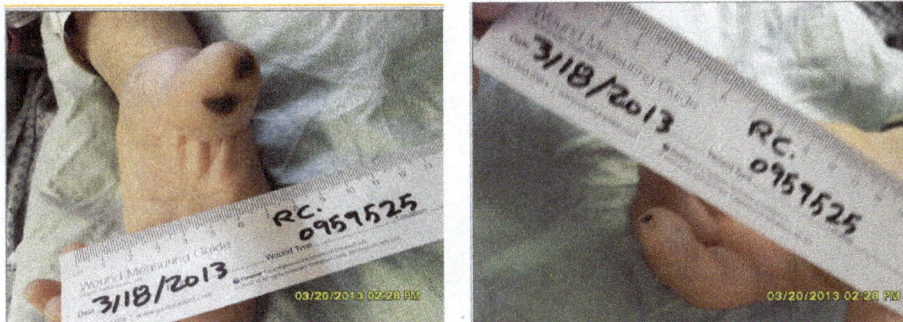

FIGURE 1: Vasculitic lesions. Multiple embolic lesions were present on the left fourth and fifth fingertips and left first toe.

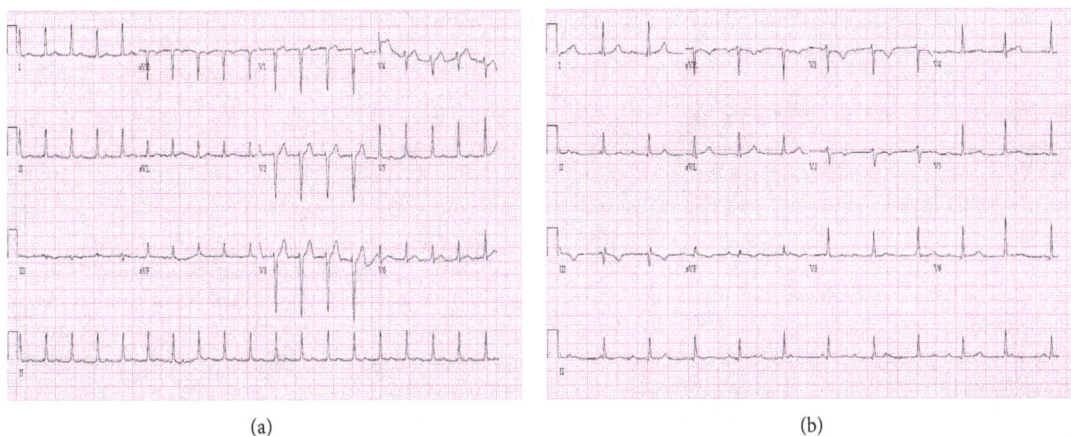

(a)   (b)

FIGURE 2: Electrocardiogram. Day 1 ECG on left and day 2 on right. Day 1 ECG reveals probable sinus tachycardia with first-degree heart block at 111 bpm. Day 2 ECG shows complete heart block with a ventricular rate of 67 bpm.

2. Case Presentation

The patient is a 36-year-old male with bicuspid aortic valve and history of IV drug use (which he initially denied). He presented to another hospital approximately one week after developing a diffuse rash, generalized muscle aches, profound weakness, fevers, and chills. At that time, he was diagnosed with an upper respiratory infection and was discharged from the emergency room on oral antibiotics. After five days he returned back to the same hospital with complaints of persistent high fevers and was admitted. During his stay, he was found to have 4/4 positive blood cultures prompting a transfer to our hospital for further evaluation and management.

His physical exam on presentation was significant for Janeway lesions as well as multiple vasculitic lesions on his fingers and toes (Figure 1) as well as a grade II/IV diastolic murmur. IE was suspected. Blood cultures were obtained and he was promptly started on intravenous Ceftriaxone and Vancomycin. At the time of admission the patient stated that he had a peripherally inserted central catheter placed three months before for treatment of non-Hodgkin's lymphoma at a neighboring hospital that was removed six days prior to presentation. He later admitted to an ICU nurse that the IV line had been inserted by a friend in a hotel room for intravenous injections of illicit drugs.

Blood cultures from the previous hospital grew *MSSA*. Repeat bacterial and fungal cultures at our institution came back negative. Initial ECG showed probable sinus tachycardia with first-degree atrioventricular block (Figure 2). Transesophageal echocardiogram (TEE) demonstrated a bicuspid aortic valve with multiple mobile echo densities along both the anterior and posterior leaflets with the largest one measuring 1.8 cm (Figure 3).

Overnight the patient was noted to have arrhythmias on telemetry and a repeat ECG showed new complete heart block (Figure 2). The patient was then taken to the operating room (OR) emergently where he had an aortic valve replacement with bovine pericardial prosthesis, pericardial patch repair of the aorto-left atrial fistula with a St. Jude Medical bovine pericardial patch, and removal of infected debris from his tricuspid valve and mitral valve. Intraoperative histopathological results of the aortic valve indicated marked acute inflammation, fibroinflammatory debris, coccoid bacteria, and calcifications. The tricuspid valve was also involved with fibroinflammatory debris consistent with endocarditis. Cultures of the specimens grew out *MSSA* and antibiotics were changed to Cefazolin. The patient had an uncomplicated postoperative course and was discharged one week later with a plan of a six-week course of intravenous Cefazolin and close outpatient follow-up.

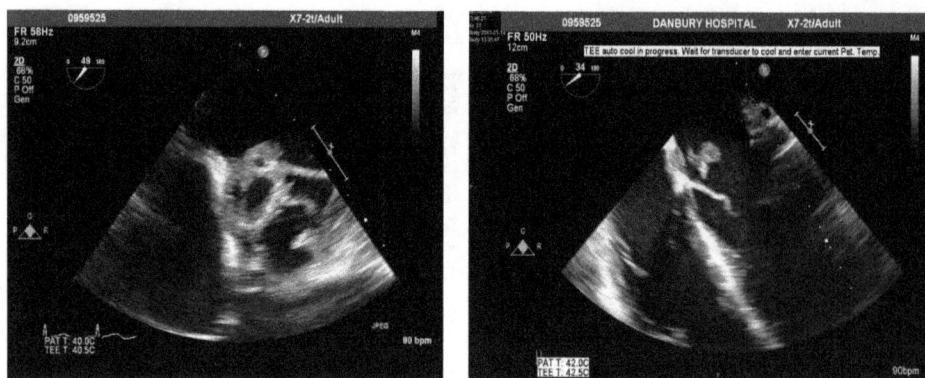

FIGURE 3: Transesophageal echocardiogram. Mass seen on anterior leaflet measuring 1.2 × 1.8 cm with perforation of the leaflet. Bicuspid aortic valve with severe aortic regurgitation and abscess cavity and fistula extending from right coronary cusp to left atrium.

The patient missed his initial two follow-ups with his infectious disease (ID) doctors and there was concern for recurrent IVDA which he denied. After multiple attempts to reach him he started to follow up and became routine in his treatment. In the outpatient setting he also had repeat blood cultures taken at 3 weeks which came back negative. Six weeks after discharge he complained to his cardiologist of night sweats, fatigue, and shortness of breath. A repeat transthoracic echocardiogram was performed showing new vegetations over the bioprosthetic aortic valve with an abscess cavity and fistulization into the right atrium, moderate/severe tricuspid insufficiency, presence of ventricular septal defects, and new vegetations in the mitral valve. He was started empirically on Cefazolin with a continuous antimicrobial infusion to maintain adequate minimum inhibitory concentration and Rifampin. Repeat blood cultures (bacterial and fungal) were negative. He was taken back to the operating room where he had a redo aortic valve replacement with a Carpentier-Edwards ThermaFix bovine pericardial bioprosthesis, closure of the VSD, and subaortic fistula into the right atrium and into the left atrium using a St. Jude Medical bovine pericardial patch. The aortic bioprosthetic valve grossly was a tricuspid porcine valve measuring 3.7 cm (diameter) × 1.5 cm (thickness) with a tan white smooth surface with green sutures attached. Histopathological examination of the valve and fistula showed fibroconnective tissue with associated foci of inflammatory exudates, cultures and staining of which were negative for bacteria and fungi. He was eventually discharged on oral Ciprofloxacin and Rifampin for a total 6-week course.

One week after discharge he developed symptoms of heart failure including shortness of breath and nocturnal dyspnea. He had a repeat echocardiogram that showed a prosthetic valve vegetation with a large aneurysmal membrane between the prosthesis and mitral annulus and evidence of left ventricular outflow tract left atrial fistula with severe regurgitation. A ventricular septal defect was present with left ventricular outflow tract right atrial flow and another vegetation was seen over the anterior mitral valve. Blood cultures (bacterial and fungal) were taken at the time both of which were negative and he was empirically started on Vancomycin, Gentamycin, Cefepime, Rifampin, and Micafungin. The patient was then taken back to the OR for the final time where he had a St. Jude mechanical aortic valve replacement with debridement of the other valves. Intraoperative histological analysis showed fibroconnective tissue that was negative for bacterial and fungal staining and cultures as well as negative for 16sRNA and 18sRNA. The patient was then stabilized and discharged on Rifampin plus Vancomycin for a total course of 6 weeks and Gentamicin for 2 weeks. Upon discharge he followed with his doctors regularly and did not have any further cardiac complications.

3. Discussion

This was a highly complex case due to the severe pathology with multiple valve involvement as well as the patients' social and behavioral issues. His management was particularly challenging as he initially failed to present to the infusion center and antibiotic course was interrupted while he was likely using the IV access for IVDU. The patient did not comply with outpatient follow-up consistently and he was initially not willing to take Warfarin; thus a mechanical valve was not an option.

The second time he presented, it was assumed that he had a persistent *MSSA* infection versus reinfection; therefore he was empirically started on Cefazolin with Rifampin and discharged on oral Ciprofloxacin plus Rifampin once cultures came back negative. Although persistent infection was the most likely culprit, this antibiotic regimen minus the Gentamycin lacked the synergistic strength that may have been required to kill his persistent infection. Also although Ciprofloxacin does provide gram-negative coverage, it is not the best choice if *Pseudomonas aeruginosa* is in the pathogen differential. Baddour et al. demonstrated that although not common, 95% of those infected with *P. aeruginosa* had a positive history of IVDU. Another difficult choice was to discharge the patient on oral antibiotics due to concern of recurrent IVDU through the peripherally inserted central catheter. This was a conscious decision which took into account his history and lack of initial follow-up. It is not necessarily the preferred method but Ciprofloxacin and Rifampin have been shown to achieve good bioavailability in the oral form [6]. Ultimately he came back for a third time and was initially treated with Cefepime, Vancomycin, Gentamycin, Rifampin, and Micafungin. His cultures came back negative and he received a 2-week course of Gentamycin with a 6-week course of Vancomycin with Rifampin. He was subsequently compliant with all his follow-ups and treatment recommendations. One year after the last surgery he remains free of endocarditis and he has been able to abstain from illegal drug use.

The social aspects and intricacies of treating IV drug users for endocarditis result often in a difficult and unstable physician-patient relationship. Creating rapport with such patients requires a significant investment of time and energy and it is absolutely essential for treatment success.

Conflict of Interests

The authors declare that there is no conflict of interests regarding the publication of this paper.

References

[1] A. S. Bayer, "Infective endocarditis," *Clinical Infectious Diseases*, vol. 17, no. 3, pp. 313–320, 1993.

[2] D. P. Levine, L. R. Crane, and M. J. Zervos, "Bacteremia in narcotic addicts at the Detroit Medical Center. II. Infectious endocarditis: a prospective comparative study," *Reviews of infectious diseases*, vol. 8, no. 3, pp. 374–396, 1986.

[3] L. E. Wilson, D. L. Thomas, J. Astemborski, T. L. Freedman, and D. Vlahov, "Prospective study of infective endocarditis among injection drug users," *Journal of Infectious Diseases*, vol. 185, no. 12, pp. 1761–1766, 2002.

[4] N. Yener, G. L. Oktar, D. Erer, M. M. Yardimci, and A. Yener, "Bicuspid aortic valve," *Annals of Thoracic and Cardiovascular Surgery*, vol. 8, pp. 264–267, 2002.

[5] C. C. Lamas and S. J. Eykyn, "Bicuspid aortic valve—a silent danger: analysis of 50 cases of infective endocarditis," *Clinical Infectious Diseases*, vol. 30, no. 2, pp. 336–341, 2000.

[6] L. M. Baddour, W. R. Wilson, A. S. Bayer et al., "Infective endocarditis: diagnosis, antimicrobial therapy, and management of complications: a statement for healthcare professionals from the Committee on Rheumatic Fever, Endocarditis, and Kawasaki Disease, Council on Cardiovascular Disease in the Young, and the Councils on Clinical Cardiology, Stroke, and Cardiovascular Surgery and Anesthesia, American Heart Association: endorsed by the Infectious Diseases Society of America," *Circulation*, vol. 111, pp. e394–e434, 2005.

19

Spontaneous Coronary Artery Dissection/Intramural Haematoma in Young Women with ST-Elevation Myocardial Infarction: "It Is Not Always a Plaque Rupture Event"

George Kassimis,[1] **Athanasios Manolis,**[1] **and Jonathan N. Townend**[2]

[1]*Department of Cardiology, Asklepeion General Hospital, Athens, Greece*
[2]*Department of Cardiology, Queen Elizabeth Hospital, Birmingham, UK*

Correspondence should be addressed to George Kassimis; gksup@yahoo.gr

Academic Editor: Man-Hong Jim

Spontaneous coronary artery dissection (SCAD) is an unusual, but increasingly recognized, cause of ST-elevation myocardial infarction (STEMI), especially among younger patients without conventional risk factors for coronary artery disease (CAD). Although dissection of the coronary intima or media is a hallmark finding, hematoma formation within the vessel wall is often present. It remains unclear whether dissection or hematoma is the primary event, but both may cause luminal stenosis and occlusion. The diagnosis of SCAD is made principally with invasive coronary angiography, although adjunctive intracoronary imaging modalities may increase the diagnostic yield. In STEMI patients, the decision whether to pursue primary percutaneous coronary intervention (PCI) or appropriate conservative medical therapy is based on clinical presentation, the extent of the dissection, the critical anatomy involvement, and the amount of ischaemic myocardium at risk. In this case report, we present two cases of young women with SCAD and STEMI, successfully treated with primary PCI. We briefly illustrate the characteristic aspects of the angiographic presentation and intravascular ultrasound-guided treatment. SCAD should always be considered in young STEMI patients without conventional risk factors for CAD with primary angioplasty to be required in patients with ongoing myocardial ischemia.

1. Introduction

We present two cases of young women with spontaneous coronary artery dissection (SCAD) and ST-elevation myocardial infarction (STEMI) successfully treated with primary percutaneous coronary intervention (PCI).

2. Case 1

A 50-year-old postmenopausal woman with no cardiovascular risk factors was admitted with an anterior STEMI. The coronary angiogram (CA) demonstrated the right coronary artery (RCA) dominant and normal (Figure 1(a)); the left main stem and circumflex vessels all appeared normal, but there was a very unusual appearance in the mid left anterior descendent (LAD), of an almost subtotally occluded long tubular segment of LAD disease after a large diagonal branch (Figure 1(b)) with TIMI 2 coronary flow, which did not respond to 200 micrograms of intracoronary nitroglycerine.

There was a strong suspicion that this was an intramural haematoma (IH), rather than a plaque rupture event, and after predilatation with a 2/20 mm balloon at 8 atm, we performed intravascular ultrasound (IVUS) imaging. This clearly demonstrated that proximally and distally to the abnormal findings the vessel was entirely normal with no evidence of atheroma. However, there was a very long segment of about 70–80 mm in length of IH, which was compressing the true lumen (Figures 1(c) and 1(d)). After further predilatation with a 2.5/20 mm balloon at 10 atm and further 200 micrograms of intracoronary nitrate the flow picked up and the ST segments then settled and the patient became pain-free (Figure 1(e)). We electively did not stent the LAD due to

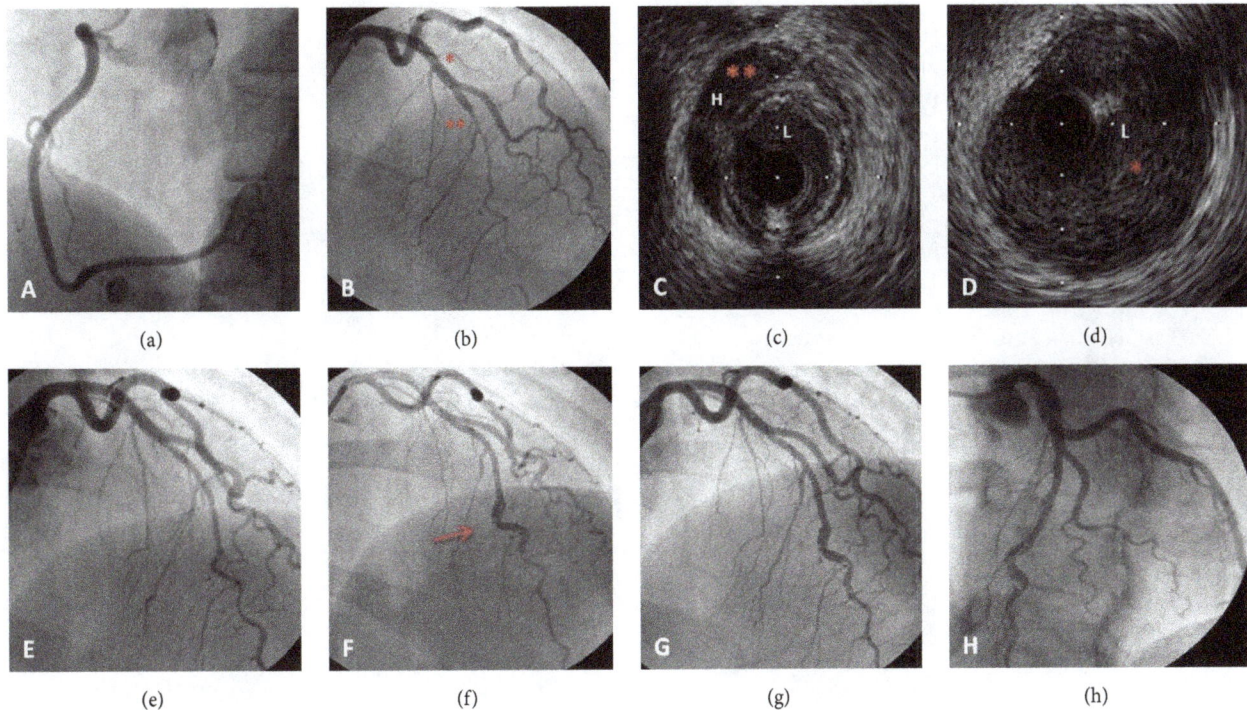

(a)   (b)   (c)   (d)

(e)   (f)   (g)   (h)

FIGURE 1: (a) Left anterior oblique (LAO) projection showing a favourable angiographic appearance of the RCA. (b) Right anterior oblique (RAO) cranial projection showing a long tubular stenosis of the mid-LAD, with abrupt demarcation (∗∗) from normal proximal segments (∗), which did not respond to intracoronary nitroglycerine. (c) IVUS examination showed near-circumferential hematoma (H) extending deep into the media and reducing the lumen (L). No atheroma was visualised. (d) IVUS examination of the proximal segments revealed normal vessel appearance and preserved lumen (L) caliber. (e) Final angiographic appearance of the mid-LAD, in RAO cranial projection. (f–h) At 6-month follow-up, RAO cranial projection of mid-LAD showing good coronary flow but with still evidence of significant vessel dissection in its distal course.

the extensive length of the IH and the potential complications of stenting for IH including propagation of the haematoma both distally and proximally and because of the evidence from previous reports that, in many cases, spontaneous resolution and healing will occur with good luminal diameters. A postprocedural echocardiogram showed good left ventricular (LV) systolic function with no regional wall motion abnormality. The patient was discharged on dual antiplatelet therapy (DAPT) for twelve months and bisoprolol 2.5 mg o.d.

Six months later she was electively admitted for a follow-up CA to reevaluate the IH of LAD. The area of interest has been partially normalised; however there was still evidence of a significant dissection in its distal course (Figures 1(f)–1(h)). The patient was however asymptomatic and there was TIMI 3 flow in the LAD. We felt it would not be sensible to pass at this stage a coronary wire for intravascular imaging, as we feared that this might affect the LAD dissection and as such we stopped at this point. From a clinical point of view this lady remains very well without angina.

3. Case 2

A 52-year-old postmenopausal woman with no cardiovascular risk factors was admitted with an inferior STEMI associated with temporary complete heart block. Urgent CA

demonstrated an unobstructed left coronary system (Figures 2(a) and 2(b)) with an almost subtotally occluded long tubular abnormality within the RCA (Figures 2(c) and 2(d)), which did not respond to intracoronary nitroglycerine, with TIMI 2 flow. Primary PCI was successfully performed, with two zotarolimus eluting stents 2.75/30 mm and 3/30 mm implanted (distal to proximal) (Figures 2(e)–2(h)) and postdilated with a 3.25 mm noncompliant balloon at 16 atm (Figures 2(i)–2(k)) with an excellent angiographic result (Figure 2(l)). Intracoronary imaging was not performed, because the vessel was dissected till the ostium of the RCA, and there was a risk of exacerbating the disruption with the imaging catheter causing ostial vessel occlusion.

A postprocedural echocardiogram showed preserved LV systolic function. The patient was discharged on DAPT for twelve months and metoprolol 25 mg b.i.d. This lady remains completely asymptomatic 6 months after procedure.

4. Discussion

These cases highlight a condition that is a relatively rare cause of STEMI. Previous studies show that SCAD is commonest in the fifth decade, with a striking female predominance, particularly in the peripartum period, with 25–31% of reported cases occurring during this time. Other predisposing factors

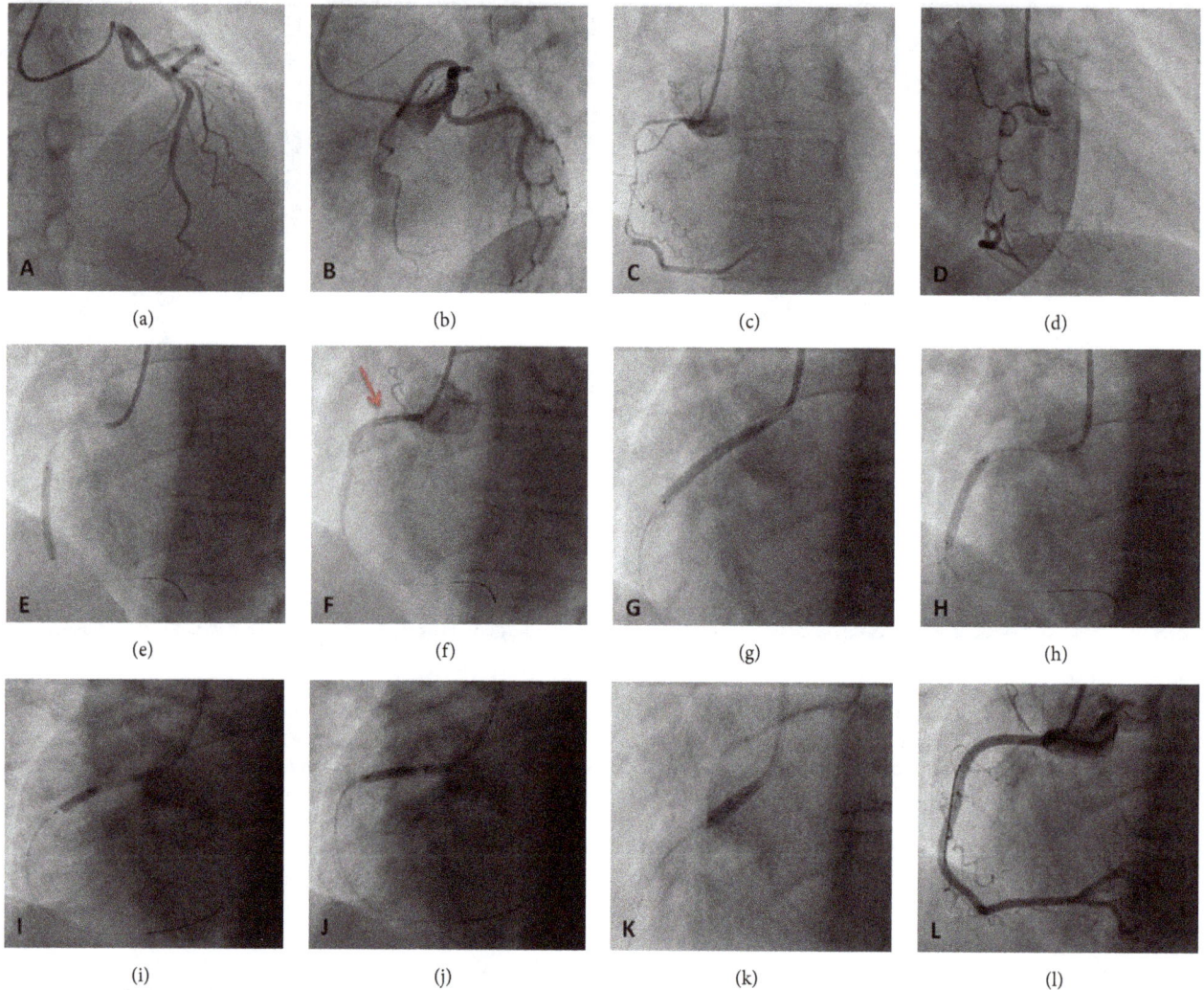

FIGURE 2: (a, b) RAO cranial and spider projections showing normal left coronary system. (c, d) LAO and RAO projections showing a very long tubular stenosis of the RCA, with abrupt demarcation from normal distal segments, which did not respond to intracoronary nitroglycerine and balloon predilation. (e) After the implantation of the first ZES 2.75/30 mm, there was a propagation of the dissection flap proximally (white line; red arrow (f)), successfully sealed with a second ZES 3/30 mm implanted proximally (g). (h) Postdilation with the stent balloon at the overlap of the 2 stents and with noncompliant balloon 3.25 mm proximally at 16 atm (i–k) with an excellent final angiographic result (l).

include connective-tissue and vasculitic disorders, cocaine abuse, and heavy isometric exercise and in some cases it has been described in association with oral contraceptive use in previously healthy individuals [1].

Urgent CA is indicated in STEMI patients and the definitive diagnosis of IH can be confirmed by IVUS or optical coherence tomography (OCT). However, this procedure is not always feasible, because of significant luminal compression by the extraluminal haematoma, and needs special care, as it can exacerbate the disruption of the vessel and cause vessel occlusion [2].

The two main pathological subsets have been described: with and without an intimal tear. An intimal tear may precipitate bleeding into the wall, with free communication between the true and false coronary lumens. Alternatively, a primary disruption of the "vasa vasorum" with subsequent bleeding and intramedial hemorrhage has been proposed as the underlying mechanism in patients in whom an intimal tear could not be identified. The resulting IH has no communication with the coronary lumen and causes luminal encroachment [1].

A simple angiographic classification to improve the diagnosis of SCAD was described by Saw [3]. Lesions with the hallmark of multiple lumen and/or contrast wall stain were classified as type 1 SCAD. Lesions with long, smooth tubular stenosis (representing IH as in our two cases) were classified as type 2 SCAD, which is seen in 2/3 of SCAD. Finally, lesions with focal or tubular stenosis (because of IH) that mimic atherosclerosis were classified as type 3 SCAD. The LAD is the most frequently involved vessel [1, 3].

The current gold-standard CA is excellent to assess luminal narrowing; however, it is poor in assessing the arterial wall, where the key abnormalities occur with SCAD. Intravascular imaging allows excellent visualizing of the arterial wall structure and composition. IVUS has a lower spatial resolution (150–200 μm) but has deeper penetration allowing for the full vessel and extent of the IH to be visualized as in our first case. IVUS can delineate true and false lumens and detect IH, which appears as a homogenous collection behind the intimal-medial membrane. OCT, on the other hand, is a much higher resolution (10–20 μm) modality and can visualize true lumen, false lumen, and even intimal tears and entry dissection points exceedingly well. However, it has poorer penetration than IVUS and may not visualize the full extent of the IH [4]. IVUS and OCT can also confirm guidewire position in the true lumen and assess optimal stent apposition and expansion [5].

Considerable controversy surrounds the aetiology of SCAD. Most likely this process occurs as a result of vascular shear stress and the presence of abnormal connective-tissue structure. Eosinophilic infiltrates observed in some cases may damage collagen and lead to cystic medial necrosis, and progesterone induced microstructural changes may be of importance in peripartum and contraceptive-associated SCAD [1]. Coronary artery tortuosity is highly prevalent in the SCAD population and is associated with recurrent SCAD [6, 7]. Angiographic features of SCAD are associated with extracoronary vasculopathy, including fibromuscular dysplasia (FMD), which could be a potentially causative factor [8, 9].

There is a lack of evidence supporting the value of specific pharmacological regimens or the value of systematic coronary revascularization over conservative management in SCAD-STEMI patients. Classically, thrombolytics and glycoprotein IIb/IIIa inhibitors are considered to be contraindicated, because they may promote additional intramural bleeding. The use of aspirin and clopidogrel following SCAD presentation is advocated by some but remains unsupported by clinical trials. The value of prasugrel or ticagrelor in these patients remains unknown. Beta-blockers are considered the mainstay of therapy, by reducing oxygen consumption and local shear stress, with the potential to stabilize the condition acutely and prevent late recurrence. Statins, while being a mainstay agent in typical atherosclerotic STEMI, are untested in SCAD [1].

Primary PCI should be considered in STEMI patients with proximal dissections in large vessels associated with ongoing ischemia and/or with reduced TIMI flow. However, PCI in patients with SCAD is associated with significant technical difficulties including propagation of intramural haematoma which may lead to further luminal compromise in remote segments including the left main stem. For this reason, it should perhaps be avoided if flow is good and there is no evidence of ongoing ischaemia or infarction. Residual distal coronary dissection and hematoma may sometimes be left untreated and will often heal with good late appearances [1, 9]. Whether drug-eluting stents (DES) provide any specific advantage over bare metal stents (BMS) in the management of SCAD remains unclear; however, as in our second case, DES may be preferred for long dissected segments in order to reduce the risk of restenosis [1]. Alternatively, BMS short spot

stenting could be deployed with OCT guidance at the entry point of the IH as recently described [10].

Surgery should be considered in unstable patients with left main or 3-vessel involvement and also in patients with ischemia after a failed PCI [1]. However, a conservative strategy has also been proposed especially for selected patients with SCAD following initial clinical stabilization [11, 12]. Although long-term survival after an index SCAD episode appears better, compared to that for typical acute coronary syndrome, rates of major adverse cardiac events are similar [13].

Conflict of Interests

The authors declare no conflict of interests.

References

[1] A. Yip and J. Saw, "Spontaneous coronary artery dissection—a review," *Cardiovascular Diagnosis & Therapy*, vol. 5, no. 1, pp. 37–48, 2015.

[2] M. Paulo, J. Sandoval, V. Lennie et al., "Combined use of OCT and IVUS in spontaneous coronary artery dissection," *JACC: Cardiovascular Imaging*, vol. 6, no. 7, pp. 830–832, 2013.

[3] J. Saw, "Coronary angiogram classification of spontaneous coronary artery dissection," *Catheterization and Cardiovascular Interventions*, vol. 84, no. 7, pp. 1115–1122, 2013.

[4] F. Alfonso, M. Paulo, and J. Dutary, "Endovascular imaging of angiographically invisible spontaneous coronary artery dissection," *JACC: Cardiovascular Interventions*, vol. 5, no. 4, pp. 452–453, 2012.

[5] K. Poon, B. Bell, O. C. Raffel, D. L. Walters, and I.-K. Jang, "Spontaneous coronary artery dissection: utility of intravascular ultrasound and optical coherence tomography during percutaneous coronary intervention," *Circulation: Cardiovascular Interventions*, vol. 4, no. 2, pp. e5–e7, 2011.

[6] M. F. Eleid, R. R. Guddeti, M. S. Tweet et al., "Coronary artery tortuosity in spontaneous coronary artery dissection: angiographic characteristics and clinical implications," *Circulation: Cardiovascular Interventions*, vol. 7, no. 5, pp. 656–662, 2014.

[7] G. Kassimis, N. Patel, and A. Banning, "Sequential spontaneous coronary dissection/mural haematoma within all three coronary arteries over a nine-year period," *Hellenic Journal of Cardiology*, vol. 55, no. 1, pp. 58–60, 2014.

[8] J. Saw, D. Ricci, A. Starovoytov, R. Fox, and C. E. Buller, "Spontaneous coronary artery dissection: prevalence of predisposing conditions including fibromuscular dysplasia in a tertiary center cohort," *JACC Cardiovascular Interventions*, vol. 6, no. 1, pp. 44–52, 2013.

[9] F. Alfonso, R. Hernandez, J. Goicolea et al., "Coronary stenting for acute coronary dissection after coronary angioplasty: implications of residual dissection," *Journal of the American College of Cardiology*, vol. 24, no. 4, pp. 989–995, 1994.

[10] K. Satogami, Y. Ino, T. Kubo et al., "Successful stenting with optical frequency domain imaging guidance for spontaneous coronary artery dissection," *Journal of the American College of Cardiology: Cardiovascular Interventions*, vol. 8, no. 6, pp. e83–e85, 2015.

[11] F. Alfonso, M. Paulo, V. Lennie et al., "Spontaneous coronary artery dissection: long-term follow-up of a large series of

patients prospectively managed with a 'conservative' therapeutic strategy," *JACC: Cardiovascular Interventions*, vol. 5, no. 10, pp. 1062–1070, 2012.

[12] M. S. Tweet, M. F. Eleid, P. J. Best et al., "Spontaneous coronary artery dissection: revascularization versus conservative therapy," *Circulation: Cardiovascular Interventions*, vol. 7, no. 6, pp. 777–786, 2014.

[13] M. S. Tweet, S. N. Hayes, S. R. Pitta et al., "Clinical features, management, and prognosis of spontaneous coronary artery dissection," *Circulation*, vol. 126, no. 5, pp. 579–588, 2012.

20

Malignant Perivascular Epithelioid Cardiac Sarcomas: A Case Report and a Review of the Literature

Candice Baldeo,[1] **Abdul wahab Hritani,**[1] **Robert Ali,**[1] **Sana Chaudhry,**[1] **and Fawad N. Khawaja**[2]

[1]*Department of Internal Medicine, University of Florida, Jacksonville, FL 32209, USA*
[2]*Department of Cardiothoracic Surgery, University of Florida, Jacksonville, FL 32209, USA*

Correspondence should be addressed to Candice Baldeo; candice.baldeo@jax.ufl.edu

Academic Editor: Ramazan Akdemir

Cardiac tumors, either benign or malignant, are difficult to diagnose due to their rarity, variety, and nonspecific presentation. Since primary cardiac sarcoma remains an unusual diagnosis, the literature on its presentation, diagnosis, and optimal management remains scarce. To our knowledge the following case of cardiac perivascular epithelioid cell tumor is the fourth reported case found in the literature. Although complete surgical resection remains the gold standard for cardiac sarcomas, our case demonstrates that not all of them can be completely resected.

1. Introduction

The prevalence of primary cardiac tumors is 0.001–0.03% in autopsy series, with malignant tumors accounting for 25% of cases [1]. Seventy-five percent of primary tumors are benign in origin, with myxoma being the most frequent in over 50% of cases. From the 25% of malignant cardiac tumors, the most frequent are cardiac sarcomas [1].

Resection remains the primary mode of treatment for primary cardiac sarcomas (PCSs). However, PCS usually has a high recurrence rate of up to 50% even after resection, and the prognosis remains dismal [2]. Early diagnosis and initiation of treatment, resection and/or chemotherapy with radiation therapy, may decrease recurrence and have mortality benefit.

2. Case Description

A 64-year-old Caucasian female with a past medical history significant for hypertension and hyperlipidemia presented to our institution with progressive shortness of breath on exertion, bilateral lower extremity edema, and a chronic dry cough for the past 3 months. She also complained of a decreased appetite and a 12-pound weight loss over the past 2 months. She denied orthopnea or paroxysmal nocturnal dyspnea. She had no previous smoking history and no significant surgical or family history. Physical examination revealed sinus tachycardia, bilateral pitting pedal edema, and basilar crackles in both lungs. Laboratory diagnosis showed leukocytosis (13.2), microcytic anemia (10.5 Hb, MCV 78.5), and thrombocytosis (524).

Chest X-ray displayed cardiomegaly with increased interstitial pulmonary markings and small bilateral pleural effusions (see Figure 1). On lateral chest X-ray there was loss of the retrosternal airspace (see Figure 2). Low voltage QRS with sinus tachycardia was noted on the EKG. Computed tomography (CT) of the chest without contrast revealed a 9.9 cm × 11.5 cm × 14.2 cm heterogeneous mass located along the anterior pericardium which was significantly displacing the heart superiorly and posteriorly (see Figure 3). This mass also exhibited internal necrosis and calcifications. Transthoracic echocardiogram (TTE) showed a preserved ejection fraction with a large mass which was compressing the anterior right ventricle.

Cardiac magnetic resonance imaging (CMRI) showed that the mass was cystic and solid in nature and again arising near anterior pericardium (see Figure 4). A CT guided core

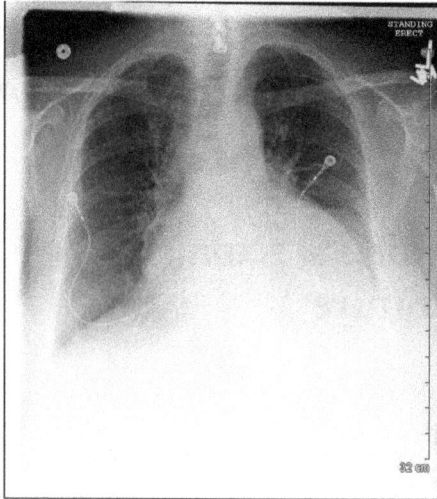

FIGURE 1: PA CXR showing cardiomegaly, interstitial edema, and small bilateral effusions.

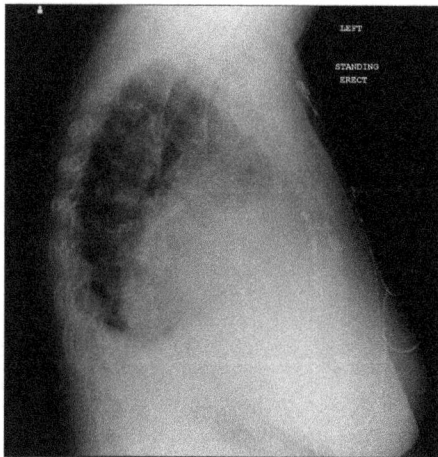

FIGURE 2: Lateral CXR showing cardiomegaly with loss of retrosternal airspace.

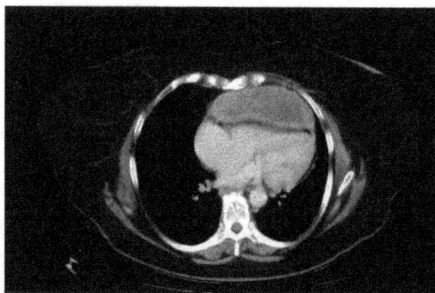

FIGURE 3: CT of chest showing 9.9 × 11.5 × 14.2 cm heterogeneous mass, with internal necrosis and calcification, associated with the anterior pericardium and displacing the heart superiorly and posteriorly.

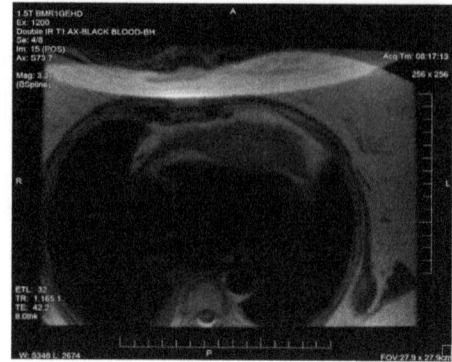

FIGURE 4: Cardiac MRI showing cystic solid mass arising in the pericardium.

needle biopsy was performed and sent to pathology where it revealed spindle and epithelioid sarcoma. Immunostains on tumor biopsy were positive for SMA and calretinin (focal in epithelioid nests) and negative for cytokeratins (Ck-AE1/AE3 and CK5/6), TTF-1, mammaglobin, breast gross cystic disease fluid protein-15, estrogen/progesterone receptors, CD34, and desmin. Left heart catheterization showed no significant abnormalities.

After discussion with the patient and her family, the decision was made to perform surgery for a complete resection of the tumor. However, at surgery it was discovered that the mass was actually arising from the pericardium and wedged underneath it. Attempts to debulk the tumor demonstrated that it had already infiltrated the myocardium. Thus, the cardiac tumor was deemed unresectable.

Pathology results of the partial tumor excision showed high-grade sarcoma with features favoring malignant perivascular epithelioid cell tumor (see Figure 5). The debulked tumor fragments (measuring collectively 12.2 × 10.8 × 4.0 cm) were grey to yellow white solid with pink-brown ragged cystic areas. Histologically, the tumor was formed of poorly differentiated high-grade spindle and epithelioid cell sarcoma with moderate nuclear pleomorphic and scattered multinucleated tumor giant cells. Mitoses were brisk with abnormal figures (>30 mitoses/10 HPF). The tumor architecture ranged from compact fascicles to cords and strands in loose edematous to myxoid and sclerotic stroma. There was prominent perivascular tumor cells condensation around thin wall blood vessels. Large areas of geographic necrosis were present in about 45% of sampled tumor. Additional stains on the debulked tumor tissue revealed focal strong positivity for desmin, SMA, HMB-45, melan A, and S100 and strong diffuse positivity for CD99 (membranous) and BCl-2. The immunostain results were in favor of PEComa.

Postoperatively, the patient required vasopressor support and intubation for respiratory failure. Vasopressors were weaned over the following 48 hours and she was eventually extubated. She refused any further chemotherapy or radiotherapy and opted for home with hospice care. She died 6 months following surgery.

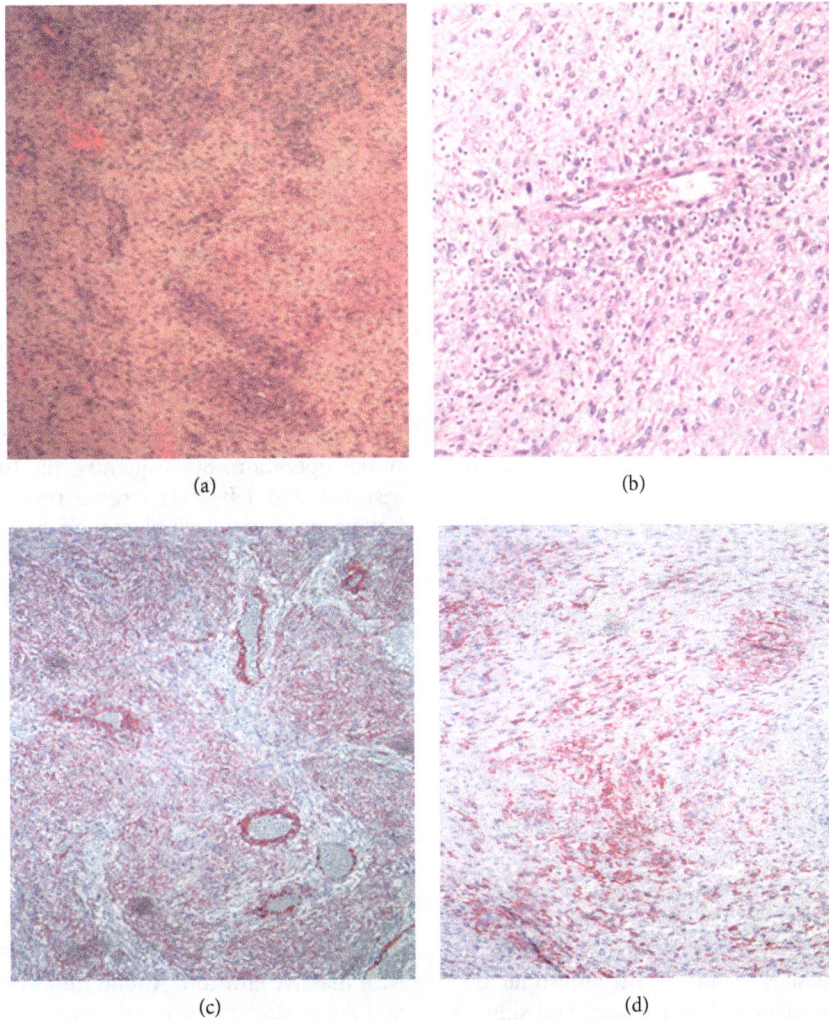

FIGURE 5: Perivascular condensation of tumor cells (H&E stain (a) ×2.5 and (b) ×20). Diffuse positivity for SMA ((c) ×10) and HMB-45 ((d) ×10).

3. Discussion

Primary cardiac sarcomas may occur in any chamber of the heart. Clinical presentation is often nonspecific and depends upon the location of the tumor. Patients can present with generalized symptoms including subjective fevers, weight loss, generalized weakness, and fatigue. Additionally, tumors can infiltrate the myocardial wall and lead to cardiomyopathy and heart failure symptoms as in our case. Furthermore, tumor infiltration into the neural pathways can cause arrhythmias and atrioventricular block. Also, intracavitary tumors, that is, when they protrude inside the atrium or the ventricle, can result in cerebrovascular accidents and pulmonary emboli when they become detached. In some rare cases, the first manifestation of a cardiac tumor is sudden cardiac death [2].

Generally, clinical history and echocardiography can help the diagnosis in most cases. Lab findings can be nonspecific and include leukocytosis, anemia, thrombocytosis, and elevated ESR. Echocardiography represents a substantial imaging technique for the detection of cardiac tumors with high sensitivity and specificity (90% and 95%, resp.) [1]. Newer techniques that may aid in the differential diagnosis of cardiac tumors from other cardiac masses include contrast echocardiography, 3D echocardiography, cardiac MRI, and cardiac CT. Definitive diagnosis is established by histopathology [1].

Surgery remains the backbone of management for cardiac sarcomas [3]. The most important factor dictating prognosis is the ability to achieve a complete surgical resection of the tumor. It has been observed that the median survival increases to 27 months with complete resection compared to 10 months where complete resection is not possible [4]. Surgery not only alleviates symptoms but also confirms diagnosis and avoids future embolic and hemodynamic complications [5]. However, complete macroscopic resection is possible in only 33% of patients [5]. Even in patients with apparent complete excision, high recurrence rates have been reported. After surgical intervention, adjuvant radiotherapy for local recurrence and chemotherapy for control of systemic disease are advised [5].

The response of soft tissue sarcomas to radiation has been well documented and currently adjuvant radiation is recommended along with surgical resection to improve overall survival [3]. Chemotherapy is currently reserved for metastatic tumors and the agents of choice are doxorubicin and ifosfamide, with response rates ranging from 55 to 66% [3]. In cardiac sarcomas, the use of chemotherapeutics may extend to the treatment of the primary tumor if surgery is ineffective [3].

Unfortunately, survival from the time of diagnosis varies from 7 months to a maximum of 2 years and there is insufficient evidence to define optimal treatment [2, 6, 7]. On long-term follow-up, the majority of patients die of distant metastases [2, 6, 7]. The average survival of patients treated purely conservatively with chemotherapy and radiotherapy is just under a year [2]. Simple, incomplete resection (debulking) extends survival by only a few months [2, 6, 7].

Heart transplantation can occasionally be considered as a final treatment option in individual cases, provided distant metastases can be ruled out [2, 8]. One significant risk of this procedure is the danger of exacerbation of undetected micrometastases by the necessary immunosuppression [2].

4. Perivascular Epithelioid Cell Tumor (PEComa)

Perivascular epithelioid cell tumor (PEComa) is recognized as a very rare mesenchymal tumor composed of histologically and immunohistochemically distinctive perivascular epithelioid cells [9, 10]. Perivascular epithelioid cell tumors have now been reported in almost every body site, and the growing list of reported sites includes gastrointestinal site, gynecologic site, genitourinary site, extremities, and skin, as well as single reports in the heart, breast, oral cavity, orbit, and skull base [9]. PEComas with a size >8 cm and mitotic counts of 1/50 HPF are categorized as malignant, such as our case [10]. Precise rates for survival, metastasis, and recurrence specific to primary malignant perivascular epithelioid cell tumor are still not available.

A number of the morphologic features of PEComas, including the admixture of spindled and epithelioid forms, the occasionally prominent nucleoli, and the presence of multinucleated cells, are also seen in melanoma and clear cell sarcoma. PEComas can histopathologically be confused with carcinomas, smooth muscle tumours, adipocytic tumours, and gastrointestinal stromal tumours (GIST) [11].

Based on our literature research, this perivascular epithelioid cell tumor is the fourth reported case found in the heart [9]. The previous cases were 2 young males (aged 29 years and 20 years, resp.) and a 10-year-old girl, and the tumors were overtly malignant only in the adult cases.

Geramizadeh and colleagues [10] described a case of a 20-year-old man who presented with chest pain, palpitation, and dyspnea for 4 days. A TTE showed a cardiac mass and decreased ejection fraction. Spiral chest computed tomography (CT) scan with contrast showed a giant mass located in the posterior part of the pericardial cavity surrounded by pericardial effusion. At surgery, the mass was detected at the posterior aspect of the heart with adhesion to the right and left ventricle and right atrium and was completely resected. On gross examination, the tumor was 15 × 14 × 6 cm. Pathology showed that the mass was a malignant perivascular epithelioid cell tumor (PEComa). The patient refused to receive chemotherapy or radiation and survived 6 months after surgery.

Tazelaar et al. described a case of a 29-year-old man with a seven-year history of atrial fibrillation presented with symptoms of mitral stenosis [12]. Thoracotomy revealed a left atrial tumor growing through the interatrial septum to involve right atrium and extending throughout the left lateral wall into the pericardial sac. Grossly, the tumor appeared to extend very near the pulmonary veins. Because of its infiltrative nature, only incisional biopsies were taken at initial operation. Subsequently, the tumor was completely resected and left atrial reconstruction performed with a bovine graft and reimplantation of pulmonary veins. The patient died shortly thereafter of heart failure thought to be due to nontumorous coronary artery thromboemboli. At postmortem examination, no residual primary or metastatic tumor was found.

Tai et al. reported a case of cardiac PEComa in a 10-year-old girl who had presented with 8 years of cardiac murmur and 2 weeks of increasing dyspnea. Chest computed tomography showed a solid mass located in the left atrioventricular groove. At surgery a 5.5 × 3 × 4.8-cm bulging mass was detected in the left atrioventricular groove. The base of the neoplasm was fixed in the posterolateral wall of the left cardiac ventricle. The slightly firm tumor was well defined with a smooth external surface. The tumor protruded from the cardiac wall into the pericardial cavity with massive effusion. A total tumorectomy was performed, and the postoperative course was uneventful. The patient is alive and well without evidence of disease 18 months after surgery [9].

5. Conclusion

When a cardiac tumor is confirmed, it is crucial for oncologists and surgeons to collaborate. These tumors are of a particular concern due to the fact that overt signs and symptoms occur rather late in the course, precluding effective tumor eradication as in our case. Perhaps if neoadjuvant therapy was attempted, complete surgical resection may have been possible.

Conflict of Interests

The authors declare that there is no conflict of interests regarding the publication of this paper.

Acknowledgment

The authors would like to thank Dr. Makary from Pathology Department at University of Florida, Jacksonville, for providing pathology slides.

References

[1] I. A. Paraskevaidis, C. A. Michalakeas, C. H. Papadopoulos, and M. Anastasiou-Nana, "Cardiac tumors," *ISRN Oncology*, vol. 2011, Article ID 208929, 5 pages, 2011.

[2] A. Hoffmeier, J. R. Sindermann, H. H. Scheld, and S. Martens, "Cardiac tumors—diagnosis and surgical treatment," *Deutsches Ärzteblatt international*, vol. 111, no. 12, pp. 205–211, 2014.

[3] A. Pakala, R. Gupta, and R. Lazzara, "Primary pericardial sarcoma: a case report and a brief review," *Cardiology Research and Practice*, Article ID 853078, 4 pages, 2011.

[4] R. Pathak, S. Nepal, S. Giri, S. Ghimire, and M. R. Aryal, "Primary cardiac sarcoma presenting as acute left-sided heart failure," *Journal of Community Hospital Internal Medicine Perspectives*, vol. 4, no. 3, Article ID 23057, 2014.

[5] H. Khan, S. Chaubey, J. Edlin, and O. Wendler, "Primary cardiac synovial sarcoma. A rare tumor with poor prognosis," *Asian Cardiovascular & Thoracic Annals*, vol. 22, no. 7, pp. 835–838, 2014.

[6] S. Neragi-Miandoab, J. Kim, and G. J. Vlahakes, "Malignant tumours of the heart: a review of tumour type, diagnosis and therapy," *Clinical Oncology*, vol. 19, no. 10, pp. 748–756, 2007.

[7] R. R. Brandt, R. Arnold, R. M. Bohle, T. Dill, and C. W. Hamm, "Cardiac angiosarcoma: case report and review of the literature," *Zeitschrift für Kardiologie*, vol. 94, no. 12, pp. 824–828, 2005.

[8] P. Überfuhr, B. Meiser, A. Fuchs et al., "Heart transplantation: an approach to treating primary cardiac sarcoma?" *Journal of Heart and Lung Transplantation*, vol. 21, no. 10, pp. 1135–1139, 2002.

[9] Y. Tai, L. Wei, and H. Shi, "Perivascular epithelioid cell tumor of the heart in a child," *Pediatric and Developmental Pathology*, vol. 13, no. 5, pp. 412–414, 2010.

[10] B. Geramizadeh, A. Salehzadeh, M. Ghazinoor, A. Moaref, and R. Mollazadeh, "Perivascular epithelioid cell tumor of the pericardium: a case report," *Cardiovascular Pathology*, vol. 17, no. 5, pp. 339–341, 2008.

[11] A. L. Folpe and D. J. Kwiatkowski, "Perivascular epithelioid cell neoplasms: pathology and pathogenesis," *Human Pathology*, vol. 41, no. 1, pp. 1–15, 2010.

[12] H. D. Tazelaar, K. P. Batts, and J. R. Srigley, "Primary extrapulmonary sugar tumor (PEST): a report of four cases," *Modern Pathology*, vol. 14, no. 6, pp. 615–622, 2001.

21

Left Ventricular Thrombus as a Complication of Clozapine-Induced Cardiomyopathy: A Case Report and Brief Literature Review

Shahbaz A. Malik,[1] Sarah Malik,[1] Taylor F. Dowsley,[2] and Balwinder Singh[3]

[1]Department of Internal Medicine, University of North Dakota School of Medicine and Health Sciences, Fargo, ND 58102, USA
[2]Department of Cardiology, Sanford Health, Fargo, ND 58102, USA
[3]Department of Psychiatry and Behavioral Science, University of North Dakota School of Medicine and Health Sciences, Fargo, ND 58102, USA

Correspondence should be addressed to Balwinder Singh; balwinder.singh@med.und.edu

Academic Editor: Tayfun Sahin

A 48-year-old male with history of schizoaffective disorder on clozapine presented with chest pain, dyspnea, and new left bundle branch block. He underwent coronary angiography, which revealed no atherosclerosis. The patient's workup was unrevealing for a cause for the cardiomyopathy and thus it was thought that clozapine was the offending agent. The patient was taken off clozapine and started on guideline directed heart failure therapy. During the course of hospitalization, he was also discovered to have a left ventricular (LV) thrombus for which he received anticoagulation. To our knowledge, this is the first case report of clozapine-induced cardiomyopathy complicated by a LV thrombus.

1. Introduction

Clozapine is the most effective antipsychotic agent available for use in treatment resistant schizophrenia [1]. Despite its efficacy, the drug has been associated with serious adverse effects such as fatal agranulocytosis and cardiovascular complications (such as myocarditis and dilated cardiomyopathy) [1]. The former is monitored with the help of regular laboratory testing and by enrolling patients in the clozapine registry. However, the cardiovascular side effects still elude early detection. We present this case of dilated, nonischemic cardiomyopathy found in a patient taking clozapine to help bring this potential and gravely morbid complication to light, hopefully, increasing awareness among practitioners.

2. Case Presentation

A 48-year-old Caucasian male presented to the emergency department (ED) via local ambulance service, with complaints of new onset chest pain and shortness of breath with activity for past two weeks. The chest pain was present all over the chest, described as a "heavy sensation," and had significantly improved by the time he arrived to the ED with some residual "achiness." The pain was nonpleuritic and did not vary with postural changes. He denied any fevers, chills, cough, hemoptysis, calf tenderness, or leg swelling. He had no history of recent viral illnesses, infections, or long distance travel and no family history for premature coronary heart disease or sudden cardiac death. He had no prior reported history of coronary artery disease (CAD). He did have a history of schizoaffective disorder for which he was on aripiprazole (15 mg daily), lamotrigine (200 mg daily), benztropine (1 mg 3 times a day), and clozapine (100 mg twice a day). He had no history of smoking or recreational drug use.

History at the time of presentation was limited due to patient's psychiatric condition, as the patient would answer questions in a bizarre fashion.

His vitals in the ED revealed a heart rate of 101 beats/min, blood pressure of 95/58 mmHg, and weight of 160 lbs, and saturation was 95% on room air. Positive findings on physical

TABLE 1: Laboratory and biochemical analyses.

Laboratory parameters (units)	Patient's results (reference range)
Complete blood count	
White cell count (K/μL)	8.2 (4–11)
Hemoglobin (g/dL)	13.1 (13.5–17.5)
Hematocrit (%)	38.3 (40–50)
MCV (fL)	83.6 (80–98)
Platelet count (K/μL)	175 (normal 140–400)
Chemistry	
Serum glucose (mg/dL)	126 (70–100)
Sodium (mEq/L)	140 (135–145)
Potassium (mEq/L)	3.5 (3.5–5.3)
Chloride (mEq/L)	104 (99–110)
Magnesium (mg/dL)	1.9 (1.8–2.4)
BUN (mg/dL)	16 (6–22)
Creatinine (mg/dL)	1.2 (0.8–1.3)
Total bilirubin (mg/dL)	1.9 (0.2–1.2)
Alanine aminotransferase (AST) (U/L)	6 (0–55)
Aspartate aminotransferase (AST) (U/L)	12 (0–35)
Alkaline phosphatase (U/L)	73 (30–150)
Iron studies	
Total iron (mcg/dL)	30 (65–175)
Iron saturation (%)	10 (20–50)
Ferritin (ng/mL)	88 (21–275)
Total iron binding capacity (mcg/dL)	307 (250–400)
Cardiac markers	
Troponin (ng/mL)	0.01 (0.00–0.08)
Troponin I (ng/mL)	0.019 (0.00–0.028)
Creatine kinase (CK) (U/L)	48 (30–200)

examination were elevated jugular venous pulsations, fine crackles at bilateral lung bases. Cardiovascular exam revealed a regular rhythm, elevated rate, and normal heart tones without any obvious S3. Pulses were palpable and symmetrical in bilateral upper and lower extremities with no peripheral edema. The patient was alert, oriented to self and time, only. On mental status examination, his thought process was tangential.

A 12-lead electrocardiogram showed sinus tachycardia of 103 beats/min and a new onset left bundle branch block (LBBB), with prolonged corrected QT interval (QTc) of 497 ms; there were no ST segment or T-wave changes. Point-of-care troponin and subsequent cardiac troponin I were both within normal range. Remaining laboratory and biochemical findings are reported in the Table 1.

Chest X-ray showed significant cardiomegaly along with prominent pulmonary vascular markings consistent with pulmonary edema. Due to his complaints of chest pain and shortness of breath along with finding of new LBBB, the patient was taken immediately to the cardiac catheterization laboratory and loaded with aspirin en route. Coronary angiography revealed an essentially normal coronary anatomy with no significant lesions or evidence of occlusive CAD. Ramus intermedius was identified. Left ventricular angiogram showed an ejection fraction (EF) of 15%. Left ventricle end diastolic pressure (LVEDP) was significantly elevated at 35 mm Hg (normal 6–12 mm Hg).

The patient was admitted to the intensive care unit (ICU) and initiated on dobutamine at 5 mcg/kg body weight/min for inotropic support. Transthoracic echocardiogram (TTE) revealed an EF of 10% with severe diffuse hypokinesis, normal left ventricular wall thickness, with evidence of elevated left atrial pressures along with markedly dilated left and right atria. Mild-to-moderate mitral regurgitation was reported. Pulmonary artery systolic pressure was elevated at 69 mm Hg. No pericardial effusion was identified. Inferior vena cava (IVC) was markedly dilated as well, showing <50% variation with breathing. Table 2 shows the results from the multiple echocardiography measurements during hospitalization.

He was initially started on diuresis with intravenous (IV) furosemide 40 mg daily that was increased to twice daily the next day. With diuresis the patient's weight gradually came down to 153 lbs (nadir at the time of discharge) and he improved symptomatically. On day 3, he was switched to per oral (PO) furosemide 40 mg daily. He initially required vasopressor support while being diuresed but was later weaned off it on day 6. Furosemide was decreased to 20 mg PO daily at that point and he was initiated on low dose metoprolol succinate at 12.5 mg daily. Lisinopril 2.5 mg daily was added on day 7. Metoprolol was increased to 25 mg daily on day 9, but lisinopril dose could not be increased further on account of blood pressures remaining in the low-normal range. Repeat TTE did not reveal any change in EF. His vitals stabilized and he started ambulating with physical therapy.

Given the relatively young age of the patient, absence of viral prodromal symptoms, unremarkable coronary angiogram excluding an ischemic etiology, normal cardiac enzymes excluding active cardiac myonecrosis, iron studies not suggestive of any iron overload condition to explain the patient's dilated cardiomyopathy, and absence of other risk factors to explain the cause for the profoundly low EF, clozapine was thought to be possible culprit of the cardiomyopathy.

Review of outside medical records indicated that the patient was on clozapine due to "command hallucinations to harm himself." Going through the clozapine registry, it was ascertained that the patient had been on 300 mg a day of clozapine (200 mg at bedtime and 100 mg in the morning) since June 2010. For unknown reasons, the dose was decreased to 200 mg a day (100 mg in the morning, 100 mg at bedtime) a few weeks prior to hospitalization. Consult liaison (CL) psychiatry team was consulted to assist in treatment planning. Given the possibility of clozapine-induced cardiomyopathy CL team tapered and discontinued clozapine. On day 7, aripiprazole was increased to 30 mg daily (admitted on 15 mg daily); lamotrigine was continued at 200 mg daily. Benztropine was later discontinued. On day 10, he was initiated on PO olanzapine 5 mg at bedtime and titrated to 10 mg on day 15.

Kidney function and hematological laboratory values remained essentially unchanged throughout the course of

TABLE 2: Echocardiography measurements during hospitalization demonstrating left ventricle dysfunction.

Parameter	Day 1	Day 6	Day 14	Day 21	Day 33
Left ventricular ejection fraction (%)	10	10	10	10	10
Left ventricular internal diameter (end diastolic) mm (millimeter)	82	81	79	73	73
Left ventricular internal diameter (end systolic) mm (millimeter)	75	70	73.8	70	68
Peak E/A ratio (early-to-late ventricular filling ratio of mitral flow)	1.66	—	—	—	—
Deceleration time (of mitral E wave) ms (meters per second)	124	—	—	—	—
Pulmonary artery peak systolic pressure in millimeter mercury	69	65	57	64	72
Left ventricle thrombus in millimeter × millimeter	—	—		26 × 20	19 × 13

the hospitalization. No cardiac arrhythmias were observed during the stay. Cardiac rehabilitation was initiated during hospitalization; his functional status gradually improved during stay. Repeat TTE at three weeks showed an EF of approximately 10% but now with a new large, echogenic, mobile, mass which measured 26 mm × 20 mm on the basal inferoseptal wall. This was representative of a LV mural thrombus. The patient's mitral regurgitation also looked worse, based on echocardiographic assessment. He was immediately started on parenteral anticoagulation with low molecular weight heparin (enoxaparin) 80 mg twice daily and then started on oral warfarin. Parenteral anticoagulation was continued until the international normalized ratio (INR) level reached a therapeutic range of greater than 2.

Cardiothoracic surgery was consulted in order to obtain an opinion in regard to the patient's mitral regurgitation. The risks of surgery for mitral valve repair outweighed the benefit in their opinion and thus no surgery was recommended. A repeat TTE on day 33 showed the size of the LV thrombus had decreased to approximately 19 mm × 13 mm (Table 2). Mitral regurgitation remained the same. During all this time, his vitals remained stable.

3. Outcome and Follow-Up

The patient improved clinically and by the end of the hospitalization course, his dyspnea improved and he was able to walk over thousand feet with cardiac rehabilitation and physical therapy. He was discharged on day 37, on metoprolol succinate at 25 mg daily, lisinopril 2.5 mg daily, and warfarin. Furosemide was switched to torsemide 20 mg daily on the day of discharge. In terms of the patient's psychiatric medications, he was sent home on aripiprazole 30 mg daily, lamotrigine 200 mg daily, and olanzapine 10 mg. He was scheduled to follow-up with an outpatient primary care provider, cardiologist, and a psychiatrist on discharge. The patient continues to follow with cardiology regularly with not much improvement in ejection fraction at three months of follow-up. This has prompted consideration for cardiac resynchronization therapy, in the near future.

4. Discussion

In this report, we described a case of a young male with schizoaffective disorder with no prior history of coronary heart disease presenting with a new onset heart failure and

cardiomyopathy. Hypertensive heart disease and genetic and toxic etiologies were ruled out on the basis of the patient's medical history and physical examination. History was also negative for the use of chemotherapeutic agents (notably anthracyclines) or other medications such as antiretroviral drugs, phenothiazines, or chloroquine that could have led to the development of cardiomyopathy. Ischemic cause was excluded based on coronary angiography, whereas infectious and metabolic etiologies were ruled out based on laboratory analyses. In the absence of any other obvious cause for the patient's cardiomyopathy, clozapine was considered the culprit and the medication was discontinued. The patient's case was complicated by a LV thrombus. LV thrombi are an uncommon yet known complication of anterior wall transmural myocardial infarctions (10%) [2]. Furthermore, severe mitral regurgitation has been thought to have a protective role in LV thrombus formation in patients with reduced ejection fraction [3]. Thus, to our knowledge, this is the first case report of cardiomyopathy related to clozapine that was further complicated by an LV thrombus, despite presence of mitral regurgitation. It is unclear whether clozapine itself could be implicated in the thrombus formation, as there have been reports of possible association of clozapine with venous thromboembolic phenomenon [4]. However, it is just as likely that the thrombus was related to poor LV function and the cardiomyopathy itself.

Schizophrenia is currently understood as a psychiatric illness with progressive clinical, neuropsychological, neurophysiological, and neurostructural deterioration [5]. It typically involves recurrent or chronic psychosis. It has been ranked by the World Health Organization as one of the top ten illnesses contributing to the global burden of disease [6]. Approximately 1% of the world's adult population suffers from schizophrenia [7]. Clozapine is the treatment of choice for patients with treatment resistant schizophrenia [8–10]. For patients with schizophrenia, it is the only antipsychotic agent with a demonstrated significant reduction in suicidality and it usually produces few or no extrapyramidal symptoms (such as tardive dyskinesia or dystonia caused by typical antipsychotics) [4, 11]. Despite its efficacy, the drug has been associated with serious adverse effects such as fatal agranulocytosis and toxic megacolon and cardiovascular complications including myocarditis and dilated cardiomyopathy. As a result, it is not considered a first-line treatment and is reserved for patients with treatment resistant schizophrenia/schizoaffective disorder [12–14].

Characteristics of patients with clozapine-induced cardiomyopathy were detailed in a systematic review from 2014, which included reviewing data from 26 cases of clozapine-induced cardiomyopathy [15]. They reported a mean age of 33.5 years, a mean dose of 360 mg, and average time to symptoms onset of 14.4 months and most commonly reported echocardiographic findings as being reduced ejection fraction with global dysfunction [15]. Specific mention of dilated cardiomyopathy was in 39% of individual case reports per the systematic review [15]. Approximately 80% of clozapine treated patients in whom cardiomyopathy was reported were less than 50 years of age, according to a manufacturer adverse event database [16].

The incidence of dilated cardiomyopathy in the general population has been reported to be 7.5–10.0 per 100,000 population [17]. A recent cohort study performed in Australia describes the incidence of clozapine-induced myocarditis and cardiomyopathy to be 3.88% and 4.65% (or 2.26 per 100 patient years), respectively [18]. The rate of cardiomyopathy in clozapine treated patients in the US was shown to be 8.9 per 100,000 person-years according to national databases reporting adverse drug effects [19]. On the other hand, the incidence of clinically severe clozapine-induced cardiomyopathy was reported as 51.5 per 100,000 patient-years [20]. Time to onset of clozapine-induced cardiomyopathy has varied between reports. One case report noted it at 3 weeks [21]. Another case report detailed the discovery on postmortem exam after the patient had been on clozapine for 4 years [22]. A case series described three men developing symptoms secondary to severe left ventricular dysfunction from clozapine use on average one year before diagnosis [23]. The clinical manifestations of clozapine-induced cardiomyopathy range from subclinical presentation [24] to fulminant pulmonary edema and cardiogenic shock [25, 26]. Common presenting symptoms include shortness of breath, palpitations, cough, fatigue, chest pain, and sometimes atypical symptoms such as worsening psychiatric mental status [27, 28]. Diagnosis of clozapine-induced cardiomyopathy has typically been on clinical exam, electrocardiography, and echocardiography. There are two reports in literature detailing the diagnosis on postmortem examination [22, 29].

Mechanism of association of clozapine with cardiomyopathy is still elusive and lacks consensus in the literature. Cardiomyopathy is not as closely related to other antipsychotics as it is to clozapine [20]. One hypothesis suggests that there may be a direct toxicity similar to anthracycline-induced cardiomyopathy [25]. Second explanation is that cardiomyopathy may evolve from clozapine associated myocarditis. Some authors have suggested that exposure to prior antipsychotics, illicit drugs, or alcohol may plays a factor [13].

Treatment of clozapine-induced cardiomyopathy involves cessation of the drug [15]. Guideline directed therapy for heart failure should be instituted [15]. Other treatment goals include prevention of additional cardiac injury related to recreational drug such as alcohol and amphetamines. Alternative antipsychotics such as olanzapine have been used in most other cases [15]. Several reports have noted that there was an improvement in cardiac function on echocardiogram after cessation of clozapine [15, 20]. However, an interesting case report suggested efficacy of beta blockers in association with an angiotensin-converting enzyme inhibitor to decrease the risk of cardiac deterioration and possibility of resuming drug in patients with psychiatric symptoms refractory to other antipsychotics [30]. In general, patients with an ejection fraction of <25% at the time of diagnosis have a poor prognosis including the highest risk of mortality with limited recovery [15]. Patients with an ejection fraction of 25–40% generally show significant improvement [15]. Patients with an ejection fraction of >40% usually show near complete recovery of cardiac function at 6 months, after cessation of clozapine and with normal heart failure treatment [15]. It should be noted that one study demonstrated that 80% of patients withdrawn from clozapine for medical reasons developed a psychotic relapse [31]. Therefore, clozapine cessation should be done under supervision of a psychiatrist and appropriate alternative medication should be substituted to prevent relapse.

Conflict of Interests

None of the authors have any disclosures or conflict of interests.

References

[1] J. Nielsen, P. Damkier, H. Lublin, and D. Taylor, "Optimizing clozapine treatment," *Acta Psychiatrica Scandinavica*, vol. 123, no. 6, pp. 411–422, 2011.

[2] A. Kalra and I.-K. Jang, "Prevalence of early left ventricular thrombus after primary coronary intervention for acute myocardial infarction," *Journal of Thrombosis and Thrombolysis*, vol. 10, no. 2, pp. 133–136, 2000.

[3] V. G. Kalaria, M. R. Passannante, T. Shah, K. Modi, and A. B. Weisse, "Effect of mitral regurgitation on left ventricular thrombus formation in dilated cardiomyopathy," *American Heart Journal*, vol. 135, no. 2, pp. 215–220, 1998.

[4] A. M. Walker, L. L. Lanza, F. Arellano, and K. J. Rothman, "Mortality in current and former users of clozapine," *Epidemiology*, vol. 8, no. 6, pp. 671–677, 1997.

[5] I. Vera, L. Rezende, V. Molina, and J. Sanz-Fuentenebro, "Clozapine as treatment of first choice in first psychotic episodes. What do we know?" *Actas Españolas de Psiquiatría*, vol. 40, no. 5, pp. 281–289, 2012.

[6] C. Murray and A. Lopez, Eds., *The Global Burden of Disease: A Comprehensive Assessment of Mortality and Disability from Diseases, Injuries and Risk Factors in 1990 and Projected to 2020*, Harvard University Press, Cambridge, Mass, USA, 1996.

[7] L. Voruganti, L. Cortese, L. Oyewumi, Z. Cernovsky, S. Zirul, and A. Awad, "Comparative evaluation of conventional and novel antipsychotic drugs with reference to their subjective tolerability, side-effect profile and impact on quality of life," *Schizophrenia Research*, vol. 43, no. 2-3, pp. 135–145, 2000.

[8] J. Kane, G. Honigfeld, J. Singer, and H. Meltzer, "Clozapine for the treatment-resistant schizophrenic. A double-blind comparison with chlorpromazine," *Archives of General Psychiatry*, vol. 45, no. 9, pp. 789–796, 1988.

[9] J. M. Kane, "Treatment-resistant schizophrenic patients," *Journal of Clinical Psychiatry*, vol. 57, supplement 9, pp. 35–40, 1996.

[10] S. W. Lewis, T. R. E. Barnes, L. Davies et al., "Randomized controlled trial of effect of prescription of clozapine versus other second-generation antipsychotic drugs in resistant schizophrenia," *Schizophrenia Bulletin*, vol. 32, no. 4, pp. 715–723, 2006.

[11] J. Hennen and R. J. Baldessarini, "Suicidal risk during treatment with clozapine: a meta-analysis," *Schizophrenia Research*, vol. 73, no. 2-3, pp. 139–145, 2005.

[12] D. M. Coulter, A. Bate, R. H. B. Meyboom, M. Lindquist, and I. R. Edwards, "Antipsychotic drugs and heart muscle disorder in international pharmacovigilance: data mining study," *British Medical Journal*, vol. 322, no. 7296, pp. 1207–1209, 2001.

[13] P. M. Wehmeier, P. Heiser, and H. Remschmidt, "Myocarditis, pericarditis and cardiomyopathy in patients treated with clozapine," *Journal of Clinical Pharmacy and Therapeutics*, vol. 30, no. 1, pp. 91–96, 2005.

[14] E. Wooltorton, "Antipsychotic clozapine (Clozaril): myocarditis and cardiovascular toxicity," *Canadian Medical Association Journal*, vol. 166, no. 9, pp. 1185–1186, 2002.

[15] M. Alawami, C. Wasywich, A. Cicovic, and C. Kenedi, "A systematic review of clozapine induced cardiomyopathy," *International Journal of Cardiology*, vol. 176, no. 2, pp. 315–320, 2014.

[16] P. G. Fontana and B. Sümegi, *Association of Clozaril (Clozapine) with Cardiovascular Toxicity*, Novartis Pharmaceuticals Canada, Dorval, Canada, 2002.

[17] G. Friman, L. Wesslen, J. Fohlman, J. Karjalainen, and C. Rolf, "The epidemiology of infectious myocarditis, lymphocytic myocarditis and dilated cardiomyopathy," *European Heart Journal*, vol. 16, pp. 36–41, 1995.

[18] D. L. Youssef, P. Narayanan, and N. Gill, "Incidence and risk factors for clozapine-induced myocarditis and cardiomyopathy at a regional mental health service in Australia," *Australasian Psychiatry*, 2015.

[19] L. La Grenade, D. Graham, and A. Trontell, "Myocarditis and cardiomyopathy associated with clozapine use in the United States," *The New England Journal of Medicine*, vol. 345, no. 3, pp. 224–225, 2001.

[20] J. G. Kilian, K. Kerr, C. Lawrence, and D. S. Celermajer, "Myocarditis and cardiomyopathy associated with clozapine," *The Lancet*, vol. 354, no. 9193, pp. 1841–1845, 1999.

[21] K. L. D. Phan and S. F. Taylor, "Clozapine-associated cardiomyopathy," *Psychosomatics*, vol. 43, article 248, 2002.

[22] J. D. Hoehns, M. M. Fouts, M. W. Kelly, and K. B. Tu, "Sudden cardiac death with clozapine and sertraline combination," *Annals of Pharmacotherapy*, vol. 35, no. 7-8, pp. 862–866, 2001.

[23] C. Rostagno, S. Domenichetti, F. Pastorelli, and G. F. Gensini, "Clozapine associated cardiomyopathy: a cluster of 3 cases," *Internal and Emergency Medicine*, vol. 6, no. 3, pp. 281–283, 2011.

[24] V. Chow, T. Yeoh, A. C. Ng et al., "Asymptomatic left ventricular dysfunction with long-term clozapine treatment for schizophrenia: a multicentre cross-sectional cohort study," *Open Heart*, vol. 1, no. 1, Article ID e000030, 2014.

[25] D. B. Merrill, G. W. Dec, and D. C. Goff, "Adverse cardiac effects associated with clozapine," *Journal of Clinical Psychopharmacology*, vol. 25, no. 1, pp. 32–41, 2005.

[26] R. J. Leo, J. L. Kreeger, and K. Y. Kim, "Cardiomyopathy associated with clozapine," *Annals of Pharmacotherapy*, vol. 30, no. 6, pp. 603–605, 1996.

[27] R. Sagar, N. Berry, R. Sadhu, and S. Mishra, "Clozapine-induced cardiomyopathy presenting as panic attacks," *Journal of Psychiatric Practice*, vol. 14, no. 3, pp. 182–184, 2008.

[28] C. A. Pastor and M. Mehta, "Masked clozapine-induced cardiomyopathy," *Journal of the American Board of Family Medicine*, vol. 21, no. 1, pp. 70–74, 2008.

[29] J. Reinders, W. Parsonage, D. Lange, J. M. Potter, and S. Plever, "Clozapine-related myocarditis and cardiomyopathy in an Australian metropolitan psychiatric service," *Australian and New Zealand Journal of Psychiatry*, vol. 38, no. 11-12, pp. 915–922, 2004.

[30] C. Rostagno, G. Di Norscia, G. F. Placidi, and G. F. Gensini, "Beta-blocker and angiotensin-converting enzyme inhibitor may limit certain cardiac adverse effects of clozapine," *General Hospital Psychiatry*, vol. 30, no. 3, pp. 280–283, 2008.

[31] R. R. Conley, "Optimizing treatment with clozapine," *Journal of Clinical Psychiatry*, vol. 59, supplement 3, pp. 44–48, 1998.

22

Multiple Coronary Artery Microfistulas Associated with Apical Hypertrophic Cardiomyopathy: Left and Right Coronary Artery to the Left Ventricle

Jeong-Woo Choi, Kyehwan Kim, Min Gyu Kang, Jin-Sin Koh, Jeong Rang Park, and Jin-Yong Hwang

Division of Cardiology, Department of Internal Medicine, Gyeongsang National University Hospital, Jinju 52727, Republic of Korea

Correspondence should be addressed to Jeong Rang Park; parkjrang@gmail.com

Academic Editor: Ramazan Akdemir

A 76-year-old woman underwent coronary angiography for chest pain. On the coronary angiogram, no significant coronary artery atherosclerotic stenosis was observed. Multiple coronary artery microfistulas, draining from the left anterior descending artery to the left ventricle and from the posterior descending artery of the right coronary artery to the left ventricle, were observed. Apical wall thickening and fistula flow from the left anterior descending artery were demonstrated by using transthoracic echocardiography. We describe a rare case of multiple coronary artery microfistulas from the left and right coronary artery to the left ventricle combined with apical hypertrophic cardiomyopathy.

1. Introduction

Coronary artery fistula (CAF) has been known as a rare entity of cardiac anomaly. The incidence of CAF has been reported to be about 0.1–0.2% [1]. A recent retrospective study reported a prevalence of up to 2% in patients who had undergone diagnostic angiography [2, 3]. However, CAFs from both coronary arteries that drain into the left ventricle (LV) are rare. Moreover, apical hypertrophic cardiomyopathy (AHCM) coexisting with CAF has been rarely reported [4–8]. We report a rare case of CAF associated with AHCM that presented with chest pain.

2. Case

A 76-year-old woman without histories of cardiovascular risks such as ischemic heart disease and heart failure and use of medications was referred to our hospital because of chest pain. Her chest pain was characterized by a squeezing sensation that was unrelated to exercise and lasted for less than half an hour. She denied any family history of heart disease. Her initial blood pressure was 110/60 mm Hg; heart rate was 68 beats per minute and regular. Auscultation revealed no evidence of cardiac murmur or crackle. On the chest radiograph, no remarkable findings such as cardiomegaly and pulmonary congestion were found. Electrocardiography revealed an ST depression in leads V5 and V6 and left ventricular hypertrophy (Figure 1). Biochemical laboratory test results, including for cardiac enzyme and B-type natriuretic peptide, were within the reference range.

In order to exclude ischemic heart disease, invasive coronary angiography was performed. No significant luminal stenosis was observed in both the left and right coronary arteries. After contrast medium injection through the orifice of the left coronary artery, remarkable tortuosity of the left coronary artery and a plexiform network of vessels in the LV wall were observed (Figure 2(a)). The LV cavity directly communicated with the diagonal branch of the left anterior descending (LAD) artery through multiple microfistulas. After diastole, the LV was filled with contrast, enough for yielding findings on ventriculography (Figure 2(b)). The right coronary angiogram showed that the posterior descending artery of the right coronary artery was also directly drained into the LV (Figure 2(c)).

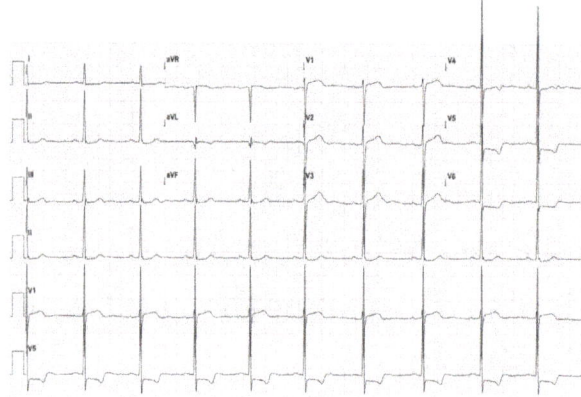

FIGURE 1: Electrocardiography. Baseline electrocardiogram showing left ventricular hypertrophy and ST-T changes in precordial leads 4–6.

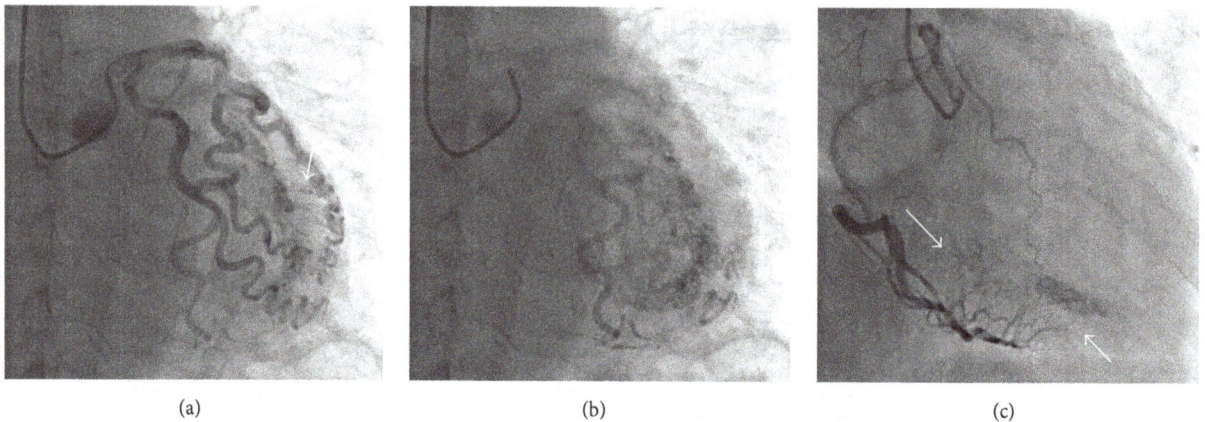

(a)   (b)   (c)

FIGURE 2: Coronary angiography. (a) A plexiform small coronary artery fistula (arrow) from the left coronary artery to the left ventricle. The left coronary artery was tortuous but showed no significant stenosis. (b) After left coronary angiography, contrast medium was drained into the left ventricle, thereby showing the endocardial border of the left ventricle. (c) Angiogram of the right coronary artery showing multiple microfistulas.

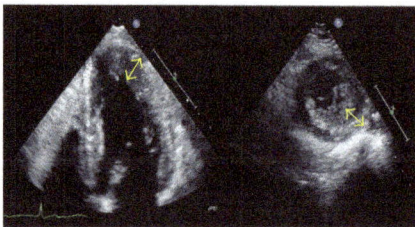

FIGURE 3: Two-dimensional echocardiography. Hypertrophy of the apical lateral wall was observed in the apical four chamber view (left) and short axis view (right).

On two-dimensional echocardiography, the ratio of the apical lateral wall thickness (12 mm) to the left ventricular lateral free wall thickness (7 mm) was greater than 1.5 times (Figure 3). Apical obliteration, aneurysmal change, or intraventricular pressure gradient was not found. Doppler echocardiography demonstrated that color signal of perpendicular to epicardium through multiple CAFs, which directly communicated with the LV at diastole (Figure 4). Pulsed

wave Doppler imaging revealed the diastolic flow of the CAFs, identified by placing a sample volume in the suspicious multiple fistulas of the myocardium (Figure 4). The size of the LV was within the normal range, as were the end-diastolic dimension of 52 mm and end-diastolic volume of 57 mL. The ratio of the mitral inflow E velocity to the annular e' velocity was 6.1. No evidence of pulmonary hypertension was found.

She received calcium channel and beta-blockers. She had no chest pain during follow-up at 18 months.

3. Discussion

CAF is an uncommon congenital anomaly that arises from one or more coronary arteries and enters into the cardiac chamber. The incidence of CAF is low at 0.08% to 2% [1, 2], even though it varied according to time reported and ethnicity. Recently, owing to the development of cardiac imaging tools and easier access for invasive coronary angiography, the incidence of CAF has increased. However, the incidence of multiple CAFs originating from both coronary arteries is only 3–5% of all CAF cases [9], and cases with coexisting AHCM are rare. CAF termination most frequently

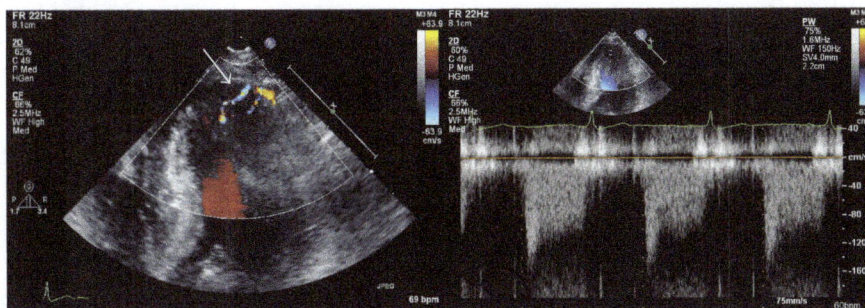

FIGURE 4: Doppler echocardiography. Color signal visible through the multiple coronary artery fistulas, which directly communicated with the left ventricle, as seen in the apical four-chamber view (left). Pulsed wave Doppler image confirming the diastolic flow of the coronary artery fistulas (right).

occurs in the right ventricle, right atrium, and pulmonary artery, being low-pressure chambers [1]. The incidence of CAF draining into the LV is only 3–17% [9]. Wearn et al. categorized CAFs into three anatomical types as follows [1, 10]: Type I, arterioluminal: the fistula drains directly from the coronary arteries to the lumen of a heart chamber; Type II, arteriosinusoidal: the fistula drains from the coronary arteries via the myocardial sinusoids into the lumen of a ventricle; the communication is through the myocardial sinusoidal network; Type III, arteriocapillary: the fistula drains into the capillaries and then through the Thebesian system into a cardiac chamber. The microfistulas in our patient may be classified as the arteriosinusoidal type. The pathogenesis of CAFs is congenital in most cases. CAFs develop because of an "embryologic arrest" of normal closure of the intertrabecular spaces that connect the coronary arteries, veins, and cardiac trabeculae [1]. However, the relationship between AHCM and CAFs has not been clarified. The apical hypertrophy could be the result of chronic LV volume overload through CAFs or could be the cause of multiple CAFs, possibly due to the disarray of myocardial cells. One retrospective study [2] reported 20 patients with micro-CAFs, of whom 18 (90%) had concentric LV hypertrophy, not apical hypertrophy. They suggested that volume overload over a long period can induce reactive myocardial hypertrophy. However, in our case, the LV volume was within the normal range and localized asymmetric hypertrophy in the apical lateral wall was observed, although the shunt was relatively large. Therefore, we thought that AHCM and CAFs may be related with congenital, myocardial disarray. Magnetic resonance imaging or cardiac biopsy could help to determine the pathophysiological mechanism underlying the interrelationship between CAFs and cardiomyopathies. However, we did not recommend cardiac magnetic resonance imaging for the patient because it has no additional affect to clinical management.

More than half of patients with CAFs have been reported to be possibly completely asymptomatic [1]. The reported clinical presentations are angina, atypical chest pain, syncope, dyspnea, palpitation, congestive heart failure, arrhythmia, and rarely sudden cardiac death due to rupture of an aneurysm [1]. Anginal symptoms could result from the coronary steal phenomenon. Especially in patients with CAFs with hypertrophy, aggravated imbalance of oxygen demand/supply in the myocardium can lead to chest pain and myocardial ischemia. Clinical suspicion and diagnosis of CAFs are difficult. Presence of myocardial ischemia may be confirmed by using a treadmill test and myocardial perfusion single-photon emission computed tomography [9, 11, 12], but these methods have limited diagnostic capabilities. Still, in most cases, CAFs are identified during routine coronary angiography and emergent catheterizations [12]. With the development of the resolution of coronary computed tomography, noninvasive methods for diagnosis of CAFs including microfistulas have become available [13, 14]. Therefore, we think that the role of echocardiography emerged to be more important in determining whether invasive coronary angiography is required. Dresios et al. [4] reinforced the role of Doppler echocardiography in multimodalities for cardiac imaging.

No guideline has been established for the management of patients with micro-CAFs. Conventional medical management is essential. Beta-blockers, calcium channel blockers, or nitrate is usually recommended for ischemia. Our patient was treated medically and remained asymptomatic.

In conclusion, we report a rare case of multiple microfistulas of both coronary arteries that drained into the LV associated with AHCM. In addition, close inspection of color and flow patterns on Doppler echocardiography is important in screening for the cause of chest pain in AHCM.

Ethical Approval

The identity of the patient was absolutely preserved.

Conflict of Interests

The authors declare that there is no conflict of interests regarding the publication of this paper.

References

[1] S. A. Said, A. A. Thiadens, M. J. Fieren, E. J. Meijboom, T. van der Werf, and G. B. Bennink, "Coronary artery fistulas," *Netherlands Heart Journal*, vol. 10, pp. 65–78, 2002.

[2] Y. Mizuguchi, A. Takahashi, T. Yamada, N. Taniguchi, S. Nakajima, and T. Hata, "Unexpectedly abundant coronary

Thebesian system: possible cause of chest pain and abnormal electrocardiogram results," *International Journal of Cardiology*, vol. 168, no. 5, pp. 4909–4912, 2013.

[3] S. Nawa, Y. Miyachi, T. Shiba et al., "Clinical and angiographic analysis of congenital coronary artery fistulae in adulthood is there any new trend?" *Japanese Heart Journal*, vol. 37, no. 1, pp. 95–104, 1996.

[4] C. Dresios, S. Apostolakis, S. Tzortzis, K. Lazaridis, and A. Gardikiotis, "Apical hypertrophic cardiomyopathy associated with multiple coronary artery-left ventricular fistulae: a report of a case and review of the literature," *European Journal of Echocardiography*, vol. 11, no. 4, p. E9, 2010.

[5] O. Alyan, O. Ozeke, and Z. Golbasi, "Coronary artery-left ventricular fistulae associated with apical hypertrophic cardiomyopathy," *European Journal of Echocardiography*, vol. 7, no. 4, pp. 326–329, 2006.

[6] G.-R. Hong, S. H. Choi, S.-M. Kang et al., "Multiple coronary artery-left ventricular microfistulae in a patient with apical hypertrophic cardiomyopathy: a demonstration by transthoracic color Doppler echocardiography," *Yonsei Medical Journal*, vol. 44, no. 4, pp. 710–714, 2003.

[7] S. Caputo, G. Capozzi, G. Santoro et al., "Multiple right coronary artery fistulae in a patient with diffuse hypertrophic cardiomyopathy: a case report," *Journal of the American Society of Echocardiography*, vol. 18, no. 8, article 884, 2005.

[8] I. K. Moon, D. C. Seo, J. W. Wee, B. W. Park, and M. S. Hyon, "Thebesian vein combined with apical hypertrophic cardiomyopathy," *Soonchunhyang Medical Science*, vol. 19, no. 2, pp. 120–122, 2013.

[9] R. E. Hobbs, H. D. Millit, P. V. Raghavan, D. S. Moodie, and W. C. Sheldon, "Coronary artery fistulae: a 10-year review," *Cleveland Clinic Quarterly*, vol. 49, no. 4, pp. 191–197, 1982.

[10] J. T. Wearn, S. R. Mettier, T. G. Klumpp, and L. J. Zschiesche, "The nature of the vascular communications between the coronary arteries and the chambers of the heart," *American Heart Journal*, vol. 9, no. 2, pp. 143–149, 1933.

[11] E. J. Kim, H. S. Seo, H. H. Lee et al., "A clinically silent case of prominent thebesian system: diagonal branch of left anterior descending coronary artery to left ventricular communication," *Korean Circulation Journal*, vol. 34, no. 1, pp. 107–111, 2004.

[12] K. Oshiro, M. Shimabukuro, Y. Nakada et al., "Multiple coronary LV fistulas: demonstration of coronary steal phenomenon by stress thallium scintigraphy and exercise hemodynamics," *American Heart Journal*, vol. 120, no. 1, pp. 217–219, 1990.

[13] S. S. Saboo, Y.-H. Juan, A. Khandelwal et al., "MDCT of congenital coronary artery fistulas," *American Journal of Roentgenology*, vol. 203, no. 3, pp. W244–W252, 2014.

[14] G. R. Mitchell, G. Morgan-Hughes, and C. Roobottom, "Coronary arterial microfistulae: a CT coronary angiography perspective," *Journal of Cardiovascular Computed Tomography*, vol. 4, no. 4, pp. 279–280, 2010.

23

Takotsubo Cardiomyopathy: A New Perspective in Asthma

Fady Y. Marmoush,[1] **Mohamad F. Barbour,**[1] **Thomas E. Noonan,**[1,2] **and Mazen O. Al-Qadi**[1]

[1]*Memorial Hospital of Rhode Island, Alpert Medical School, Brown University, Pawtucket, RI 02860, USA*
[2]*Harvard Medical School, USA*

Correspondence should be addressed to Fady Y. Marmoush; fady_marmoush@brown.edu

Academic Editor: Filippo M. Sarullo

Takotsubo cardiomyopathy (TCM) is an entity of reversible cardiomyopathy known for its association with physical or emotional stress and may mimic myocardial infarction. We report an exceedingly rare case of albuterol-induced TCM with moderate asthma exacerbation. An interesting association that may help in understanding the etiology of TCM in the asthmatic population. Although the prognosis of TCM is excellent, it is crucial to recognize beta agonists as a potential stressor.

1. Introduction

Takotsubo cardiomyopathy (TCM) has been recognized more recently as an entity of reversible cardiomyopathy. It is also known as stress-induced cardiomyopathy for its strong association with physical or emotional stress. The clinical presentations and electrocardiographic changes are nonspecific. Furthermore, cardiac biomarkers are frequently elevated which makes the differentiation between TCM and acute myocardial infarction challenging. We are reporting a case of albuterol-induced TCM associated with moderate asthma exacerbation due to excess albuterol use. This case report along with few other reports in the literature sheds light on an unrecognized etiology for TCM in patients with asthma exacerbation.

2. Case Description

An 80-year-old woman with past medical history of asthma, hypertension, and hyperlipidemia presented with progressively increasing shortness of breath and wheezing associated with left-sided, constant, nonradiating chest pain that was not exertional and started few hours prior to her presentation. She used her rescue albuterol inhaler several times. She denied any fever, chills, or cough. She has never smoked in the past. Her only medication for asthma is albuterol inhalation as needed. Her chest pain resolved spontaneously several minutes before arrival to the emergency room. On examination, she had nontoxic appearance and was in mild distress. She was afebrile and the blood pressure was 145/64 mmHg and she had a pulse of regular 100 beats per minute and respiratory rate of 22 breaths per minute. Oxygen saturation was 93% on ambient air. Chest exam was remarkable for prolonged expiratory phase and scattered expiratory wheezes but no rhonchi or accessory muscle use. Laboratory findings on admission showed white blood cell count 6,200/mm^3, hemoglobin 13 g/dL, and troponin I mildly elevated at 0.05 ng/mL (normal reference < 0.030 ng/mL). B natriuretic peptide was 55 pg/mL. Chest radiograph was normal. Electrocardiogram (EKG) was remarkable for left atrial enlargement and new left bundle branch block (LBBB). Initial management for asthma exacerbation included intravenous methyl-prednisone and albuterol/ipratropium along with continuation of aspirin. Though the shortness of breath improved after a few hours, the patient experienced recurrent chest pain relieved with nitroglycerine. The second troponin rose to 0.422 ng/mL and peaked at 1.112 ng/mL on serial measurements with no changes on EKG. Management for acute coronary syndrome was initiated including aspirin, clopidogrel, statins, and intravenous heparin. Echocardiography demonstrated ejection fraction of 60–65% with hypokinesis of the left ventricular apex and distal septum. Cardiac

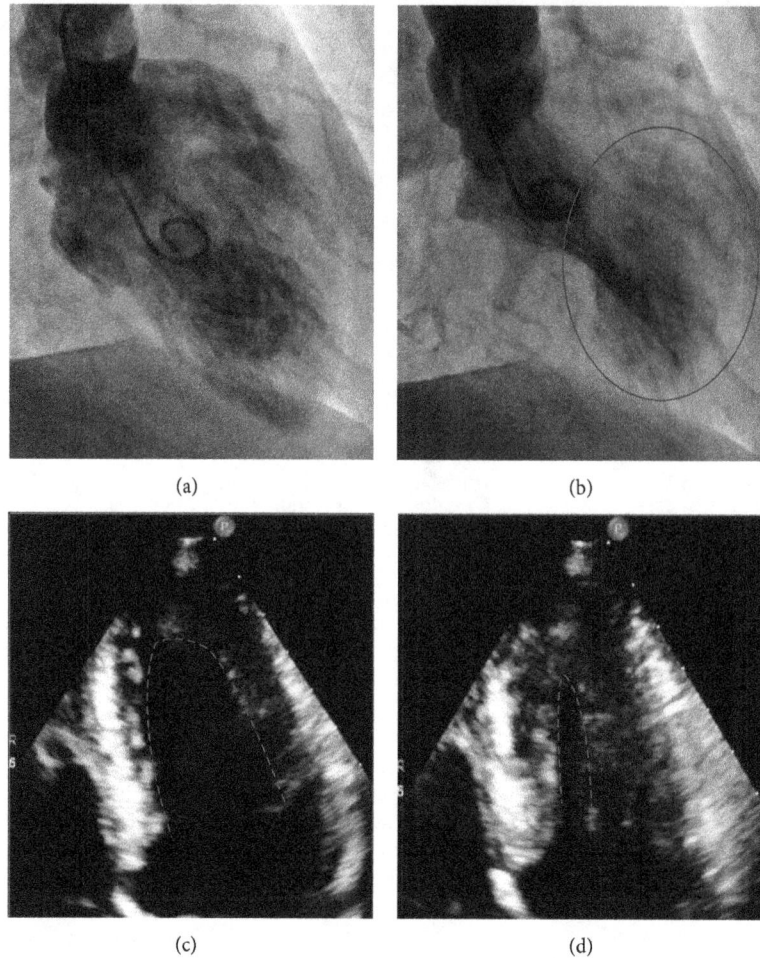

FIGURE 1: Left ventricular catheterization shows (a) the end of diastole and (b) apical ballooning at the end of systole. Transthoracic echocardiogram shows (c) LV end of diastole and (d) LV end of systole (no apical ballooning).

catheterization was performed revealing normal epicardial coronary arteries with evidence of apical ballooning (Figures 1(a) and 1(b)). Based on these findings, she was diagnosed with TCM. Eventually, the troponin trended down with no recurrence of chest pain or dyspnea during hospitalization. Three months later, the patient had persistence of left bundle branch block and repeat echocardiography (Figures 1(c) and 1(d)) showed complete resolution of apical ballooning with preserved ejection fraction.

3. Discussion

Stress-induced cardiomyopathy also known as Takotsubo cardiomyopathy (TCM) was first reported in Japan in 1990 by Sato et al. Tako-tsubo is a Japanese term that describes the octopus trap, referring to the apical ballooning morphology of the left ventricular apex associated with the condition. TCM is an acute but reversible subtype of cardiomyopathy that may mimic acute myocardial infarction with no evidence of obstructive epicardial coronary artery disease. It is usually preceded by acute physical or emotional stress such as grief, exacerbation of chronic illnesses (e.g., asthma), or use of

exogenous catecholamines. TCM has a distinctive morphology of hypokinesis of the left ventricular mid- and apical segments with hyperkinesis of the basal segments leading to distal ballooning of the apex [1]. In a single-center study, approximately 2.2% of patients presenting with ST segment elevation had TCM [2].

We report an exceedingly rare case of albuterol-induced TCM. To our knowledge, there were only 5 similar cases reported in literature [3–7]. Although our patient presented with asthma exacerbation which may count as an acute stressor, there was no evidence of severe stress as in status asthmaticus or respiratory failure as previously reported in two cases [5, 6]. The likely mechanism of TCM in our case is mediated through the β agonist action of albuterol. Although $\beta 2$ agonists are highly selective, they may lose their selectivity at high doses [8]. Furthermore, Paur et al. showed that there is a myocardial depressive effect through catecholamines-specific $\beta 2$ adrenergic receptor inhibitory signaling in a rat model with regional preference to the apex given the ventricular apical-basal $\beta 2$ adrenergic receptor gradient [9]. Moreover, TCM has been described after the use of other β agonists [10].

Another postulated mechanism for TCM is microvascular spasm with subsequent myocardial apical stunning [11, 12], which explains the extent of myocardial dysfunction beyond a single coronary territory and may explain the presence of left bundle branch block. Although coronary microvascular spasm is less likely to explain TCM in asthmatics [13–15], our patient had persistence of left bundle branch block in the absence of reduced ejection fraction which may indicate an underlying microvascular ischemia contributing to the presentation.

Spasm of multiple epicardial vessels or aborted infarction of a long wrap around left anterior descending artery is not supported by angiographic and intravascular ultrasonographic studies.

Our patient fits into the demographic profile of TCM described in literature [1, 2, 12, 16–20]. Most patients were postmenopausal women (82% to 100% of patients). Chest pain was observed in 50–70% of cases while the majority had typically mild elevations in troponin levels as our patient had. Our case shows evidence of new left bundle branch block which was described to occur in 9% of patients with TCM on presentation, in particular, our patient's age group [21]. Given the nonspecific clinical features, the diagnosis of TCM is usually made after excluding acute coronary events. In addition, the modified Mayo Clinic criteria for diagnosis of TCM are frequently used. Patients must meet all four criteria: (a) transient left ventricular midsegments hypokinesis or akinesis (with or without apical involvement) that extends beyond a single vessel distribution, with or without a stressor; (b) absence of occlusive coronary disease; (c) evidence of myocardial injury (new EKG abnormalities or elevation in troponin); and (d) exclusion of pheochromocytoma or myocarditis. Treatment of TCM is supportive and includes the standard therapy for cardiomyopathy (angiotensin converting enzyme inhibitor and beta blockers). Diuretics are used to manage pulmonary edema and other manifestations of volume overload. Mechanical circulatory support devices (e.g., intra-aortic balloon pump) can be used in cases complicated by cardiogenic shock. When left ventricular thrombus is present, anticoagulation is indicated.

The prognosis of TCM is excellent with most patients recovering completely within 4–8 weeks. Recurrence may occur in 1.5% of patients and can be reduced by angiotensin converting enzyme inhibitors [22]. The effect of beta blockers on recurrence is less defined. Fatality from TCM is rare and occurs in less than 3% of patients [23].

4. Conclusion

Although the prognosis of TCM is excellent, it is crucial to recognize beta agonists as a potential stressor, especially in patients with acute asthma attacks. Despite increasing awareness of beta agonist-induced TCM, the diagnosis of TCM remains that of exclusion.

Conflict of Interests

The authors declare that there is no conflict of interests regarding the publication of this paper.

References

[1] K. Tsuchihashi, K. Ueshima, T. Uchida et al., "Transient left ventricular apical ballooning without coronary artery stenosis: a novel heart syndrome mimicking acute myocardial infarction," *Journal of the American College of Cardiology*, vol. 38, no. 1, pp. 11–18, 2001.

[2] K. A. Bybee, A. Prasad, G. W. Barsness et al., "Clinical characteristics and Thrombolysis in Myocardial Infarction frame counts in women with transient left ventricular apical ballooning syndrome," *The American Journal of Cardiology*, vol. 94, no. 3, pp. 343–346, 2004.

[3] I. Mendoza and G. M. Novaro, "Repeat recurrence of takotsubo cardiomyopathy related to inhaled beta-2-adrenoceptor agonists," *World Journal of Cardiology*, vol. 4, no. 6, pp. 211–213, 2012.

[4] B. Patel, D. Assad, C. Wiemann, and M. Zughaib, "Repeated use of albuterol inhaler as a potential cause of Takotsubo cardiomyopathy," *American Journal of Case Reports*, vol. 15, pp. 221–225, 2014.

[5] S. L. Rennyson, J. M. Parker, J. D. Symanski, and L. Littmann, "Recurrent, severe, and rapidly reversible apical ballooning syndrome in status asthmaticus," *Heart & Lung*, vol. 39, no. 6, pp. 537–539, 2010.

[6] D. A. Stanojevic, V. M. Alla, J. D. Lynch, and C. B. Hunter, "Case of reverse takotsubo cardiomyopathy in status asthmaticus," *Southern Medical Journal*, vol. 103, no. 9, article 964, 2010.

[7] F. Venditti, B. Bellandi, and G. Parodi, "Fatal Tako-Tsubo cardiomyopathy recurrence after β2-agonist administration," *International Journal of Cardiology*, vol. 161, no. 1, pp. e10–e11, 2012.

[8] M. Cazzola, M. G. Matera, and C. F. Donner, "Inhaled β2-adrenoceptor agonists: cardiovascular safety in patients with obstructive lung disease," *Drugs*, vol. 65, no. 12, pp. 1595–1610, 2005.

[9] H. Paur, P. T. Wright, M. B. Sikkel et al., "High levels of circulating epinephrine trigger apical cardiodepression in a β2-adrenergic receptor/Gi-dependent manner: a new model of takotsubo cardiomyopathy," *Circulation*, vol. 126, no. 6, pp. 697–706, 2012.

[10] W. J. Mosley II, A. Manuchehry, C. McEvoy, and V. Rigolin, "Takotsubo cardiomyopathy induced by dobutamine infusion: a new phenomenon or an old disease with a new name," *Echocardiography*, vol. 27, no. 3, pp. E30–E33, 2010.

[11] K. Dote, H. Sato, H. Tateishi, T. Uchida, and M. Ishihara, "Myocardial stunning due to simultaneous multivessel coronary spasms: a review of 5 cases," *Journal of Cardiology*, vol. 21, no. 2, pp. 203–214, 1991.

[12] S. Kurisu, H. Sato, T. Kawagoe et al., "Tako-tsubo-like left ventricular dysfunction with ST-segment elevation: a novel cardiac syndrome mimicking acute myocardial infarction," *American Heart Journal*, vol. 143, no. 3, pp. 448–455, 2002.

[13] S. Haruta, M. Okayama, T. Uchida, K. Hirosawa, and H. Kasanuki, "Airway hyperresponsiveness in patients with coronary spastic angina—relationship between coronary spasticity and airway responsiveness," *Circulation Journal*, vol. 71, no. 2, pp. 234–241, 2007.

[14] G. Tacoy, S. A. Kocaman, S. Balcioglu et al., "Coronary vasospastic crisis leading to cardiogenic shock and recurrent ventricular fibrillation in a patient with long-standing asthma," *Journal of Cardiology*, vol. 52, no. 3, pp. 300–304, 2008.

[15] M. Gianni, F. Dentali, A. M. Grandi, G. Sumner, R. Hiralal, and E. Lonn, "Apical ballooning syndrome or takotsubo cardiomyopathy: a systematic review," *European Heart Journal*, vol. 27, no. 13, pp. 1523–1529, 2006.

[16] K. A. Bybee, T. Kara, A. Prasad et al., "Systematic review: transient left ventricular apical ballooning: a syndrome that mimics ST-segment elevation myocardial infarction," *Annals of Internal Medicine*, vol. 141, no. 11, pp. 858–865, 2004.

[17] Y. Abe, M. Kondo, R. Matsuoka, M. Araki, K. Dohyama, and H. Tanio, "Assessment of clinical features in transient left ventricular apical ballooning," *Journal of the American College of Cardiology*, vol. 41, no. 5, pp. 737–742, 2003.

[18] Y. J. Akashi, K. Nakazawa, M. Sakakibara, F. Miyake, H. Koike, and K. Sasaka, "The clinical features of *takotsubo* cardiomyopathy," *QJM*, vol. 96, no. 8, pp. 563–573, 2003.

[19] W. J. R. Desmet, B. F. M. Adriaenssens, and J. A. Y. Dens, "Apical ballooning of the left ventricle: first series in white patients," *Heart*, vol. 89, no. 9, pp. 1027–1031, 2003.

[20] S. Kawai, H. Suzuki, H. Yamaguchi et al., "Ampulla cardiomyopathy ('Takotusbo' cardiomyopathy)—reversible left ventricular dysfunction: with ST segment elevation," *Japanese Circulation Journal*, vol. 64, no. 2, pp. 156–159, 2000.

[21] G. Parodi, C. Salvadori, S. Del Pace et al., "Left bundle branch block as an electrocardiographic pattern at presentation of patients with Tako-tsubo cardiomyopathy," *Journal of Cardiovascular Medicine*, vol. 10, no. 1, pp. 100–103, 2009.

[22] K. Singh, K. Carson, Z. Usmani, G. Sawhney, R. Shah, and J. Horowitz, "Systematic review and meta-analysis of incidence and correlates of recurrence of takotsubo cardiomyopathy," *International Journal of Cardiology*, vol. 174, no. 3, pp. 696–701, 2014.

[23] D. Donohue and M.-R. Movahed, "Clinical characteristics, demographics and prognosis of transient left ventricular apical ballooning syndrome," *Heart Failure Reviews*, vol. 10, no. 4, pp. 311–316, 2005.

24

Left Ventricular Aneurysm Presenting as a Late Complication of Childhood Chemotherapy

Braghadheeswar Thyagarajan, Lubna Bashir Munshi, and Martin Miguel Amor

Department of Internal Medicine, Monmouth Medical Center, Long Branch, NJ 07740, USA

Correspondence should be addressed to Braghadheeswar Thyagarajan; bthyag@barnabashealth.org

Academic Editor: Filippo M. Sarullo

Cardiotoxicity is a well known adverse effect of chemotherapy. Multiple cardiac injuries have been reported including cardiomyopathy, pericarditis, myocarditis, angina, arrhythmias, and myocardial infarction. A left ventricular aneurysm due to chemotherapy is a rare and a dangerous complication which is particularly challenging in diagnosis requiring a high index of suspicion and periodic imaging. We present a case of a young Caucasian male with a past medical history of Acute Lymphocytic Leukemia status after chemotherapy during his childhood diagnosed with left ventricular aneurysm several years later.

1. Introduction

Cardiotoxicity is a well known adverse effect in children who receive chemotherapy for cancer [1]. Multiple cardiac injuries have been reported including cardiomyopathy, congestive heart failure, pericarditis, myocarditis, angina, arrhythmias, and myocardial infarction [2, 3]. The incidence of postmyocardial infarction left aneurysm varies from 3.5 to 5% in autopsy studies and 22 to 35% in the echocardiographic and radionuclide studies [4]. We present a case of a young Caucasian male with a past medical history of Acute Lymphocytic Leukemia status after chemotherapy during his childhood diagnosed with left ventricular aneurysm several years later.

2. Case Report

This is a case of a 27-year-old Caucasian male with past medical history significant for ALL who was brought into the ED by the EMS after an episode of cardiac arrest.

The patient's history starts when he was 5 years of age when he was diagnosed with Acute Lymphoblastic Leukemia. He underwent chemotherapy with vincristine, doxorubicin, and steroids at the time of diagnosis. At the end of two years, it was diagnosed that his ALL has progressed to involve the central nervous system and he was given chemotherapy for

an additional two years which also included methotrexate. During this time the patient had complaints of constipation and after two weeks of no bowel movements, the patient was found straining in the toilet when he clenched his chest due to pain and fainted. He was taken to the hospital where he had a blood work and echocardiogram which were unremarkable. The patient recovered completely with no further similar episodes in his childhood. It is unclear whether the patient had an acute coronary syndrome or any arrythmias at that time. The patient eventually lost follow-up with his primary care doctor. There is no other past medical history and no positive family history for cardiac diseases. The patient also denied smoking, drinking of alcohol, and illicit drug use which was confirmed with the patient later.

On the day of admission, the patient was performing his usual duties in his workplace which included lifting of heavy objects. When the patient was walking after his work, he suddenly collapsed down on the floor. His friend who was present at the side witnessed this event. There was no breathing or palpable pulse. CPR was started and the paddles of the AED were connected which showed a shockable rhythm. The patient was shocked for four times and chest compression was given in between. When the patient was brought to the emergency department of the hospital he had an EKG (Figure 1) which showed normal

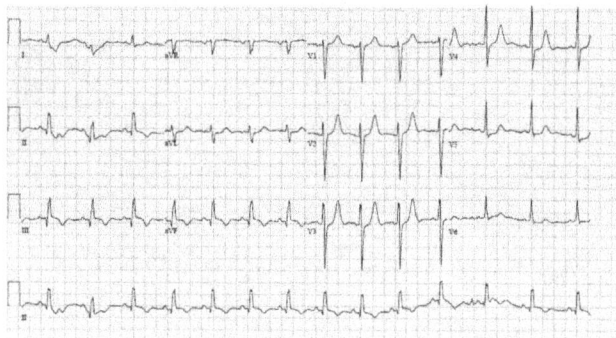

FIGURE 1: EKG showing normal sinus rhythm, Q waves in the inferior wall leads concerning old myocardial infarction.

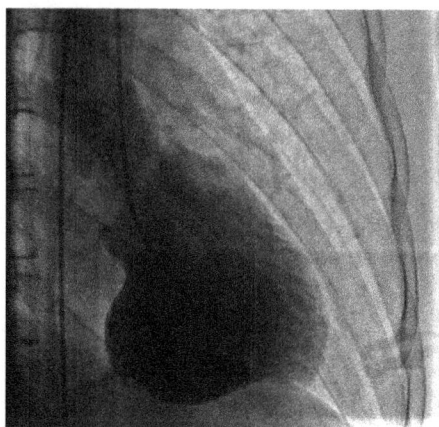

FIGURE 2: Left ventriculography with contrast showing left ventricular aneurysm.

sinus rhythm, Q waves in the inferior wall leads concerning old myocardial infarction versus a direct damage to the RCA territory myocardium due to chemotherapy effect. His vitals at the time of admission were blood pressure 86/47, heart rate 88, and respiratory rate 16 and he was afebrile. His labs were unremarkable with negative troponins. He was unresponsive at this time and his lungs and heart were clear to auscultation. He was intubated in the emergency department for airway protection and the patient was immediately admitted to the Intensive Care Unit.

Eventually the patient got stabilized and was extubated. He had an echocardiogram which showed a LVEF of 36.9%, large basal and mid inferior aneurysm, akinesis of the inferior and inferolateral wall, moderate global hypokinesis of the left ventricle, and trace mitral regurgitation. He had a left and right cardiac catheterization along with left ventriculography (Figures 2, 3, and 4) which showed no evidence of disease in his left main, left anterior descending, and right coronary artery and left circumflex. His left ventriculography showed a normal sized ventricle, LVEF of 35 to 40%, and a large inferior wall aneurysm with the inferior base and midportion being akinetic. After the cardiac catheterization, the patient was transferred to a tertiary medical center for further care and he eventually received an Implantable Cardioverter Defibrillator

with no surgical intervention and was managed medically with beta blocker and ACE inhibitor. Six months later after this event, the patient has been doing well with no further episodes of arrhythmias and has improved EF.

3. Discussion

ALL is the most common cancer diagnosed in children and represents approximately 25% of cancer diagnoses among children younger than 15 years. ALL occurs at an annual rate of 35 to 40 cases per 1 million people in the United States [5, 6]. Over the past 25 years, there has been a gradual increase in the incidence of ALL [3, 4, 7]. The 5-year survival rate for ALL has increased over the same time from 60% to approximately 90% for children younger than 15 years and from 28% to more than 75% for adolescents aged 15 to 19 years [8]. CNS involvement is approximately 3% in ALL [7].

Our patient received treatment with vincristine, doxorubicin, and steroids. And due to the involvement of CNS he had to receive treatment with intrathecal methotrexate for two years. Cardiotoxicity is a well known adverse effect in children who receive chemotherapy for cancer [1]. Doxorubicin has a direct cardiotoxic effect which is myocardial depression [9]. The incidence of congestive heart failure due to doxorubicin is dose dependent, ranging from 0.2% incidence of CHF in a dose of $150 \, mg/m^2$ to 8.7% in a dose of $600 \, mg/m^2$ [10]. The mechanism by which doxorubicin damages the cardiac myocyte is due to the formation of free oxygen radical and cardiac myocytes that are sensitive to these radicals are more prone to damage [11]. Another mechanism is by the effect of doxorubicin on mitochondrial performance which is by the interference with oxidative phosphorylation and inhibition of ATP synthesis. Free radicals released are thought to be responsible for many secondary effects such as lipid peroxidation, the oxidation of proteins and DNA, and depletion of glutathione and pyridine nucleotide reducing equivalents in the cell. These changes cause loss of mitochondrial integrity and function. And this causes an oncotic or necrotic cell death further leading to death of cardiac myocytes leading to cardiomyopathy [12]. It is shown that vincristine could protect the cardiac myocytes from the damage of oxidative stress from doxorubicin [13]. It is also shown that there is increased risk of myocardial infarction for about 25 years after treatment with doxorubicin [14]. High-dose methotrexate decreases levels of S-adenosylmethionine (a methyl donor) and increases sulfur-containing excitatory amino acids. These metabolic events have the potential to cause neurologic injury (e.g., demyelination) and overactivity (e.g., seizures). There is no information to support a role for these compounds in patients with cardiac toxicity. However, methotrexate inhibits the remethylation of homocysteine and causes acute and chronic elevations in homocysteine levels. Homocysteine also has important prothrombotic effects on the coagulation system due to its mechanism of getting rapidly autooxidized in plasma, and this process forms reactive oxygen species, such as superoxide and hydrogen peroxide. Chronic elevations of homocysteine levels can cause premature vascular disease, including stroke,

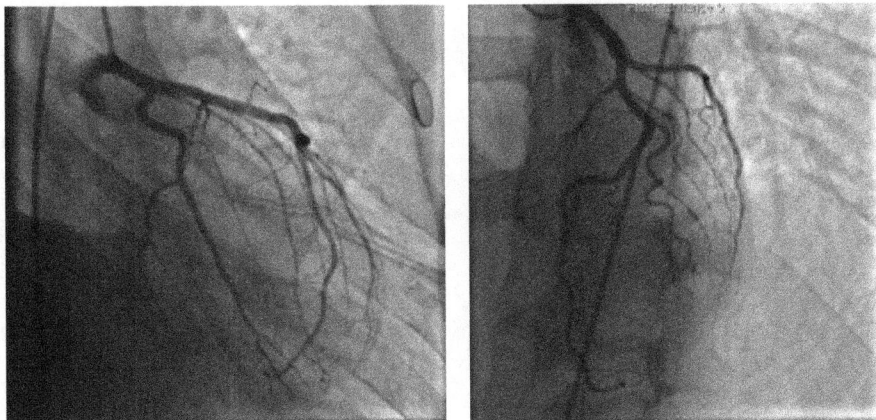

FIGURE 3: Normal LAD and LCX.

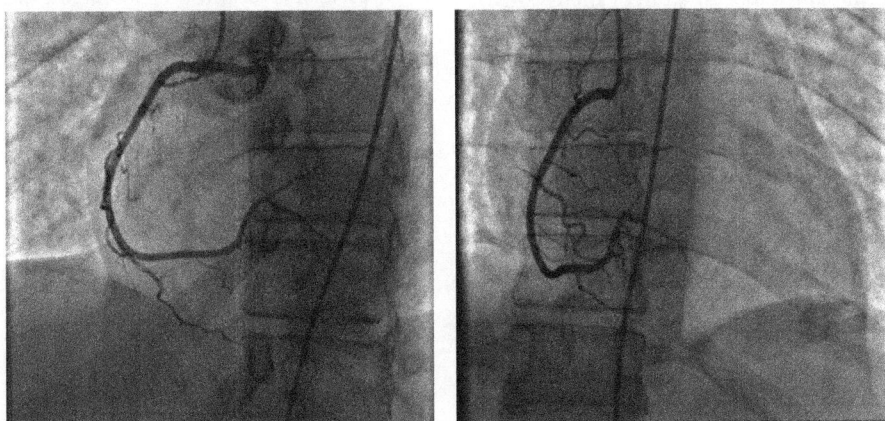

FIGURE 4: Normal RCA.

myocardial infarction, and venous thromboembolism [15]. In our patient, who was treated with both doxorubicin and methotrexate during his childhood, the cardiotoxic effects could have been due to one drug or a combination of both.

Left ventricular aneurysm is defined as a distinct area of abnormal left ventricular diastolic contour with systolic dyskinesia or paradoxical bulging as visualised by ventriculography [16]. Left ventricular aneurysm usually results from myocardial infarction. Other rare etiologies of LVA include hypertrophic cardiomyopathy, Chagas' disease, sarcoidosis, congenital LVA and idiopathic dilated cardiomyopathy [17–20]. The incidence of left ventricular aneurysm is about 22% in anterior wall MI and the time period in which they usually occur is within 3 months after AMI [21] with only 3% of the LV aneurysm being inferior [22]. In an extensive review of medical literature we were not able to find any cases of left ventricular aneurysm as a direct consequence of doxorubicin or methotrexate. But there are articles about doxorubicin causing cardiomyopathy similar to the dilated type [23], isolated case reports where the cardiomyopathy was caused 17 years after the chemotherapy [24], and also articles about heart failure as a late complication due to doxorubicin [25]. As mentioned earlier in the discussion, doxorubicin can also lead to myocardial infarction due to damage of the myocytes;

it is unclear in our patient whether he suffered myocardial infarction in childhood, when he had an episode of chest pain during straining episode of bowel movement. The patient at that time had no EKG changes and his echocardiogram was unremarkable. Unfortunately the patient never had a cardiac cath. during his childhood. The left ventricular aneurysm developed by the patient currently could have been a primary consequence because of the direct effect of chemotherapy on cardiac myocytes versus a secondary consequence because of a myocardial infarction or cardiomyopathy due to the toxicity of doxorubicin, irrespective of which our patient suffered a lethal cardiac arrhythmia due to his aneurysm.

A left ventricular aneurysm can cause a variety of complications such as arrythmias, angina pectoris, congestive heart failure, thromboembolism, and rupture. One-third of the patients develop arrhythmias and the arrhythmogenic focus is usually between the normal myocardium and the myocardium of the aneurysm [26]. Our patient suffered ventricular fibrillation which has a very high mortality. Contrast ventriculography is considered as gold standard for the diagnosis of left ventricular aneurysm; 2D echocardiogram also has high specificity and sensitivity [26]. Surgical management is only indicated for ventricular aneurysm associated with intractable ventricular tachyarrhythmias and/or pump failure [27]. In other scenarios, the management is with ICD to prevent VT/VF, medical management with beta blockers or calcium channel blocker along with anticoagulation in the presence of a thrombus [17]. Our patient, did not have intractable ventricular tachyarrhythmia or pump failure requiring emergent surgery. He eventually had an ICD placed and was medically managed as outpatient. Six months after this event, the patient did not have further episodes of arrhythmias and his ejection fraction also improved.

4. Conclusion

Chemotherapy during childhood can cause lethal cardiac complications even after decades of completing the treatment. Periodic monitoring with imaging studies such as 2D echocardiogram should be done in these patients to assess the ventricular function and formation of aneurysm or detect dilated cardiomyopathy so that appropriate preventive measures can be taken to reduced mortality. The need for the same should be stressed with the patients as well as their parents.

Conflict of Interests

The authors declare that there is no conflict of interests regarding the publication of this paper.

References

[1] S. E. Lipshultz, P. Sambatakos, M. Maguire et al., "Cardiotoxicity and cardioprotection in childhood cancer," *Acta Haematologica*, vol. 132, no. 3-4, pp. 391–399, 2014.

[2] M. L. Lindsey, R. A. Lange, H. Parsons, T. Andrews, and G. J. Aune, "The tell-tale heart: molecular and cellular responses to childhood anthracycline exposure," *American Journal of Physiology—Heart and Circulatory Physiology*, vol. 307, no. 10, pp. H1379–H1389, 2014.

[3] M. T. Nolan, R. M. Lowenthal, A. Venn, and T. H. Marwick, "Chemotherapy-related cardiomyopathy: a neglected aspect of cancer survivorship," *Internal Medicine Journal*, vol. 44, no. 10, pp. 939–950, 2014.

[4] B. M. Friedman and M. I. F. A. C. P. Dunn, "Postinfarction ventricular aneurysms," *Clinical Cardiology*, vol. 18, no. 9, pp. 505–511, 1995.

[5] "Childhood cancer," in *SEER Cancer Statistics Review, 1975–2010*, N. Howlader, A. M. Noone, M. Krapcho et al., Eds., section 28, National Cancer Institute, Bethesda, Md, USA, 2013.

[6] ICCC, "Childhood cancer," in *SEER Cancer Statistics Review, 1975–2010*, N. Howlader, A. M. Noone, M. Krapcho et al., Eds., section 29, National Cancer Institute, Bethesda, Md, USA, 2013.

[7] National Cancer Institute, *PDQ Childhood Acute Lymphoblastic Leukemia Treatment*, National Cancer Institute, Bethesda, Md, USA, 2015, http://cancer.gov/cancertopics/pdq/treatment/child-ALL/HealthProfessional.

[8] M. A. Smith, S. F. Altekruse, P. C. Adamson, G. H. Reaman, and N. L. Seibel, "Declining childhood and adolescent cancer mortality," *Cancer*, vol. 120, no. 16, pp. 2497–2506, 2014.

[9] E. T. H. Yeh, A. T. Tong, D. J. Lenihan et al., "Cardiovascular complications of cancer therapy: diagnosis, pathogenesis, and management," *Circulation*, vol. 109, no. 25, pp. 3122–3131, 2004.

[10] M. Volkova and R. Russell, "Anthracycline cardiotoxicity: prevalence, pathogenesis and treatment," *Current Cardiology Reviews*, vol. 7, no. 4, pp. 214–220, 2011.

[11] K. J. A. Davies and J. H. Doroshow, "Redox cycling of anthracyclines by cardiac mitochondria. I. Anthracycline radical formation by NADH dehydrogenase," *The Journal of Biological Chemistry*, vol. 261, no. 7, pp. 3060–3067, 1986.

[12] K. B. Wallace, "Adriamycin-induced interference with cardiac mitochondrial calcium homeostasis," *Cardiovascular Toxicology*, vol. 7, no. 2, pp. 101–107, 2007.

[13] K. Chatterjee, J. Zhang, R. Tao, N. Honbo, and J. S. Karliner, "Vincristine attenuates doxorubicin cardiotoxicity," *Biochemical and Biophysical Research Communications*, vol. 373, no. 4, pp. 555–560, 2008.

[14] A. J. Swerdlow, C. D. Higgins, P. Smith et al., "Myocardial infarction mortality risk after treatment for Hodgkin disease: a collaborative British cohort study," *Journal of the National Cancer Institute*, vol. 99, no. 3, pp. 206–214, 2007.

[15] A. Perez-Verdia, F. Angulo, F. L. Hardwicke, and K. M. Nugent, "Acute cardiac toxicity associated with high-dose intravenous methotrexate therapy: case report and review of the literature," *Pharmacotherapy*, vol. 25, no. 9, pp. 1271–1276, 2005.

[16] J. D. Rutherford, E. Braunwald, and P. E. Cohn, "Chronic ischemic heart disease," in *Heart Disease: A Textbook of Cardiovascular Medicine*, E. Braunwald, Ed., p. 1364, WB Saunders, Philadelphia, Pa, USA, 1988.

[17] M. S. Maron, J. J. Finley, J. M. Bos et al., "Prevalence, clinical significance, and natural history of left ventricular apical aneurysms in hypertrophic cardiomyopathy," *Circulation*, vol. 118, no. 15, pp. 1541–1549, 2008.

[18] M. Takeno, S. Seto, F. Kawahara et al., "Chronic Chagas' heart disease in a Japanease-Brazilian traveler. A case report," *Japanese Heart Journal*, vol. 40, no. 3, pp. 375–382, 1999.

[19] H. Kosuge, M. Noda, T. Kakuta, Y. Kishi, M. Isobe, and F. Numano, "Left ventricular apical aneurysm in cardiac sarcoidosis," *Japanese Heart Journal*, vol. 42, no. 2, pp. 265–269, 2001.

[20] X. Shudong, W. Bifeng, Z. Xiaolian, and H. Xiaosheng, "Left ventricular aneurysm in patients with idiopathic dilated cardiomyopathy: clinical analysis of six cases," *Netherlands Heart Journal*, 2010.

[21] C. A. Visser, G. Kan, R. S. Meltzer, J. J. Koolen, and A. J. Dunning, "Incidence, timing and prognostic value of left ventricular aneurysm formation after myocardial infarction: a prospective, serial echocardiographic study of 158 patients," *The American Journal of Cardiology*, vol. 57, no. 10, pp. 729–732, 1986.

[22] J. Stehlik, R. L. Maholic, and R. Thaman, "Images in cardiovascular medicine. Massive left ventricular aneurysm," *Circulation*, vol. 109, no. 17, pp. e203–e204, 2004.

[23] K. Chatterjee, J. Zhang, N. Honbo, and J. S. Karliner, "Doxorubicin cardiomyopathy," *Cardiology*, vol. 115, no. 2, pp. 155–162, 2010.

[24] S. Kumar, R. Marfatia, S. Tannenbaum, C. Yang, and E. Avelar, "Doxorubicin-induced cardiomyopathy 17 years after chemotherapy," *Texas Heart Institute Journal*, vol. 39, no. 3, pp. 424–427, 2012.

[25] S. L. Gottlieb, W. A. Edmiston Jr., and L. J. Haywood, "Late, late doxorubicin cardiotoxicity," *Chest*, vol. 78, no. 6, pp. 880–882, 1980.

[26] H. A. Ba'albaki and S. D. Clements Jr., "Left ventricular aneurysm: a review," *Clinical Cardiology*, vol. 12, no. 1, pp. 5–13, 1989.

[27] T. J. Ryan, J. L. Anderson, E. M. Antman et al., "ACC/AHA guidelines for the management of patients with acute myocardial infarction: executive summary. A report of the American College of Cardiology/American Heart Association task force on practice guidelines (Committee on Management of Acute Myocardial Infarction)," *Circulation*, vol. 94, no. 9, pp. 2341–2350, 1996.

25

Radiation Therapy-Induced Cardiovascular Disease Treated by a Percutaneous Approach

Luigi Fiocca,[1] Micol Coccato,[1] Vasile Sirbu,[1] Angelina Vassileva,[1]
Giulio Guagliumi,[1] Giuseppe Musumeci,[1] Amedeo Terzi,[1] Gianluca Canu,[1]
Elisa Cerchierini,[2] Diego Cugola,[1] and Orazio Valsecchi[1]

[1]Cardiovascular Department, Papa Giovanni XXIII Hospital, 24127 Bergamo, Italy
[2]Anesthesia and Intensive Care Department, Papa Giovanni XXIII Hospital, 24127 Bergamo, Italy

Correspondence should be addressed to Luigi Fiocca; luigifiocca@gmail.com

Academic Editor: Kenei Shimada

We report the case of a 51-year-old woman, treated with radiotherapy at the age of two years, for a pulmonary sarcoma. Subsequently she developed severe aortic stenosis and bilateral ostial coronary artery disease, symptomatic for dyspnea (NYHA III functional class). Due to the prohibitive surgical risk, she underwent successful stenting in the right coronary artery and left main ostia with drug eluting stents and, afterwards, transcatheter aortic valve replacement with transfemoral implantation of a 23 mm Edwards SAPIEN XT valve. The percutaneous treatment was successful without complications and the patient is in NYHA II functional class at 2 years' follow-up, fully carrying out normal daily activities.

1. Introduction

Cardiovascular diseases in patients who undergo thoracic radiotherapy represent a significant reason for long-term mortality. Vascular disease after radiotherapy usually occurs through an accelerated development of age related atherosclerosis, often involving coronary ostia, resulting in an increased risk of myocardial infarction or sudden cardiac death [1]. Early fibrosis, involving cardiac valves, is common after radiotherapy, with important prognostic consequences [2–4].

Surgery management of these patients is troublesome, due to anatomical sequelae of radiation exposure, with adherence and pulmonary fibrosis that increase the surgical risk.

Percutaneous treatment of coronary and structural disease is nowadays widely applied, representing a valid option for high surgical risk patients.

Transcatheter aortic valve implantation (TAVI) is increasingly popular as an alternative for symptomatic patients affected by severe aortic stenosis that are at high risk for surgery [5–7].

2. Case Report

A 51-year-old woman with pulmonary fibrosarcoma diagnosed at age 2, treated with repeated cycles of radiotherapy, presented with exertional dyspnea.

She had late sequelae of radiotherapy including mediastinal and left pulmonary fibrosis, with severe restrictive lung disease (Figure 1). She underwent a cardiologic evaluation for worsening dyspnea, which revealed a markedly impaired functional capacity (NYHA III functional class). Transthoracic and transesophageal echocardiogram revealed mildly impaired left ventricular function (ejection fraction 45%), severe aortic stenosis (mean gradient 40 mmHg, indexed valve area $0.5 \text{ cm}^2/\text{m}^2$), and moderate aortic and mitral regurgitation. An angio-CT scan showed thickening and calcification of the aortic valve and a porcelain aorta, supporting the diagnosis of radiation-induced cardiovascular disease (Figure 1).

Afterwards, she was admitted to our cardiology department for an invasive evaluation. Coronary angiography showed focal critical ostial left main (LM) stenosis (with

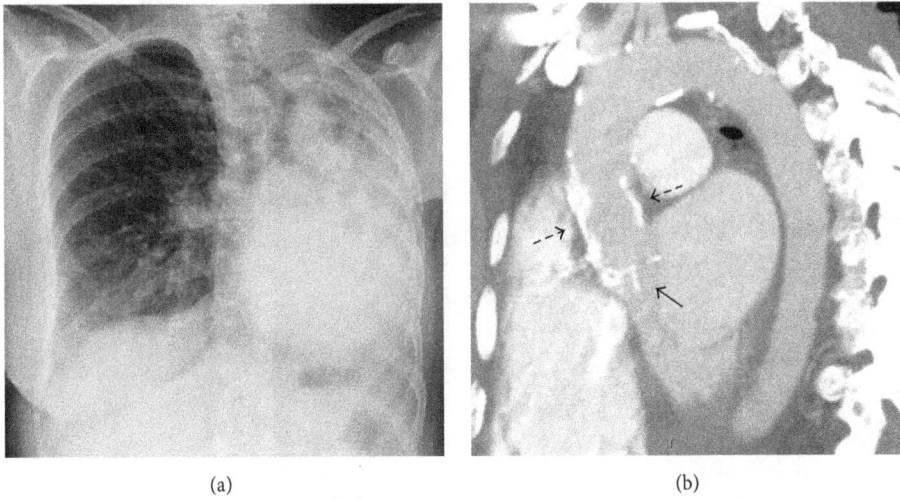

FIGURE 1: (a) Chest X-ray demonstrating left fibrothorax with ipsilateral mediastinum and trachea displacement. (b) CT scan demonstrating thickening and calcification of the aortic valvular leaflets (arrow) and diffuse calcification of the ascending aorta (dashed arrows).

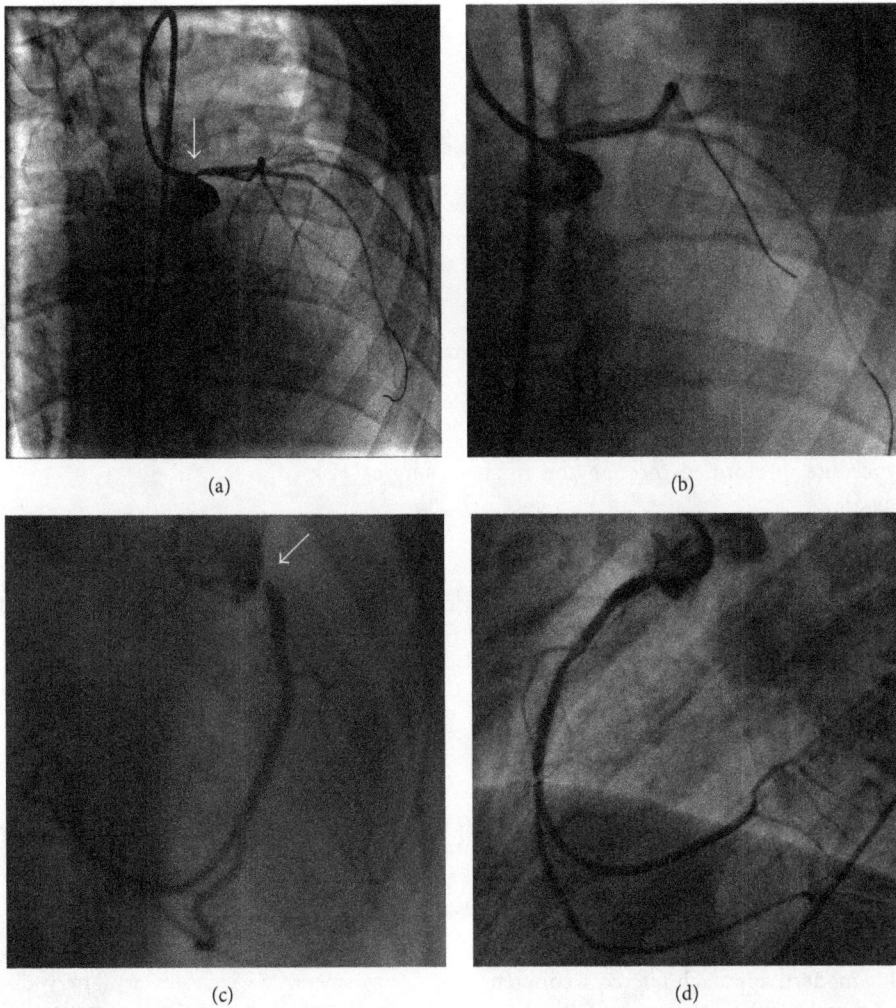

FIGURE 2: (a) Left coronary artery showing critical ostial left main stenosis (arrow). (b) Final result of the left main direct stenting with everolimus eluting stent. (c) Tight ostial lesion of the right coronary artery (RCA; arrow). (d) Final result after direct stenting of ostial RCA with sirolimus eluting stent.

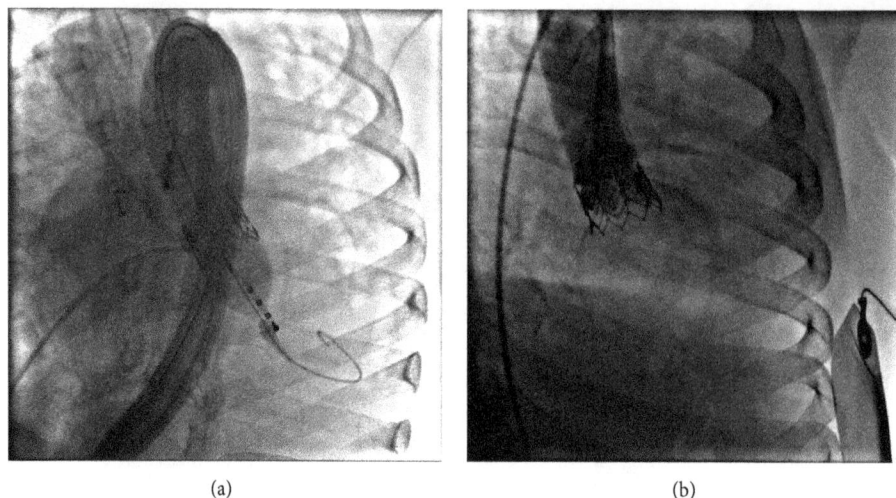

(a)   (b)

FIGURE 3: (a) Transcatheter aortic valve implantation (Edwards SAPIEN XT 23 mm). (b) Aortography after TAVI procedure.

damping pressure) and critical ostial right coronary artery (RCA) disease (Figure 2). Severe, diffuse calcification of the ascending aorta was also present. The cardiac catheterization showed severe aortic valve stenosis (peak-to-peak gradient 70 mmHg) and pulmonary artery hypertension (mean pulmonary artery pressure 35 mmHg, capillary wedge pressure 20 mmHg).

Considering the high surgical risk due to severe restrictive lung disease, severe calcification of the ascending aorta, and postradiation thoracic adherence, the heart team planned a staged percutaneous approach. The patient underwent a successful coronary angioplasty with drug eluting stent implantation on ostial RCA and LM (sirolimus eluting stent 3.0 × 13 mm on RCA, everolimus eluting stent 3,5 × 12 mm on LM, Figure 2). According to angio-CT sizing, a 23 mm Edwards SAPIEN XT valve (Edwards Lifesciences, Irvine, CA) was selected for the procedure. One month later, she underwent TAVI procedure, performed through the right femoral artery (Figure 3).

After the procedure, the echocardiogram showed a markedly decreased transaortic valvular gradient (mean gradient 10 mmHg) with a mild periprosthetic regurgitation, improved left ventricular systolic function, and mild mitral regurgitation. The patient was discharged on aspirin, clopidogrel up to twelve months, ivabradine, and furosemide.

At 24 months' follow-up, she is in NYHA II functional class, fully carrying out normal daily activities. Echocardiogram confirms the good performance of the prosthetic valve and normal left ventricular systolic function.

3. Discussion

This case report describes a fully percutaneous treatment of the cardiovascular consequences of thoracic exposure to radiation therapy. This modern approach offered a concrete chance to this young woman, who otherwise should have undergone a very high risk surgical intervention.

The risk of long-term radiotherapy damage depends on the radiation dose and the field of exposure [8]. The pathogenesis of radiation-induced coronary artery disease (CAD)

is complex and not yet fully understood; radiation exposure may act as an independent risk factor of arteriosclerosis. Radiation-induced valvular disease is uncommon [8]; valve lesions are diagnosed on average 11.5 years after radiation exposure and symptoms occur at least 5 years later [9].

The pathophysiology of radiation-induced valvular disease is not completely clarified: cellular injury, combined with pressure-related trauma, may cause valvular fibrosis and calcification [10, 11]: irradiation seems to trigger a degenerative process that lasts for years.

Most radiation effects are dose related and it is probable that modern techniques with lower radiation exposure and smaller treatment volumes may reduce these risks.

TAVI is a highly effective procedure for selected patients who are at high surgical risk. The lack of long-term outcomes limits the use of TAVI to the elderly. In this case, the young age represented a concern, overweighted by the prohibitive surgical risk.

Conflict of Interests

No conflict of interests relevant to this paper was reported by any of the authors.

Acknowledgment

The authors are grateful to Dr. Giorgio Fasolini, Radiologist at the Department of Diagnostic Imaging of Papa Giovanni XXIII Hospital, Bergamo, for his valuable contribution.

References

[1] F. Orzan, A. Brusca, M. R. Conte, P. Presbitero, and M. C. Figliomeni, "Severe coronary artery disease after radiation therapy of the chest and mediastinum: clinical presentation and treatment," *British Heart Journal*, vol. 69, no. 6, pp. 496–500, 1993.

[2] F. A. Stewart, I. Seemann, S. Hoving, and N. S. Russell, "Understanding radiation-induced cardiovascular damage and

strategies for intervention," *Clinical Oncology*, vol. 25, no. 10, pp. 617–624, 2013.

[3] S. L. Galper, J. B. Yu, P. M. Mauch et al., "Clinically significant cardiac disease in patients with Hodgkin lymphoma treated with mediastinal irradiation," *Blood*, vol. 117, no. 2, pp. 412–418, 2011.

[4] R. A. Aqel and G. J. Zoghbi, "Radiation therapy-related cardiovascular disease," *Journal of Heart and Lung Transplantation*, vol. 25, no. 2, pp. 257–258, 2006.

[5] M. Thomas, G. Schymik, T. Walther et al., "Thirty-day results of the SAPIEN aortic bioprosthesis European outcome (SOURCE) registry: a European registry of transcatheter aortic valve implantation using the edwards SAPIEN valve," *Circulation*, vol. 122, no. 1, pp. 62–69, 2010.

[6] R. R. Makkar, G. P. Fontana, H. Jilaihawi et al., "Transcatheter aortic-valve replacement for inoperable severe aortic stenosis," *The New England Journal of Medicine*, vol. 366, pp. 1696–1704, 2012.

[7] S. R. Kapadia, E. M. Tuzcu, R. R. Makkar et al., "Long-term outcomes of inoperable patients with aortic stenosis randomly assigned to transcatheter aortic valve replacement or standard therapy," *Circulation*, vol. 130, pp. 1483–1492, 2014.

[8] M. C. Hull, C. G. Morris, C. J. Pepine, and N. P. Mendenhall, "Valvular dysfunction and carotid, subclavian, and coronary artery disease in survivors of Hodgkin lymphoma treated with radiation therapy," *Journal of the American Medical Association*, vol. 290, no. 21, pp. 2831–2837, 2003.

[9] R. G. Carlson, W. R. Mayfield, S. Normann, and J. A. Alexander, "Radiation-associated valvular disease," *Chest*, vol. 99, pp. 538–545, 1991.

[10] M. D. Brand, C. A. Abadi, G. P. Aurigemma, H. L. Dauerman, and T. E. Meyer, "Radiation-associated valvular heart disease in Hodgkin's disease is associated with characteristic thickening and fibrosis of the aortic-mitral curtain," *Journal of Heart Valve Disease*, vol. 10, no. 5, pp. 681–685, 2001.

[11] N. M. Katz, A. W. Hall, and M. D. Cerqueira, "Radiation induced valvulitis with late leaflet rupture," *Heart*, vol. 86, no. 6, article e20, 2001.

26

Biventricular Noncompaction Cardiomyopathy in an Adult with Unique Facial Dysmorphisms: Case Report and Brief Review

Gaurav Rao[1] and James Tauras[2]

[1]*Division of Internal Medicine, Montefiore Medical Center, Albert Einstein College of Medicine, Bronx, NY 10467, USA*
[2]*Division of Cardiology, Weiler Hospital, Albert Einstein College of Medicine, Bronx, NY 10461, USA*

Correspondence should be addressed to Gaurav Rao; grao@montefiore.org

Academic Editor: Jesus Peteiro

Left ventricular noncompaction (LVNC) is a rare cardiomyopathy that is believed it to arise from an arrest in embryonic endomyocardial development. More recent studies suggest that it can be acquired later on in life sporadically. It may be accompanied by life-threatening complications, which are most commonly heart failure, arrhythmias, and thromboembolic events. We report a case of biventricular noncompaction cardiomyopathy in a 36-year-old man presenting for the first time with clinical heart failure as well as atrial arrhythmia. Transthoracic echocardiography (TTE) revealed LVNC with depressed ejection fraction (EF). Cardiac magnetic resonance imaging (MRI) further revealed a left atrial appendage thrombus as well as right ventricular noncompaction involvement. His physical exam was unique for a characteristic facial dysmorphisms pattern and developmental delays reminiscent of the earliest descriptions of LVNC in the pediatric population and it was rarely described in adult patients. This unique presentation underscores the importance of a better understanding of the genetics and natural course of LVNC. This will help us to elucidate the uncertainty surrounding its clinical management, discussed in a brief review of the literature following the case.

1. Introduction

Left ventricular noncompaction (LVNC) is a rare cardiomyopathy that is thought to arise during embryogenesis secondary to arrested myocardial development. This results in a thickened myocardium bilayer comprised of noncompacted myocardium, characterized by prominent deep intertrabecular recesses [1] and a thin compacted layer of myocardium [2]. Its etiology is genetic or sporadic. The most common clinical manifestations are heart failure, ventricular arrhythmias, and thromboembolic events [3]. As a younger cardiomyopathy, its natural history is still being understood with optimal management yet to be determined. We present a unique case of biventricular noncompaction and its complications in an adult with unique facial dysmorphisms resulting in multiple management implications.

2. Case Presentation

A 36-year-old man with a three-month history of intermittent lower leg extremity edema managed with furosemide by his primary care doctor presented with worsening lower leg edema, dyspnea on exertion with decreased exercise tolerance. He had no other significant medical history apart from history of cognitive, speech, and hearing impairment since an early age. He was a nonsmoker with occasional alcohol use and no recent foreign travel. There was no family history of cardiomyopathy.

In the emergency department, electrocardiogram revealed atrial flutter with 2:1 conduction with a heart rate upwards of 130 beats per minute. Physical exam was significant for facial dysmorphisms with a prominent forehead, micrognathia, high arching palate, and low set

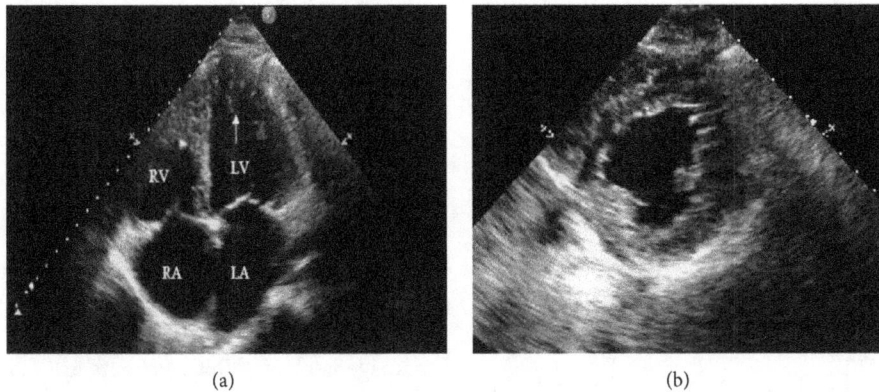

(a)   (b)

FIGURE 1: Echocardiogram of the heart. (a) Apical four-chamber view of the heart with marked trabeculations of the apex (white arrow). (b) Parasternal short axis view at the level of the papillary muscles with prominent LV inferolateral trabeculations. RA: right atrium, LA: left atrium, RV: right ventricle, and LV: left ventricle.

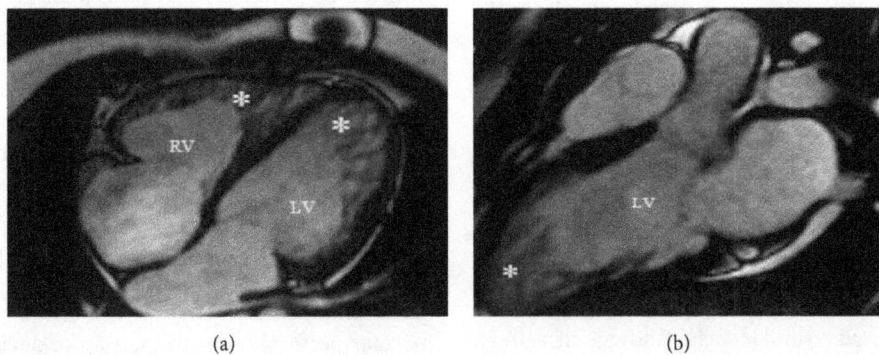

(a)   (b)

FIGURE 2: Cardiac MRI of the heart. (a) Cardiac MRI showing extensive biventricular trabeculations with (b) sagittal view demonstrating deep recesses in the left ventricle cavity (see asterisk).

ears. His jugular venous pressure (JVP) was elevated with systolic ejection murmur 3/6 heard best at apex along with bibasilar crackles on lung auscultation. Lower extremity exam was significant for pitting edema to the knees.

Laboratory data was significant for newly elevated creatinine of 1.8 mg/dL and pro-BNP of 10,500 pg/mL. The rest of laboratory tests were normal. X-ray showed cardiomegaly and vascular congestion. Transthoracic echocardiography (TTE) revealed biatrial dilatation, severe biventricular failure with LV ejection fraction (EF) of 15%, and prominent trabeculations in the left ventricle (Figure 1). Cardiac magnetic resonance imaging (MRI) showed similar findings, but it also demonstrated biventricular, extensive myocardial trabeculations compatible with noncompaction cardiomyopathy (Figure 2).

He was begun on nitroglycerin and furosemide with pulmonary artery catheter placement and transferred to the cardiac care unit. Escalating doses of metoprolol were used for rate control. Heparin infusion was also initiated for atrial fibrillation stroke risk. Transesophageal echocardiography (TEE) was done prior to a planned cardioversion the following day, which showed a left atrial appendage thrombus.

Over the following week, our patient was aggressively diuresed and intravenous diuretics were down titrated prior to transferring out of the unit. He was commenced on beta-blocker, ACE inhibitor, and long-term anticoagulation for his thrombus. He spontaneously converted to sinus rhythm. Given the improvement in patient's EF to 41% on subsequent imaging, ICD (implantable cardioverter defibrillator) evaluation would be readdressed in 3–6 months after goal directed medical therapy. Genetic testing discussions were deferred to outpatient followup as well.

3. Discussion

The American Heart Association defines LVNC as a genetic cardiomyopathy [1] while the European Society of Cardiology classifies it as an unclassified cardiomyopathy [4]. This cardiomyopathy may be genetic or sporadically acquired; however, there are still ongoing studies further exploring this.

In the genetic form, LVNC can be an isolated trait or associated with genetic diseases and other congenital defects. Increased risk in family members of affected individuals has been noted from initial studies [5] and genes responsible for some familial cases have been described. Mutations in the *G4.5* gene on the Xq28 chromosome result in a wide range of X-linked cardiomyopathies in the pediatric population such as Barth syndrome and LVNC [6–8]. However, this mutation was not found in the adult population, where autosomal dominance mode of transmission was more common [7–9]. This suggests that presentation of LVNC in adulthood is genetically distinct from pediatric cases. LVNC can be linked to mutations in genes that code for signaling pathway regulators [10], cytoskeletal [11], nuclear membrane, and mitochondrial proteins [12]. Genetic overlap between LVNC and other cardiomyopathies including dilated and hypertrophic cardiomyopathy has been reported as well [7]. These mutations result in a failure of myocytes to compact, resulting in a spongiform appearance with the persistence of deep intertrabecular recesses.

Sporadic forms of LVNC can be acquired later in life. There is emerging data to suggest that increased LV trabeculation fulfilling the criteria for LVNC can be brought on in the setting of increased left ventricular mechanical loading. This can be seen in highly trained athletes [13], pregnancy [14], and sickle cell anemia [15]. Due to limitations in genetic testing, it is unclear if there is a genetic predisposition to the disease in these cases with modifying genes that are able to influence the LVNC phenotype [16]. However, given the common genetic overlap between dilated and hypertrophic cardiomyopathies, which morphologically develop later in life, the hypothesis that this may occur similarly in LVNC should be considered [17].

As noted in our patient, an association between similar facial dysmorphisms of a prominent forehead, low set ears, micrognathia, and high-arching palate and LVNC was first described by Chin et al. [5] in 1990 in a pediatric population. Ichida et al. also describe similar facial findings in a third of the pediatric study population [18]. These patients also had developmental delays as in our patient. Given the strong genetic association in the pediatric population, a link between facial dysmorphisms and development delays in association with LVNC suggests a genetic syndrome, although the chromosome responsible has not been identified.

No associated facial dysmorphisms were seen in two large adult populations with LVNC [2, 3], which can be expected given the studies suggesting that LVNC presenting in adults is genetically distinct from the pediatric population, as described earlier. Our patient's presentation of LVNC in adulthood with associated facial dysmorphisms is unique and rare, suggesting an overlap between the pediatric and adult genetic spectra of LVNC. A possible variable penetrance of the gene mutation or a delayed genetic susceptibility to mechanical loading may also explain this observation, allowing our patient to remain asymptomatic until adulthood.

Our patient was diagnosed initially on echocardiography, which is the first diagnostic tool for LVNC. Several diagnostic criteria have been applied, but the most commonly used one remains a noncompacted/compacted ratio of >2.0 in end-systole [19], although there is no gold standard. Another modality for diagnosis is cardiac magnetic resonance imaging (CMR), which as per the criteria in Petersen et al. [20] uses a ratio of >2.3 in diastole to accurately distinguish nonpathological from pathological noncompaction.

Although left ventricle involvement is much more common, particularly apical, anterior, and inferolateral segments [2, 5], right ventricular (RV) noncompaction has been reported more so in cases where CMR was used in addition to echocardiography for diagnosis [21]. As in our patient, who did not have RV trabeculations on initial echocardiography, the potential role of CMR over echocardiography in evaluation of the RV noncompaction has been suggested before [22] given its enhanced 3-dimensional assessment. Thus, the prevalence of RV involvement may have been underestimated in the past. CMR aids in the diagnosis of biventricular involvement in LVNC although its implications on management are unclear.

There are no specific guidelines or treatment for the management of LVNC. Patients are managed according to their specific clinical need and corresponding guideline. Our patient had all the common clinical complications of LVNC. He presented with heart failure, which is the most common reason for presentation in adults [2, 3]. He was started on an ACE inhibitor and a beta-blocker. His atrial fibrillation, which is common in LVNC, was managed with a rate control strategy prior to spontaneous conversion and he was placed on long-term anticoagulation for his atrial thrombus. The role of anticoagulation is unclear in patients with LVNC and normal LV function. Expert recommendations for primary prophylaxis exist in the setting of arrhythmias, systolic dysfunction [23], or proven atrial or ventricular thrombi as in our patient.

The benefit of ICD placement in this population is unknown as well. The deep recesses of the heart may predispose patients with LVNC to complications, such as ventricular perforation in the setting of device placement. One single study suggests that it is an effective therapy in LVNC for primary and secondary prevention of life-threatening arrhythmias [24]. More studies are needed to determine the safety and efficacy of ICD use in this population. It was considered in our patient but, given his conversion to sinus rhythm without ventricular arrhythmic episodes as well as improvement in EF on subsequent imaging, we felt that a trial of goal directed medical treatment was warranted first. Expert opinions suggest echocardiographic screening of family members as well as genetic testing.

In conclusion, LVNC has a genetic origin that can be found in isolated form or in association with other cardiomyopathies. It can also be acquired later on in life in response to a mechanical stress, perhaps in patients who are genetically predisposed. A better understanding of its genetics and the novel gene mutations implicated may further delineate the natural course of this disease. This will help guide its diagnosis as well as its management. A consensus imaging diagnostic criteria for LVNC are necessary in the context of clinical specifications, given its prevalence in asymptomatic patients [25]. More studies are necessary to determine its optimal management.

Consent

Written informed consent was obtained from the patient for the publication of this case report and its accompanying images.

Conflict of Interests

The authors declare that they have no competing interests.

Authors' Contribution

Gaurav Rao conceived the study, acquired the data, reviewed the literature, and drafted the preliminary and final paper. James Tauras, the attending cardiologist on the heart failure consult service, reviewed the echocardiogram as well as the cardiac magnetic resonance imaging and was intellectually involved in the proofreading and revision of the paper.

References

[1] B. J. Maron, J. A. Towbin, G. Thiene et al., "Contemporary definitions and classification of the cardiomyopathies: an American Heart Association Scientific Statement from the Council on Clinical Cardiology, Heart Failure and Transplantation Committee; Quality of Care and Outcomes Research and Functional Genomics and Translational Biology Interdisciplinary Working Groups; and Council on Epidemiology and Prevention," *Circulation*, vol. 113, no. 14, pp. 1807–1816, 2006.

[2] M. Ritter, E. Oechslin, G. Sütsch, C. Attenhofer, J. Schneider, and R. Jenni, "Isolated noncompaction of the myocardium in adults," *Mayo Clinic Proceedings*, vol. 72, no. 1, pp. 26–31, 1997.

[3] E. N. Oechslin, C. H. Attenhofer Jost, J. R. Rojas, P. A. Kaufmann, and R. Jenni, "Long-term follow-up of 34 adults with isolated left ventricular noncompaction: a distinct cardiomyopathy with poor prognosis," *Journal of the American College of Cardiology*, vol. 36, no. 2, pp. 493–500, 2000.

[4] P. Elliott, B. Andersson, E. Arbustini et al., "Classification of the cardiomyopathies: a position statement from the european society of cardiology working group on myocardial and pericardial diseases," *European Heart Journal*, vol. 29, no. 2, pp. 270–276, 2008.

[5] T. K. Chin, J. K. Perloff, R. G. Williams, K. Jue, and R. Mohrmann, "Isolated noncompaction of left ventricular myocardium: a study of eight cases," *Circulation*, vol. 82, no. 2, pp. 507–513, 1990.

[6] S. B. Bleyl, B. R. Mumford, M.-C. Brown-Harrison et al., "Xq28-linked noncompaction of the left ventricular myocardium: prenatal diagnosis and pathologic analysis of affected individuals," *The American Journal of Medical Genetics*, vol. 72, no. 3, pp. 257–265, 1997.

[7] F. Ichida, S. Tsubata, K. R. Bowles et al., "Novel gene mutations in patients with left ventricular noncompaction or Barth syndrome," *Circulation*, vol. 103, no. 9, pp. 1256–1263, 2001.

[8] S. B. Bleyl, B. R. Mumford, V. Thompson et al., "Neonatal, lethal noncompaction of the left ventricular myocardium is allelic with Barth syndrome," *American Journal of Human Genetics*, vol. 61, no. 4, pp. 868–872, 1997.

[9] S. Sasse-Klaassen, B. Gerull, E. Oechslin, R. Jenni, and L. Thierfelder, "Isolated noncompaction of the left ventricular myocardium in the adult is an autosomal dominant disorder in the majority of patients," *The American Journal of Medical Genetics*, vol. 119, no. 2, pp. 162–167, 2003.

[10] G. Luxán, J. C. Casanova, B. Martínez-Poveda et al., "Mutations in the NOTCH pathway regulator MIB1 cause left ventricular noncompaction cardiomyopathy," *Nature Medicine*, vol. 19, no. 2, pp. 193–201, 2013.

[11] S. Klaassen, S. Probst, E. Oechslin et al., "Mutations in sarcomere protein genes in left ventricular noncompaction," *Circulation*, vol. 117, no. 22, pp. 2893–2901, 2008.

[12] M. Hermida-Prieto, L. Monserrat, A. Castro-Beiras et al., "Familial dilated cardiomyopathy and isolated left ventricular noncompaction associated with lamin A/C gene mutations," *The American Journal of Cardiology*, vol. 94, no. 1, pp. 50–54, 2004.

[13] S. Gati, N. Chandra, R. L. Bennett et al., "Increased left ventricular trabeculation in highly trained athletes: do we need more stringent criteria for the diagnosis of left ventricular noncompaction in athletes?" *Heart*, vol. 99, no. 6, pp. 401–408, 2013.

[14] S. Gati, M. Papadakis, N. D. Papamichael et al., "Reversible de novo left ventricular trabeculations in pregnant women: implications for the diagnosis of left ventricular noncompaction in low-risk populations," *Circulation*, vol. 130, no. 6, pp. 475–483, 2014.

[15] S. Gati, M. Papadakis, N. Van Niekerk, M. Reed, T. Yeghen, and S. Sharma, "Increased left ventricular trabeculation in individuals with sickle cell anaemia: physiology or pathology?" *International Journal of Cardiology*, vol. 168, no. 2, pp. 1658–1660, 2013.

[16] E. Arbustini, F. Weidemann, and J. L. Hall, "Left ventricular noncompaction: a distinct cardiomyopathy or a trait shared by different cardiac diseases?" *Journal of the American College of Cardiology*, vol. 64, no. 17, pp. 1840–1850, 2014.

[17] E. Oechslin and R. Jenni, "Left ventricular non-compaction revisited: a distinct phenotype with genetic heterogeneity?" *European Heart Journal*, vol. 32, no. 12, pp. 1446–1456, 2011.

[18] F. Ichida, Y. Hamamichi, T. Miyawaki et al., "Clinical features of isolated noncompaction of the ventricular myocardium: long-term clinical course, hemodynamic properties, and genetic background," *Journal of the American College of Cardiology*, vol. 34, no. 1, pp. 233–240, 1999.

[19] R. Jenni, E. Oechslin, J. Schneider, C. Attenhofer Jost, and P. A. Kaufmann, "Echocardiographic and pathoanatomical characteristics of isolated left ventricular non-compaction: a step towards classification as a distinct cardiomyopathy," *Heart*, vol. 86, no. 6, pp. 666–671, 2001.

[20] S. E. Petersen, J. B. Selvanayagam, F. Wiesmann et al., "Left ventricular non-compaction: insights from cardiovascular magnetic resonance imaging," *Journal of the American College of Cardiology*, vol. 46, no. 1, pp. 101–105, 2005.

[21] Y. Sato, N. Matsumoto, S. Matsuo et al., "Right ventricular involvement in a patient with isolated noncompaction of the ventricular myocardium," *Cardiovascular Revascularization Medicine*, vol. 8, no. 4, pp. 275–277, 2007.

[22] L. J. J. Borreguero, R. Corti, R. F. de Soria, J. I. Osende, V. Fuster, and J. J. Badimon, "Images in cardiovascular medicine. Diagnosis of isolated noncompaction of the myocardium by magnetic resonance imaging," *Circulation*, vol. 105, no. 21, pp. E177–E178, 2002.

[23] C. Stöllberger, G. Blazek, C. Dobias, A. Hanafin, C. Wegner, and J. Finsterer, "Frequency of stroke and embolism in left ventricular hypertrabeculation/noncompaction," *The American Journal of Cardiology*, vol. 108, no. 7, pp. 1021–1023, 2011.

[24] R. Kobza, R. Jenni, P. Erne, E. Oechslin, and F. Duru, "Implantable cardioverter-defibrillators in patients with left ventricular noncompaction," *Pacing and Clinical Electrophysiology*, vol. 31, no. 4, pp. 461–467, 2008.

[25] F. Zemrak, M. A. Ahlman, G. Captur et al., "The relationship of left ventricular trabeculation to ventricular function and structure over a 9.5-year follow-up: the MESA study," *Journal of the American College of Cardiology*, vol. 64, no. 19, pp. 1971–1980, 2014.

27

Respiratory Failure in an Adolescent with Primary Cardiac Sarcoma

Daniel Angeli[1] and Stephen J. Angeli[2]

[1]Department of Medicine, Montefiore Medical Center, Bronx, NY, USA
[2]Holy Name Medical Center, USA

Correspondence should be addressed to Stephen J. Angeli; essay105@yahoo.com

Academic Editor: Yoshiro Naito

We report a case of progressive respiratory failure secondary to primary cardiac sarcoma masquerading as primary lung disease. An 18-year-old female presented to our hospital emergency department with progressive cough, dyspnea, and hemoptysis. She was treated for primary lung infection without improvement and had respiratory failure with endotracheal intubation by the third hospital day. An "intermediate" plasma brain natriuretic protein (BNP) of 216 pg/mL did not raise concerns about a heart failure diagnosis and may have delayed the correct diagnosis. Computed tomography of the chest with intravenous contrast was performed on the fifth hospital day and revealed a cardiac mass. A transthoracic echocardiogram confirmed a large left atrial mass that was obstructing mitral inflow. She was transferred to a tertiary center for emergency cardiac surgery. Primary cardiac tumors are a rare and treatable cause of heart failure in adolescent and young adult patients. Presentation can be confused with primary lung disease and must be suspected early. Plasma BNP cutoff levels used in the adult population should not be extrapolated to adolescents, as levels, both normal and abnormal, are significantly lower in this group of patients.

1. Introduction

An 18-year-old female with no previous medical history presented to the emergency department with a two-week history of increasing cough, fatigue, dyspnea, and hemoptysis. There was no fever. There was no recent travel. On examination, she was afebrile with respiratory rate of 20 breaths/min. and a pulse rate of 125 beats/min. Blood pressure was 104/68 mm Hg. Auscultation of her chest revealed a few scattered rales and no cardiac murmur, but a third heart sound was heard. Laboratory studies showed a white blood count of 11.0/μL, neutrophils of 8.7/μL (80%), and hemoglobin of 15.9 gm/dL. Oxygen saturation while breathing room air was 93%. Sputum and blood cultures were normal. Her plasma brain natriuretic protein (BNP) was 216 pg/mL and procalcitonin was <0.1 ng/mL. Chest X-ray revealed diffuse bilateral infiltrates.

Initial treatment consisted of oral azithromycin and intravenous ceftriaxone for presumed community acquired pneumonia. She failed to improve and on the second hospital day intravenous vancomycin was added to her regimen. A chest X-ray showed worsening bilateral pulmonary infiltrates and enlarging bilateral pleural effusions. By the third hospital day, her condition deteriorated further and respiratory distress resulted in endotracheal intubation and mechanical respiratory assistance. She was placed in the intensive care unit. Given the failure to improve with an antibiotic regimen, and the low procalcitonin level, the diagnosis of hypersensitivity pneumonitis was considered. Intravenous methylprednisolone was added to her regimen.

Computed tomography (CT) of the chest with intravenous contrast was performed on the fifth hospital day and it revealed "(1) bilateral pleural effusions, areas of air space consolidation involving upper and lower lobes. This is concerning for multifocal pneumonia. There is also vascular congestion. (2) Low density in the left atrium and left ventricle is nonspecific, possibly due to respiratory motion degradation. Cardiac lesions cannot be excluded. Cardiac echo is suggested" (Figures 1 and 2).

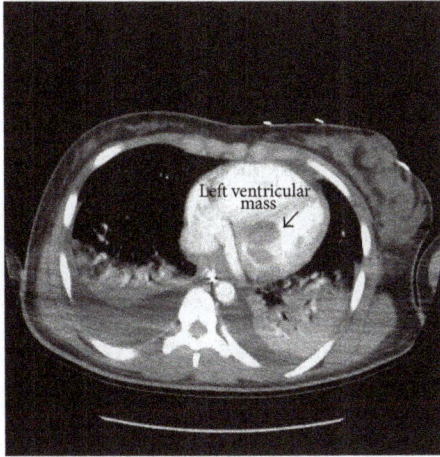

FIGURE 1: CT of the chest following intravenous contrast showing part of the mass extending into the left ventricular.

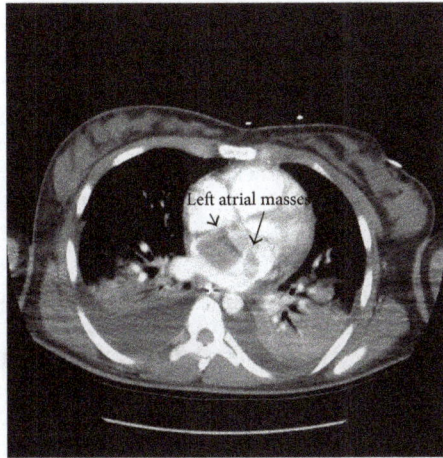

FIGURE 2: CT of the chest following intravenous contrast showing left atrial mass.

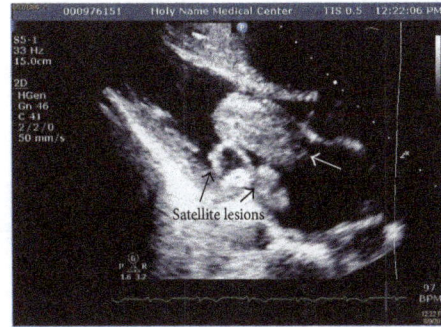

FIGURE 3: Transthoracic echocardiogram showing left atrial mass with satellite lesions and thickening of the posterior mitral leaflet.

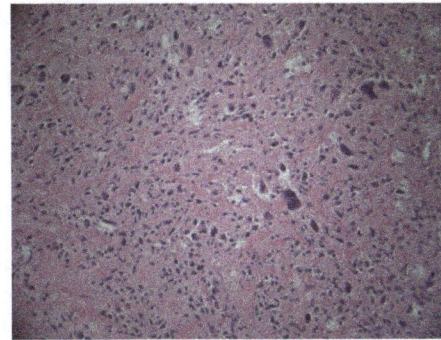

FIGURE 4: Malignant spindle cell proliferation with some very large tumor cells and areas of focal necrosis.

A bedside transthoracic echocardiogram showed a large, mobile, lobulated left atrial mass with attachment to the atrial septum. The largest component of the mass measured 5.1 × 2.9 cm and prolapsed through the mitral orifice in diastole obstructing flow. Smaller satellite lesions were present and there was thickening of the posterior mitral leaflet. Left ventricular systolic function was normal. The right heart was enlarged, and the estimated right ventricular systolic pressure was estimated at 59 mm Hg (Figure 3).

The patient was referred for emergency cardiac surgery. At operation, she was found to have a large lobulated mass within the left atrium. It was attached to the septum but appeared to be growing along the free wall of the LA towards the mitral valve annulus. The valve was distorted due to the mass with thickening of the posterior leaflet. Excision of the mass and replacement of the mitral valve with a tissue prosthesis were performed. Separate lesions within the left atrium adherent to the endocardium were also sent for pathology study. Surgical pathology revealed high-grade cardiac sarcoma (malignant fibrous histiocytoma with foci of myxoid malignant fibrous histiocytoma and foci of necrosis. The tumor invades into the atrial myocardium and involves the lateral margins of the atrial tissue present in the specimen) (Figures 4 and 5).

Her postoperative course was generally satisfactory. She has since been treated with chemotherapy.

2. Discussion

This is the case of a critically ill 18-year-old female who was diagnosed with a malignant sarcoma arising in the left atrium. She rapidly deteriorated over several days with life-threatening respiratory failure and presented a clinical puzzle to the clinicians involved in her care. Fortunately, the correct diagnosis was finally made and the patient was promptly treated. Our patient was admitted to the adult medicine service. In addition to a discussion on the features of this rare and dangerous condition, we will also discuss how adolescents and children can differ from adults in certain key measures and how an appreciation of this may have led to an earlier diagnosis.

Primary tumors of the heart are extremely rare. Based upon the data of 22 large autopsy series, the frequency of primary cardiac tumors is approximately 0.02%, corresponding to 200 tumors in 1 million autopsies. Metastatic tumors to

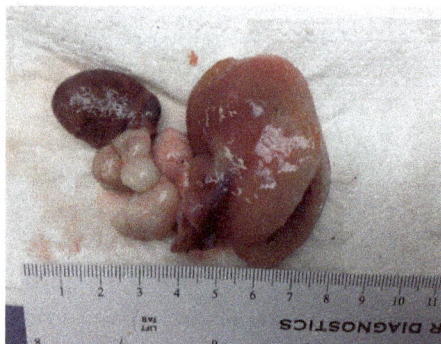

FIGURE 5: Large, multilobular mass.

the heart are far more common [1]. In adults, myxomas are the most common benign tumors and in children, rhabdomyomas and fibromas are the most common. Of primary cardiac tumors, malignant tumors constitute only 17% [2].

Cardiac tumors may produce symptoms based on their location in the heart and whether they interfere with normal cardiac function. Some cardiac tumors are found incidentally. Left atrial and left ventricular tumors can present with systemic complaints of fever, chills, and fatigue, as well as symptoms specific to the hemodynamic effects of mitral obstruction, as was the case with our patient. Other potential presenting findings may be systemic embolization, arrhythmias, chest pain, syncope, and presyncope [3].

Our patient presented with respiratory symptoms that were initially treated as community acquired pneumonia and then, when she failed to improve, as a case of environmentally mediated hypersensitivity pneumonitis. Severe pulmonary edema secondary to the presence of an obstructing left heart mass with interference of normal mitral function was later documented. The observed brain natriuretic peptide (BNP) level of 216 pg/mL is an "indeterminate" level for the adult population in which this biomarker was first studied. The young age of our patient very likely affected the magnitude of the BNP level and deserves closer examination.

BNP is a 32-amino-acid polypeptide secreted by the ventricles of the heart in response to excessive stretching of myocardial cells. BNP has been studied extensively and is now in widespread clinical use as an aid in the diagnosis of patients with dyspnea. In the adult population, dyspneic patients with heart failure have BNP values of >400 pg/mL. Values <100 pg/mL have a good negative predictive value and heart failure can be excluded. Values between 100 and 400 pg/mL are considered "gray zone" elevation and can be seen in a variety of clinical settings, and clinical judgment is generally recommended [4].

Plasma BNP levels have been shown to have wide individual variability. Such factors as age, sex, renal function, and type of heart failure can affect levels. Normal BNP is known to increase with increasing age [5]. In a multicenter study of 161 children and adolescents with symptomatic systolic heart failure (class II–IV), studying the effects of high versus low dose carvedilol, the median initial plasma BNP across all groups was 110 pg/mL [6]. In another study of 163 children

and adolescents with moderately symptomatic class II and III heart failure, the median BNP was 110 pg/mL, compared with 20 to 40 pg/mL reported in normal children. A BNP level ≥140 pg/mL in this cohort was predictive of adverse outcomes [7]. It is therefore not advisable to extrapolate the BNP cutoff values obtained in the adult population to children and adolescents. Seen in this light, it is possible that the observed BNP in this case may have raised the possibility of heart failure earlier in her course.

Depending on the location and type of tumor, surgery may or may not be necessary. Because of the risk of embolization or hemodynamic compromise, left side lesions, such as myxomas, should undergo resection. In the case of malignant cardiac tumors, surgical excision in combination with systemic chemotherapy remains the best available treatment [8].

To make the diagnosis, imaging studies are essential and will be presented briefly. Certain features of the mass are more suggestive of malignancy. These include broad-based mass, invasion of surrounding tissue, mass presence in more than a single chamber, poor definition of mass border, tissue inhomogeneity, large size >5 cm, and presence of either pericardial or pleural effusion [9].

Two-dimensional echocardiography is often the initial diagnostic modality of choice. It is readily available and has very good sensitivity of 93%. Transesophageal echocardiography is also excellent with a sensitivity of 97% [10]. In addition to morphology, echocardiography provides hemodynamic information on regurgitation and stenosis as well as estimation of right ventricular pressure. Limitations to echocardiography include limited field of view and modest ability to differentiate tumor types and interference from lung and other noncardiac tissue. Tissue characterization can be enhanced by the use of echocardiographic contrast perfusion imaging. Such modality would better differentiate the neovascularization of malignancies from the avascularity of thrombi and the sparse vascularity of stromal tumors, such as myxomas [11]. Cardiac magnetic resonance (CMR) has become the imaging modality of choice in its ability to provide high spatial resolution, wide view of the heart and surrounding structures and give accurate tissue characterization. While CMR criteria for distinguishing benign from malignant tumors are highly accurate, histologic diagnosis still remains the "gold standard." Computed tomography (CT) with electrocardiographic gating is another tool that can provide important structural information in the assessment of cardiac masses [12].

3. Conclusion

Cardiac tumors are a rare and treatable cause of heart failure in adolescent and young adult patients. Only timely diagnosis and treatment will give the patient the best chance at survival. The presentation may be confused with primary pulmonary disease and must be suspected early. An array of cardiac imaging studies, each with their respective strengths, can be used to establish the diagnosis. Caution must be employed when interpreting plasma BNP levels, taking into account the significantly lower levels seen in young patients.

Conflict of Interests

The authors declare that there is no conflict of interests regarding the publication of this paper.

References

[1] K. Reynen, "Frequency of primary tumors of the heart," *The American Journal of Cardiology*, vol. 77, no. 1, article 107, 1996.

[2] J. E. Molina, J. E. Edwards, and H. B. Ward, "Primary cardiac tumors: experience at the University of Minnesota," *Thoracic and Cardiovascular Surgeon*, vol. 38, supplement 2, pp. 183–191, 1990.

[3] R. S. Beroukhim, A. Prakash, E. R. Valsangiacomo Buechel et al., "Characterization of cardiac tumors in children by cardiovascular magnetic resonance imaging: a multicenter experience," *Journal of the American College of Cardiology*, vol. 58, no. 10, pp. 1044–1054, 2011.

[4] A. Maisel, "B-type natriuretic peptide measurements in diagnosing congestive heart failure in the dyspneic emergency department patient," *Reviews in Cardiovascular Medicine*, vol. 3, supplement 4, pp. S10–S17, 2002.

[5] M. M. Redfield, R. J. Rodeheffer, S. J. Jacobsen, D. W. Mahoney, K. R. Bailey, and J. C. Burnett Jr., "Plasma brain natriuretic peptide concentration: impact of age and gender," *Journal of the American College of Cardiology*, vol. 40, no. 5, pp. 976–982, 2002.

[6] R. E. Shaddy, M. M. Boucek, D. T. Hsu et al., "Carvedilol for children and adolescents with heart failure: a randomized controlled trial," *The Journal of the American Medical Association*, vol. 298, no. 10, pp. 1171–1179, 2007.

[7] S. R. Auerbach, M. E. Richmond, J. M. Lamour et al., "BNP levels predict outcome in pediatric heart failure patients: post hoc analysis of the pediatric carvedilol trial," *Circulation: Heart Failure*, vol. 3, no. 5, pp. 606–611, 2010.

[8] L. Linnemeier, B. D. Benneyworth, M. Turrentine, M. Rodefeld, and J. Brown, "Pediatric cardiac tumors: a 45-year, single-institution review," *World Journal for Pediatric and Congenital Heart Surgery*, vol. 6, no. 2, pp. 215–219, 2015.

[9] A. Esposito, F. de Cobelli, G. Ironi et al., "CMR in the assessment of cardiac masses: primary malignant tumors," *JACC: Cardiovascular Imaging*, vol. 7, no. 10, pp. 1057–1061, 2014.

[10] Q. Meng, H. Lai, J. Lima, W. Tong, Y. Qian, and S. Lai, "Echocardiographic and pathologic characteristics of primary cardiac tumors: a study of 149 cases," *International Journal of Cardiology*, vol. 84, no. 1, pp. 69–75, 2002.

[11] J. N. Kirkpatrick, T. Wong, J. E. Bednarz et al., "Differential diagnosis of cardiac masses using contrast echocardiographic perfusion imaging," *Journal of the American College of Cardiology*, vol. 43, no. 8, pp. 1412–1419, 2004.

[12] E. T. D. Hoey, K. Mankad, S. Puppala, D. Gopalan, and M. U. Sivananthan, "MRI and CT appearances of cardiac tumours in adults," *Clinical Radiology*, vol. 64, no. 12, pp. 1214–1230, 2009.

28

Symptomatic Trifascicular Block in Steinert's Disease: Is It Too Soon for a Pacemaker?

Glenmore Lasam,[1] **Roberto Roberti,**[2] **Gina LaCapra,**[1] **and Roberto Ramirez**[1]

[1]*Department of Internal Medicine, Overlook Medical Center, Summit, NJ 07901, USA*
[2]*Section of Cardiology, Overlook Medical Center, Summit, NJ 07901, USA*

Correspondence should be addressed to Glenmore Lasam; glenmore_md@yahoo.com

Academic Editor: Kjell Nikus

We report a case of a 62-year-old male with Steinert's disease who presented with progressive intermittent episodes of lightheadedness five years after he was diagnosed with the disease. On evaluation, he developed a new onset trifascicular block (first degree atrioventricular block, new onset right bundle branch block, and left anterior fascicular block). A dual chamber pacemaker was inserted and lightheadedness improved significantly.

1. Introduction

Steinert's disease or myotonic dystrophy type 1 may present as symptomatic trifascicular block which may progress to high degree atrioventricular block and fatal arrhythmias that could lead to sudden cardiac death. This could pose a dilemma to the clinician whether to do conservative surveillance or immediate pacemaker insertion to abate symptom.

2. Case Presentation

A 62-year-old male was diagnosed with Steinert's disease (myotonic dystrophy type 1) at the age of 50 when he presented with bilateral leg muscle weakness associated with numbness in his toes and occasional dysphagia compatible with esophageal dysmotility. The diagnosis was confirmed by genetic testing and electromyography. His sister, nephew, and niece were diagnosed with the same disease. Five years ago, he gradually developed jaw weakness and started complaining of intermittent episodes of lightheadedness and easy fatigability. He denied any syncope, chest pain, dyspnea, orthopnea, or palpitations. He had trace bipedal edema and 4/5 bilateral lower extremity motor strength. Electrocardiogram showed normal sinus rhythm, first degree atrioventricular block, left axis deviation, new onset right bundle branch block, and left anterior fascicular block (trifascicular block) which were new

findings (Figure 2) compared to five months earlier (Figure 1). Holter monitoring did not demonstrate any pauses. Transthoracic echocardiogram revealed mild left ventricular hypertrophy with normal ejection fraction. Adenosine myocardial perfusion imaging showed moderate distal anterior and distal lateral ischemia with ejection fraction of 53%. He was started on aspirin.

Three months after the onset of the trifascicular block, the lightheadedness became more frequent and, even though a repeat electrocardiogram revealed no changes, a dual chamber pacemaker was recommended due to the unstable progression of conduction disease in myotonic dystrophy. The pacemaker was successfully inserted as confirmed by electrocardiogram (Figure 3) and subsequently the lightheadedness improved.

3. Discussion

Myotonic dystrophy (DM) is an autosomal dominant disorder characterized by myotonia (delayed muscle relaxation after contraction), weakness and atrophy of skeletal muscles, and systemic manifestations including endocrine abnormalities, cataracts, cognitive impairment, and cardiac involvement [1]. There are two types of myotonic dystrophy. Classical DM, called Steinert's disease or myotonic dystrophy type 1 (DM1), has been associated with the presence of

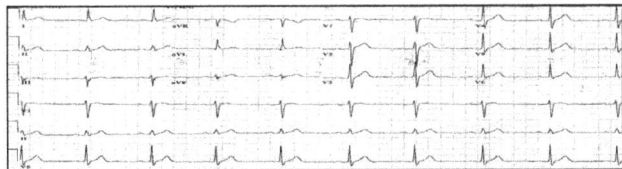

FIGURE 1: Patient's baseline 12-lead electrocardiogram. The tracing revealed sinus bradycardia (with heart rate in the 55) with normal axis.

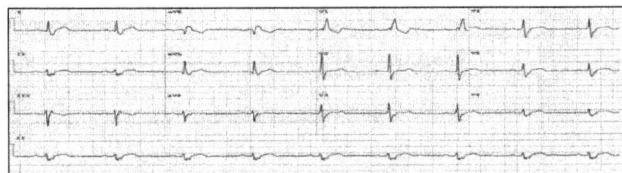

FIGURE 2: Patient's 12-lead electrocardiogram when he presented with frequent lightheadedness. The tracing revealed sinus bradycardia with first degree atrioventricular block, right bundle branch block, and left axis deviation consistent with left anterior fascicular block (new finding).

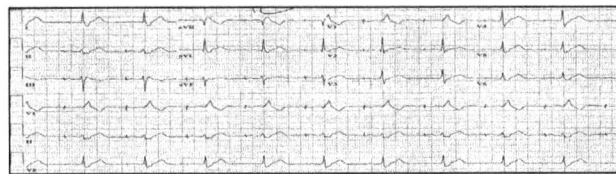

FIGURE 3: Patient's 12-lead electrocardiogram after the pacemaker insertion. The tracing revealed electronic atrial paced rhythm, left axis deviation, and right bundle branch block.

an abnormal expansion of a CTG trinucleotide repeat on chromosome 19q13.3 [2] in the *DMPK* gene that codes for myotonic dystrophy protein kinase, a protein mainly expressed in smooth, cardiac, and skeletal muscle cells [3]. Myotonic dystrophy type 2 (DM2) is caused by a dominantly transmitted CCTG repeat expansion in intron 1 of the zinc finger protein 9 (ZNF9) gene on chromosome 3q [4]. A critical element in the pathogenesis of this disease in both types is the intranuclear accumulation of the expanded RNA sequences which disrupt the regulation of alternative splicing of mRNA and perturb the expression of many genes; thus multiple systems are affected clinically. DM1 is more common, affecting approximately 1 in 8000, making it the most common adult form of muscular dystrophy while DM2 is less common affecting approximately 1 in 20000 [5].

Sixty-five percent of DM1 patients have an abnormal ECG in which conduction abnormalities are the result of myocyte hypertrophy, fibrosis, focal fatty infiltration, and also lymphocytic infiltration, which can occur anywhere along the conduction system including the His-Purkinje system [6]. Prolongation of the PR segment occurs in roughly 20–40% of patients and QRS widening occurs in 5–25% of patients [7], left bundle branch block in 4%, right bundle branch block in 3%, and nonspecific intraventricular conduction delay in 12% of patients [5]. Severe atrioventricular and intraventricular conduction defect is related to CTG repeat length and the presence of abnormal late potential (caused by slowed and fragmented conduction through damaged areas of myocardium) is directly correlated to CTG expansion and represents a substrate for malignant reentrant ventricular arrhythmias [7].

DM1, and possibly DM2, is associated with a significantly increased risk of cardiomyopathy, heart failure, conduction disorders, and arrhythmias [8]. The symptomatic presentations include palpitations, presyncope and syncope, heart failure symptoms, and sudden cardiac death [9]. Structural heart disease is also frequently observed in DM, with LV dilatation or hypertrophy observed in 20% of patients, LV systolic dysfunction in 14%, and clinical heart failure in 2% of DM1 patients based upon clinical history [10].

A 12-lead EKG is an appropriate screening test and should be performed annually after the diagnosis of DM [11]. Radionucleotide imaging and echocardiography may reveal diastolic and systolic dysfunction in either ventricle [5]. Electrophysiological study (EPS) correlating the H-V interval measurement with the electrocardiographic findings may identify predictive risk factors [12], strongly recommended in patients with clinical manifestations suggestive of ventricular tachycardia and/or with a family history of sudden death [13, 14]. In an innovative study on DM1 and cardiac disease, VT could be induced at EPS in 18% of patients in the absence of ventricular arrhythmias during Holter monitoring [14]. Among DM1 patients with major infranodal conduction delays, institution of an invasive strategy utilizing systematic electrophysiological studies with subsequent prophylactic permanent pacing indicated by malignant arrhythmias is associated with nine-year survival of almost seventy-six percent [15]. An implantable loop recorder is useful in detecting fifty percent of arrhythmias in DM1 patients and should be instituted more often in apparently asymptomatic [16] as well as high risk myotonic dystrophy patients to identify asymptomatic arrhythmias [17] which aids in the determination about antiarrhythmic devices. Cardiovascular magnetic resonance may help define the LV abnormalities of the disease including dilatation, systolic dysfunction, hypertrophy, and, occasionally, noncompaction [18, 19].

Based on the recommendation of the ACC/AHA/HRS 2008 Guidelines for device-based therapy, our patient qualified for the class IIB indication for pacemaker insertion which encompasses any degree of AV block (including first degree AV block), bifascicular block, or any fascicular block with or without symptoms (level of evidence: B) [20].

Patients with DM have an annual mortality of approximately 3.5%, one-third of which is sudden cardiac death and the systematic identification of conduction disease, and aggressive use of prophylactic pacemakers is associated with low rate of sudden cardiac death at 1.16% per year [21]. DM1 patients even when asymptomatic presenting with the Groh's criteria (prolonged PR of equal or >240 ms, wide QRS complex of equal or >120 ms, or atrial tachyarrhythmias) were at higher risk of sudden death when compared to those with normal ECGs [22]. The prophylactic implantation of pacemaker in high risk MD patients according to Groh's criteria reduced the incidence rate of sudden death to 0.2 per 100 patient-years [23].

The paroxysmal nature and the high prevalence of arrhythmias in DM patients reiterates the importance of follow-up not solely through regular ECG, but also through 24 h Holter monitoring since 32% of the patients showed conduction disturbances in the 24 h Holter monitoring that was not identified on ECG [24]. A high prevalence and changes between baseline ECG and follow-up Holter monitoring justified permanent pacemaker implantation in thirty percent of DM1 patients [25]. Current approach is to obtain 12-lead electrocardiogram each year and to consider prophylactic pacing in patients with more advanced conduction disturbances such as right bundle branch block associated with left fascicular block or bundle branch block with significant increase in PR interval, especially if there is evidence of worsening conduction over time [26]. Prophylactically inserted pacemaker in DM1 patients with HV interval of ≥70 ms even in the absence of related symptoms was monitored after implantation and was found out to have paroxysmal arrhythmias in 83.7% consisting of complete AV block, sinoatrial block, or atrial or ventricular tachyarrhythmias; thus a pacemaker including detailed diagnostic functions facilitates the diagnosis and management of frequent paroxysmal tachyarrhythmias that may remain obscure during conventional clinical surveillance [27]. Heart failure with a documented left ventricular ejection fraction of less than 50 percent should be treated with current medical treatment including angiotensin-converting enzyme inhibitors, angiotensin II receptor blockers, beta blockers, aldosterone-antagonists, and diuretics [9].

4. Conclusion

The timing of pacemaker implantation in Steinert's disease (DM1) should be individualized and tailored from the patient's presentation considering in the background the current clinical practice guideline's recommendation.

Conflict of Interests

The authors declare that they have no conflict of interests.

References

[1] D. L. Mann, D. P. Zipes, P. Libby, R. O. Bonow, and E. Braunwald, "Neurologic disorders and cardiovascular disease," in *Braunwald's Heart Disease: A Textbook of Cardiovascular Medicine*, W. J. Groh and D. P. Zipes, Eds., p. 2137, Saunders Elsevier, Philadelphia, PA, USA, 10th edition, 2015.

[2] G. Pelargonio, A. Dello Russo, T. Sanna, G. De Martino, and F. Bellocci, "Myotonic dystrophy and the heart," *Heart*, vol. 88, no. 6, pp. 665–670, 2002.

[3] D. Verhaert, K. Richards, J. A. Rafael-Fortney, and S. V. Raman, "Cardiac involvement in patients with muscular dystrophies magnetic resonance imaging phenotype and genotypic considerations," *Circulation: Cardiovascular Imaging*, vol. 4, no. 1, pp. 67–76, 2011.

[4] B. G. H. Schoser, W. Kress, M. C. Walter, B. Halliger-Keller, H. Lochmüller, and K. Ricker, "Homozygosity for CCTG mutation in myotonic dystrophy type 2," *Brain*, vol. 127, no. 8, pp. 1868–1877, 2004.

[5] E. M. McNally and D. Sparano, "Mechanisms and management of the heart in myotonic dystrophy," *Heart*, vol. 97, no. 13, pp. 1094–1100, 2011.

[6] H. H. Nguyen, J. T. Wolfe III, D. R. Holmes Jr., and W. D. Edwards, "Pathology of the cardiac conduction system in myotonic dystrophy: a study of 12 cases," *Journal of the American College of Cardiology*, vol. 11, no. 3, pp. 662–671, 1988.

[7] P. Melacini, C. Villanova, E. Menegazzo et al., "Correlation between cardiac involvement and CTG trinucleotide repeat length in myotonic dystrophy," *Journal of the American College of Cardiology*, vol. 25, no. 1, pp. 239–245, 1995.

[8] M. Lund, L. J. Diaz, M. F. Ranthe et al., "Cardiac involvement in myotonic dystrophy: a nationwide cohort study," *European Heart Journal*, vol. 35, no. 32, pp. 2158–2164, 2014.

[9] H. Petri, J. Vissing, N. Witting, H. Bundgaard, and L. Kober, "Cardiac manifestations of myotonic dystrophy type 1," *International Journal of Cardiology*, vol. 160, no. 2, pp. 82–88, 2012.

[10] D. Bhakta, M. R. Lowe, and W. J. Groh, "Prevalence of structural cardiac abnormalities in patients with myotonic dystrophy type I," *American Heart Journal*, vol. 147, no. 2, pp. 224–227, 2004.

[11] K. Khalighi, A. Kodali, S. B. Thapamagar, and S. R. Walker, "Cardiac involvement in myotonic dystrophy," *Journal of Community Hospital Internal Medicine Perspectives*, vol. 5, no. 1, Article ID 25319, 2015.

[12] S. A. D. Nishioka, M. M. Filho, S. Marie, M. Zatz, and R. Costa, "Myotonic dystrophy and heart disease. Behavior of arrhythmic events and conduction disturbances," *Arquivos Brasileiros de Cardiologia*, vol. 84, no. 4, pp. 330–336, 2005.

[13] N. R. A. Clarke, A. D. Kelion, J. Nixon, D. Hilton-Jones, and J. C. Forfar, "Does cytosine-thymine-guanine (CTG) expansion size predict cardiac events and electrocardiographic progression in myotonic dystrophy?" *Heart*, vol. 86, no. 4, pp. 411–416, 2001.

[14] A. Lazarus, J. Varin, Z. Ounnoughene et al., "Relationships among electrophysiological findings and clinical status, heart function, and extent of DNA mutation in myotonic dystrophy," *Circulation*, vol. 99, no. 8, pp. 1041–1046, 1999.

[15] K. Wahbi, C. Meune, R. Porcher et al., "Electrophysiological study with prophylactic pacing and survival in adults with myotonic dystrophy and conduction system disease," *The Journal of the American Medical Association*, vol. 307, no. 12, pp. 1292–1301, 2012.

[16] C. Stöllberger, C. Steger, P. Gabriel, and J. Finsterer, "Implantable loop recorders in myotonic dystrophy 1," *International Journal of Cardiology*, vol. 152, no. 2, pp. 249–251, 2011.

[17] D. Hadian, M. R. Lowe, L. R. Scott, and W. J. Groh, "Use of an insertable loop recorder in a myotonic dystrophy patient," *Journal of Cardiovascular Electrophysiology*, vol. 13, no. 1, pp. 72–73, 2002.

[18] J. Finsterer, C. Stöllberger, and W. Kopsa, "Noncompaction in myotonic dystrophy type 1 on cardiac MRI," *Cardiology*, vol. 103, no. 3, pp. 167–168, 2005.

[19] M. W. Ashford Jr., W. Liu, S. J. Lin et al., "Occult cardiac contractile dysfunction in dystrophin-deficient children revealed by cardiac magnetic resonance strain imaging," *Circulation*, vol. 112, no. 16, pp. 2462–2467, 2005.

[20] A. E. Epstein, J. P. DiMarco, K. A. Ellenbogen et al., "ACC/AHA/HRS 2008 guidelines for device-based therapy of cardiac rhythm abnormalities: executive summary: a report of the American College of Cardiology/American Heart Association task force on practice guidelines (writing committee to revise the ACC/AHA/NASPE 2002 guideline update for implantation of cardiac pacemakers and antiarrhythmia devices) developed in collaboration with the American Association for Thoracic Surgery and Society of Thoracic Surgeons," *Circulation*, vol. 117, pp. 2820–2840, 2008.

[21] A. H. Ha, M. A. Tarnopolsky, T. G. Bergstra, G. M. Nair, A. Al-Qubbany, and J. S. Healey, "Predictors of atrio-ventricular conduction disease, long-term outcomes in patients with myotonic dystrophy types I and II," *Pacing and Clinical Electrophysiology*, vol. 35, no. 10, pp. 1262–1269, 2012.

[22] W. J. Groh, M. R. Groh, C. Saha et al., "Electrocardiographic abnormalities and sudden death in myotonic dystrophy type 1," *The New England Journal of Medicine*, vol. 358, no. 25, pp. 2688–2697, 2008.

[23] V. Laurent, S. Pellieux, P. Corcia et al., "Mortality in myotonic dystrophy patients in the area of prophylactic pacing devices," *International Journal of Cardiology*, vol. 150, no. 1, pp. 54–58, 2011.

[24] K. Merlevede, D. Vermander, P. Theys, E. Legius, H. Ector, and W. Robberecht, "Cardiac involvement and CTG expansion in myotonic dystrophy," *Journal of Neurology*, vol. 249, no. 6, pp. 693–698, 2002.

[25] M. I. Sá, S. Cabral, P. D. Costa, T. Coelho, M. Freitas, and J. L. Gomes, "Ambulatory electrocardiographic monitoring in type 1 myotonic dystrophy," *Revista Portuguesa de Cardiologia*, vol. 26, no. 7-8, pp. 745–753, 2007.

[26] R. Breton and J. Mathieu, "Usefulness of clinical and electrocardiographic data for predicting adverse cardiac events in patients with myotonic dystrophy," *Canadian Journal of Cardiology*, vol. 25, no. 2, pp. 23–27, 2009.

[27] A. Lazarus, J. Varin, D. Babuty, F. R. Anselme, J. Coste, and D. Duboc, "Long-term follow-up of arrhythmias in patients with myotonic dystrophy treated by pacing: a multicenter diagnostic pacemaker study," *Journal of the American College of Cardiology*, vol. 40, no. 9, pp. 1645–1652, 2002.

29

Bortezomib-Induced Complete Heart Block and Myocardial Scar: The Potential Role of Cardiac Biomarkers in Monitoring Cardiotoxicity

Sachin Diwadkar,[1] **Aarti A. Patel,**[1] **and Michael G. Fradley**[1,2]

[1]*Division of Cardiovascular Medicine, University of South Florida, 2 Tampa General Circle, Tampa, FL 33606, USA*
[2]*H. Lee Moffitt Cancer Center & Research Institute, 12902 Magnolia Drive, Tampa, FL 33612, USA*

Correspondence should be addressed to Michael G. Fradley; mfradley@health.usf.edu

Academic Editor: Kjell Nikus

Bortezomib is a proteasome inhibitor used to treat multiple myeloma and mantle cell lymphoma. Traditionally, bortezomib was thought to have little cardiovascular toxicity; however, there is increasing evidence that bortezomib can lead to cardiac complications including left ventricular dysfunction and atrioventricular block. We present the case of a 66-year-old man with multiple myeloma and persistent asymptomatic elevations of cardiac biomarkers who developed complete heart block and evidence of myocardial scar after his eighth cycle of bortezomib, requiring permanent pacemaker placement. In addition to discussing the cardiovascular complications of bortezomib therapy, we propose a potential role for biomarkers in the prediction and monitoring of bortezomib cardiotoxicity.

1. Introduction

With newer chemotherapeutic agents, survival rates for many cancers have increased dramatically. Unfortunately, many of these agents have unintended cardiovascular side effects. There has been increasing focus on developing strategies with cardiac biomarkers to better predict and monitor chemotherapy-induced cardiotoxicity [1]. Although the majority of the work has focused on anthracyclines and HER2 targeted therapies, other chemotherapeutics can lead to cardiac dysfunction. Bortezomib is a proteasome inhibitor used to treat multiple myeloma and mantle cell lymphoma. Though rare, cardiac complications including heart block and heart failure have been described [2]. We report the case of a patient with persistently elevated cardiac biomarkers who developed complete heart block and myocardial scar after his eighth cycle of bortezomib therapy. This case illustrates potential bortezomib-induced cardiac complications and the possible role of cardiac biomarkers in identifying individuals at higher risk for developing bortezomib cardiotoxicity.

2. Case Report

A 66-year-old man with stage IIIA IgA lambda chain multiple myeloma receiving chemotherapy with bortezomib, lenalidomide, and dexamethasone (VRD) with no significant cardiovascular history presented for a routine pre-stem cell transplant clinic appointment. He was feeling well and had not experienced any recent chest pain, dyspnea, palpitations, syncope, or presyncope. He reported mild fatigue but continued to engage in daily 30-minute walks without limitation. In the oncology clinic, he underwent routine electrocardiogram as part of the stem cell transplant workup which revealed complete atrioventricular (AV) block with a ventricular escape rhythm of 55 beats per minute (bpm) (Figure 1). On exam, his blood pressure was 124/59 mmHg and pulse was 52 bpm. Physical exam revealed a regular rhythm with normal heart sounds and no other abnormalities. Laboratory testing showed normal electrolytes, normal kidney and liver function, and mild normocytic anemia (hemoglobin 13.0 g/dL). Cardiac biomarkers were elevated with troponin

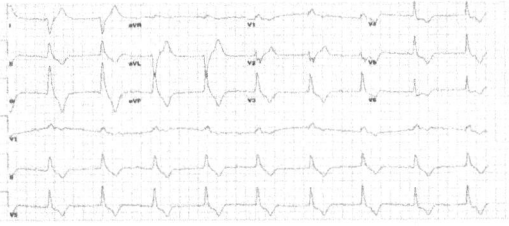

FIGURE 1: Electrocardiogram demonstrates complete heart block with a wide ventricular escape rhythm at 55 beats per minute.

I of 2.49 ng/mL, CK-MB of 20.2, and creatine phosphokinase of 549. BNP was also elevated at 333 pg/mL. Echocardiogram revealed normal left ventricular systolic function with an ejection fraction of 55% and mild hypokinesis of the mid-inferolateral myocardium. Throughout this time, the patient remained asymptomatic. The patient was transferred urgently to a tertiary care facility for further management.

The patient was first diagnosed with multiple myeloma nine months earlier after seeking medical attention for right arm weakness and paresthesia. A bone scan was consistent with extensive metastatic disease and he underwent biopsy of a right humerus lytic lesion which demonstrated a lambda restricted plasma cell population consistent with a plasmacytoma. On serologic testing, he was noted to have an IgA lambda monoclonal gammopathy and a 24-hour urine protein was notable for 19.8 g of protein of which 19.6 g represented urine free lambda excretion. Despite his significant urinary protein excretion, his kidney function (BUN, creatinine, and glomerular filtration rate) remained normal. Bone marrow biopsy confirmed multiple myeloma without evidence of amyloid deposition. He was initiated on bortezomib, cyclophosphamide, and dexamethasone (VCD). He received three cycles without significant response, so his treatment regimen was changed to VRD. Complete treatment regimen with associated clinical and laboratory parameters is presented in Table 1.

During his initial chemotherapy regimen with bortezomib, cyclophosphamide, and dexamethasone, he was noted to have elevated troponin I at 0.163 ng/mL and BNP at 1810 pg/mL. Given these findings, he was referred to cardiology clinic for evaluation of possible cardiac amyloidosis (despite negative bone marrow evaluation). Aside from hyperlipidemia, he had no personal or family history of cardiovascular disease including significant conduction system disease. In the month prior to his multiple myeloma diagnosis, he completed an exercise stress echocardiogram which was negative for ischemia. The echocardiogram revealed normal left ventricular (LV) function and wall thickness and the stress ECG showed sinus rhythm with right bundle branch block. Due to the elevated cardiac biomarkers, he underwent a repeat transthoracic echocardiogram which again demonstrated normal LV function without significant diastolic dysfunction. A repeat ECG obtained at the time showed normal sinus rhythm with normal voltage and incomplete right bundle branch block. As a result of these findings, cardiac amyloidosis was considered unlikely.

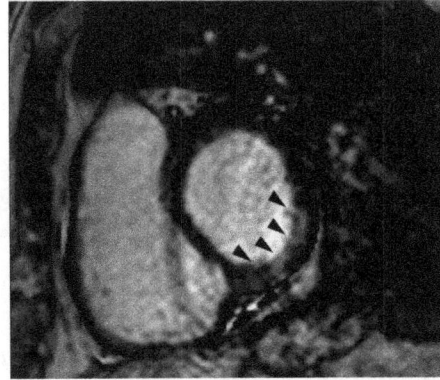

FIGURE 2: Cardiac magnetic resonance demonstrates late gadolinium enhancement (arrows) in the inferolateral left ventricle.

Upon transfer to the tertiary care hospital, the patient remained in complete AV block. A cardiac MRI was obtained, revealing normal left ventricular function (ejection fraction of 60%), with myocardial thinning and a small subendocardial perfusion defect in the midinferolateral segment with focal late gadolinium enhancement (LGE) suggestive of scar/fibrosis (Figure 2). There was no evidence on the MRI to suggest cardiac amyloidosis or other infiltrative diseases such as LV hypertrophy and/or diffuse LGE. Left heart catheterization was subsequently performed showing angiographically normal coronary arteries (Figures 3(a) and 3(b)). Throughout all of these procedures, the patient remained hemodynamically stable in complete heart block. He ultimately underwent implantation of a permanent dual-chamber pacemaker. Unfortunately, he was unable to move forward with stem cell transplant after the pacemaker implantation due to significant pulmonary fibrosis identified during vital organ testing. He elected not to receive any additional chemotherapy and eventually expired from progression of his multiple myeloma.

3. Discussion

This case demonstrates rare adverse cardiovascular effects of bortezomib and introduces the potential usefulness of biomarkers to predict cardiac dysfunction in patients undergoing active treatment with this chemotherapy. Utilizing cardiac biomarkers such as troponin I and BNP as a method to predict cardiac dysfunction during treatment with bortezomib has not been previously described.

Our patient presented with atrioventricular (AV) heart block in the setting of ongoing chemotherapy with bortezomib (8 cycles). Advanced age and cumulative dose have been shown to increase the risk of adverse cardiac events [3]. In our case, the patient was noted to have asymptomatic elevations of troponin and brain natriuretic peptide (BNP) as early as six months prior to the development of AV block on ECG. These levels were persistently elevated, with troponin I reaching levels suggestive of myocardial necrosis. Further evaluation with cardiac MRI demonstrated scar/fibrosis in the inferolateral left ventricle, and there was no significant

TABLE 1: Multiple myeloma treatment summary with relevant clinical and laboratory parameters.

	5/23/2013 Prechemotherapy	6/18/2013 VCD, 1 cycle	8/6/2013 VCD, 3 cycles Change to RVD	10/1/2013 RVD, 2 cycles	12/3/2013 RVD, 4 cycles	12/30/2013 RVD, 5 cycles
IgA (mg/dL)	1758	2358	2130	1377	885	492
M Spike (g/dL)	2.91	2.7	2.0	2.0	1.2	0.7
BUN (mg/dL)	16	22	25	19	11	11
Creatinine (mg/dL)	0.95	1.0	1.2	0.9	0.9	0.9
24-hour urine protein (g)	19.8		2.4		0.78	1.0
Blood pressure (mmHg)	127/72	119/58	108/63	120/66	107/67	117/69
Pulse (bpm)	80	60	75	63	71	69

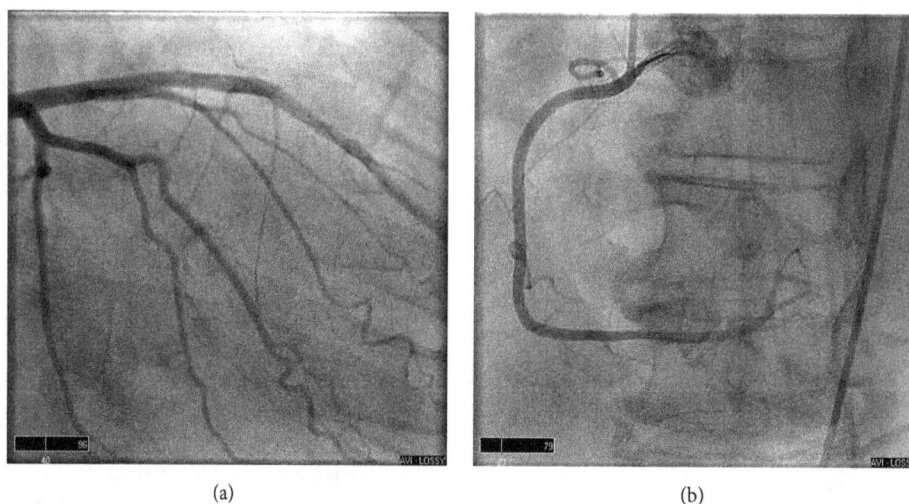

(a)

(b)

FIGURE 3: Coronary angiograms show no obstructive lesions in (a) the left anterior descending and the left circumflex artery or (b) the right coronary artery.

coronary artery disease seen on left heart catheterization. Based on a Naranjo score of 5-6, it is "possible or probable" the scar seen on MRI and the AV block was an adverse event due to bortezomib exposure [4].

Chemotherapy-induced cardiotoxicity is the likely cause for the observed findings. The patient underwent thorough cardiac evaluation to rule out common cardiac conditions that can cause the observed findings such as atherosclerotic heart disease and myocarditis. In addition, based on the echocardiogram and cardiac MRI findings, there is no evidence to suggest cardiac amyloid or other infiltrative diseases as the cause of his cardiac dysfunction. Cardiac MRI has emerged as a noninvasive method to aid in diagnosis of cardiac amyloidosis in preselected patients with studies showing sensitivity and specificity in the range of 86–88% and 86–90% in those with positive endomyocardial biopsy [5, 6]. In patients without biopsy proven amyloidosis (endomyocardial or other tissue types), those with cardiac amyloidosis demonstrate characteristic diffuse LGE patterns coupled with other markers of cardiac dysfunction such as LV hypertrophy [7]. Our patient had a negative bone

marrow biopsy for amyloidosis and cardiac MRI lacked typical features of amyloidosis, suggesting extremely low likelihood of cardiac amyloidosis.

Although the patient was exposed to multiple chemotherapeutics, we believe that bortezomib is the likely cause of his cardiac dysfunction. Cyclophosphamide can lead to left ventricular dysfunction, myopericarditis, and heart block; however, these findings generally occur during therapy or the first several weeks posttreatment [8, 9]. When our patient's cardiac dysfunction developed, it had been over five months since he had received any cyclophosphamide. Thus, cyclophosphamide-induced toxicity is quite unlikely. Lenalidomide is associated with thromboembolism but rarely with any other cardiovascular toxicity (as compared to thalidomide which can cause bradyarrhythmias) [8, 9].

Bortezomib is a dipeptide boronate proteasome inhibitor. It reversibly binds and inhibits the 20S proteasome which is the proteolytic core particle of the 26S proteasome [10]. In the United States, it is approved for the treatment of multiple myeloma and mantle cell lymphoma. The presence of cardiac dysfunction with its use ranges from 0 to 17.9% in reported studies, though a meta-analysis of these data failed to identify definite increased cardiac risk [3]. The reported adverse cardiac events included cardiomyopathy/congestive heart failure, myocardial infarction, AV block, and supraventricular tachycardia [2, 11–13]. Some data suggests that these cardiotoxicities may occur even in the absence of underlying cardiovascular disease or risk factors. For example, one observational study reported 11.6% incidence of cardiac complications in patients without prior cardiac history treated with bortezomib [2]. The lack of prospective studies has made it difficult to accurately quantitate the true risk of cardiac dysfunction associated with bortezomib however.

The exact mechanism by which bortezomib interacts with cardiac myocardium is unknown, but there are several postulated mechanisms for the development of cardiac dysfunction, including direct cardiac insult as well as indirect exacerbation of underlying cardiac disease. The ubiquitin-proteasome pathway plays an important role in regulating the cell cycle in cardiac myocytes. As a proteasome inhibitor, bortezomib impairs the activation of transcription factors such as nuclear factor kappa-beta which is essential for cell survival, regulative apoptosis gene expression, and angiogenesis [14]. Proteasome inhibition also has downstream effects on vascular smooth muscle cells leading to atherosclerotic plaque instability [15]. In patients with cardiac risk factors or prior history of coronary artery disease, bortezomib may cause plaque progression and increase the vulnerability of existing plaque leading to ischemic events. In animal studies, there has been evidence of decreased proteasome activity impairing cardiac function by accumulation of proteins inside the myocytes as well as mitochondrial abnormalities resulting in impaired contractility [16, 17]. Through one or more of these mechanisms, the end result for patients undergoing treatment with bortezomib is increased risk of cardiac dysfunction.

Although limited data currently exist, similar cardiovascular toxicities have been associated with the use of the novel irreversible proteasome inhibitor carfilzomib. The majority of the observed cardiotoxicities with this agent were new-onset left ventricular dysfunction. These findings are most common in patients who had a history of cardiac events and exposure to doxorubicin. In this population, elevated BNP levels were also commonly observed, although the clinical significance of this finding remains unclear. In addition, hypotension and arrhythmias including atrial fibrillation have been reported [18, 19]. Given these data, in patients that develop significant cardiac dysfunction due to bortezomib or another proteasome inhibitor, considerable caution should be exercised if rechallenge with the drug is deemed necessary. If the primary cardiac toxicity has not been definitely treated (e.g., with a pacemaker) and/or completely resolved, alternative agents should be considered.

There is increasing evidence that cardiac biomarkers can both predict and detect chemotherapy-induced cardiotoxicity. Most of the research has focused on troponin and BNP. Cardiac troponins (I and T) are sensitive and specific markers of myocardial injury, and BNP is a neurohormone released from the ventricular tissue in the setting of elevated filling pressure and myocardial stress. A number of studies have evaluated the role of troponin in the detection of subclinical myocardial disease and the risk of developing overt cardiac dysfunction with the use of chemotherapeutic agents, particularly anthracyclines and trastuzumab. In a study of 211 breast cancer patients receiving anthracyclines, patients with baseline elevated troponin levels were more likely to develop cardiac dysfunction during therapy [20]. In a related study, elevations in troponin as early as 12 hours after exposure to anthracyclines predict patients at higher risk for future cardiovascular events [21]. Similarly, there was an increased risk of cardiotoxicity in breast cancer patients exposed to anthracyclines and trastuzumab who demonstrated increased troponin levels [22]. Although the majority of studies suggest that BNP is useful in predicting anthracycline induced cardiac dysfunction, the data is conflicting in the trastuzumab population [22–25]. BNP may also be useful in predicting and monitoring cardiac dysfunction due to tyrosine kinase inhibitors used in the treatment of renal cell carcinoma [26].

Biomarker elevations are also predictive of mortality and adverse outcomes in other cancer populations such as those with cardiac amyloidosis or stem cell transplant recipients. Both NT pro-BNP and troponin T can be used as markers of disease prognosis in patients with cardiac amyloidosis [27, 28]. In these patients being considered for stem cell transplant, elevated levels of troponin and BNP predict early morbidity and mortality providing guidance about a patient's suitability for this procedure [29, 30].

Despite this increasingly robust biomarker data, there are no studies specifically addressing the role of biomarkers in predicting bortezomib cardiotoxicity. BNP elevations were commonly observed in patients exposed to the proteasome inhibitor carfilzomib (median increase of 407 pg/mL from baseline); however, the predictive and/or diagnostic benefit is not clear [18]. Although the incidence of cardiotoxicity is lower with bortezomib compared to other chemotherapeutics, it still may be reasonable to apply the surveillance algorithms prior to and during therapy with proteasome inhibitors in an effort to detect those at higher risk for developing cardiac dysfunction. Using biomarkers to detect subclinical toxicity may allow for earlier cardiovascular treatment and/or intervention to prevent more significant cardiac dysfunction. Nonetheless, additional studies are necessary to specifically evaluate the potential predictive and/or diagnostic role of cardiac biomarkers in bortezomib treated patients and to identify the optimal timing and frequency of monitoring.

4. Conclusion

Heart block and myocardial scar/fibrosis are rare but serious side effects associated with bortezomib administration. Although the incidence of cardiotoxicity is low in patients treated with bortezomib, these events can affect patient morbidity and mortality independent of the oncologic prognosis. Improved surveillance and early detection of cardiac disorders during therapy has the potential to improve patient outcomes and prevent the discontinuation of cancer therapy.

Conflict of Interests

The authors declare that there is no conflict of interests regarding the publication of this paper.

References

[1] P. L. Stevens and D. J. Lenihan, "Cardiotoxicity due to chemotherapy: the role of biomarkers," *Current Cardiology Reports*, vol. 17, article 49, 2015.

[2] O. Enrico, B. Gabriele, C. Nadia et al., "Unexpected cardiotoxicity in haematological bortezomib treated patients," *British Journal of Haematology*, vol. 138, no. 3, pp. 396–397, 2007.

[3] Y. Xiao, J. Yin, J. Wei, and Z. Shang, "Incidence and risk of cardiotoxicity associated with bortezomib in the treatment of cancer: a systematic review and meta-analysis," *PLoS ONE*, vol. 9, no. 1, Article ID e87671, 2014.

[4] C. A. Naranjo, U. Busto, E. M. Sellers et al., "A method for estimating the probability of adverse drug reactions," *Clinical Pharmacology and Therapeutics*, vol. 30, no. 2, pp. 239–245, 1981.

[5] B. A. Austin, W. H. W. Tang, E. R. Rodriguez et al., "Delayed hyper-enhancement magnetic resonance imaging provides incremental diagnostic and prognostic utility in suspected cardiac amyloidosis," *JACC: Cardiovascular Imaging*, vol. 2, no. 12, pp. 1369–1377, 2009.

[6] F. L. Ruberg, E. Appelbaum, R. Davidoff et al., "Diagnostic and prognostic utility of cardiovascular magnetic resonance imaging in light-chain cardiac amyloidosis," *American Journal of Cardiology*, vol. 103, no. 4, pp. 544–549, 2009.

[7] I. S. Syed, J. F. Glockner, D. Feng et al., "Role of cardiac magnetic resonance imaging in the detection of cardiac amyloidosis," *JACC: Cardiovascular Imaging*, vol. 3, no. 2, pp. 155–164, 2010.

[8] J. D. Floyd, D. T. Nguyen, R. L. Lobins, Q. Bashir, D. C. Doll, and M. C. Perry, "Cardiotoxicity of cancer therapy," *Journal of Clinical Oncology*, vol. 23, no. 30, pp. 7685–7696, 2005.

[9] E. T. H. Yeh and C. L. Bickford, "Cardiovascular complications of cancer therapy: incidence, pathogenesis, diagnosis, and management," *Journal of the American College of Cardiology*, vol. 53, no. 24, pp. 2231–2247, 2009.

[10] S. D. Demo, C. J. Kirk, M. A. Aujay et al., "Antitumor activity of PR-171, a novel irreversible inhibitor of the proteasome," *Cancer Research*, vol. 67, no. 13, pp. 6383–6391, 2007.

[11] C. A. Dasanu, "Complete heart block secondary to bortezomib use in multiple myeloma," *Journal of Oncology Pharmacy Practice*, vol. 17, no. 3, pp. 282–284, 2011.

[12] P. W. X. Foley, M. S. Hamilton, and F. Leyva, "Myocardial scarring following chemotherapy for multiple myeloma detected using late gadolinium hyperenhancement cardiovascular magnetic resonance," *Journal of Cardiovascular Medicine*, vol. 11, no. 5, pp. 386–388, 2010.

[13] A. Subedi, L. R. Sharma, and B. K. Shah, "Bortezomib-induced acute congestive heart failure: a case report and review of literature," *Annals of Hematology*, vol. 93, no. 10, pp. 1797–1799, 2014.

[14] P. G. Richardson, B. Barlogie, J. Berenson et al., "A phase 2 study of bortezomib in relapsed, refractory myeloma," *The New England Journal of Medicine*, vol. 348, no. 26, pp. 2609–2617, 2003.

[15] D. Versari, J. Herrmann, M. Gössl et al., "Dysregulation of the ubiquitin-proteasome system in human carotid atherosclerosis," *Arteriosclerosis, Thrombosis, and Vascular Biology*, vol. 26, no. 9, pp. 2132–2139, 2006.

[16] E. J. Birks, N. Latif, K. Enesa et al., "Elevated p53 expression is associated with dysregulation of the ubiquitin-proteasome system in dilated cardiomyopathy," *Cardiovascular Research*, vol. 79, no. 3, pp. 472–480, 2008.

[17] D. Nowis, M. Mączewski, U. Mackiewicz et al., "Cardiotoxicity of the anticancer therapeutic agent bortezomib," *The American Journal of Pathology*, vol. 176, no. 6, pp. 2658–2668, 2010.

[18] S. Atrash, A. Tullos, S. Panozzo et al., "Cardiac complications in relapsed and refractory multiple myeloma patients treated with carfilzomib," *Blood Cancer Journal*, vol. 5, article e272, 2015.

[19] A. K. Stewart, S. V. Rajkumar, M. A. Dimopoulos et al., "Carfilzomib, lenalidomide, and dexamethasone for relapsed multiple myeloma," *The New England Journal of Medicine*, vol. 372, no. 2, pp. 142–152, 2015.

[20] D. Cardinale, M. T. Sandri, A. Martinoni et al., "Myocardial injury revealed by plasma troponin I in breast cancer treated with high-dose chemotherapy," *Annals of Oncology*, vol. 13, no. 5, pp. 710–715, 2002.

[21] D. Cardinale, M. T. Sandri, A. Colombo et al., "Prognostic value of troponin I in cardiac risk stratification of cancer patients undergoing high-dose chemotherapy," *Circulation*, vol. 109, no. 22, pp. 2749–2754, 2004.

[22] B. Ky, M. Putt, H. Sawaya et al., "Early increases in multiple biomarkers predict subsequent cardiotoxicity in patients with breast cancer treated with doxorubicin, taxanes, and trastuzumab," *Journal of the American College of Cardiology*, vol. 63, no. 8, pp. 809–816, 2014.

[23] J. M. Horacek, R. Pudil, L. Jebavy, M. Tichy, P. Zak, and J. Maly, "Assessment of anthracycline-induced cardiotoxicity with biochemical markers," *Experimental Oncology*, vol. 29, no. 4, pp. 309–313, 2007.

[24] T. Suzuki, D. Hayashi, T. Yamazaki et al., "Elevated B-type natriuretic peptide levels after anthracycline administration," *American Heart Journal*, vol. 136, no. 2, pp. 362–363, 1998.

[25] D. Cardinale, A. Colombo, R. Torrisi et al., "Trastuzumab-induced cardiotoxicity: clinical and prognostic implications of troponin I evaluation," *Journal of Clinical Oncology*, vol. 28, no. 25, pp. 3910–3916, 2010.

[26] P. S. Hall, L. C. Harshman, S. Srinivas, and R. M. Witteles, "The frequency and severity of cardiovascular toxicity from targeted therapy in advanced renal cell carcinoma patients," *JACC: Heart Failure*, vol. 1, no. 1, pp. 72–78, 2013.

[27] A. Dispenzieri, M. A. Gertz, S. K. Kumar et al., "High sensitivity cardiac troponin T in patients with immunoglobulin light chain amyloidosis," *Heart*, vol. 100, no. 5, pp. 383–388, 2014.

[28] A. Dispenzieri, M. A. Gertz, R. A. Kyle et al., "Serum cardiac troponins and N-terminal pro-brain natriuretic peptide: a staging system for primary systemic amyloidosis," *Journal of Clinical Oncology*, vol. 22, no. 18, pp. 3751–3757, 2004.

[29] M. A. Gertz, M. Q. Lacy, A. Dispenzieri et al., "Refinement in patient selection to reduce treatment-related mortality from autologous stem cell transplantation in amyloidosis," *Bone Marrow Transplantation*, vol. 48, no. 4, pp. 557–561, 2013.

[30] A. Dispenzieri, M. A. Gertz, R. A. Kyle et al., "Prognostication of survival using cardiac troponins and N-terminal pro-brain natriuretic peptide in patients with primary systemic amyloidosis undergoing peripheral blood stem cell transplantation," *Blood*, vol. 104, no. 6, pp. 1881–1887, 2004.

30

Physiologic Functional Evaluation of Left Internal Mammary Artery Graft to Left Anterior Descending Coronary Artery Steal due to Unligated First Thoracic Branch in a Case of Refractory Angina

Fadi J. Sawaya, Henry Liberman, and Chandan Devireddy

Department of Medicine, Division of Cardiology, Emory University School of Medicine, Atlanta, GA 30308, USA

Correspondence should be addressed to Chandan Devireddy; cdevire@emory.edu

Academic Editor: Ertuğurul Ercan

Unligated side branches of the left internal mammary artery (LIMA) have been described in the literature as a cause of coronary steal resulting in angina. Despite a number of studies reporting successful side branch embolization to relieve symptoms, this phenomenon remains controversial. Hemodynamic evidence of coronary steal using angiographic and intravascular Doppler techniques has been supported by some and rejected by others. In this case study using an intracoronary Doppler wire with adenosine, we demonstrate that a trial occlusion of the LIMA thoracic side branch with selective balloon inflation can confirm physiologic significant steal and whether coil embolization of the side branch is indicated.

1. Introduction

The internal mammary artery is the graft of choice in coronary artery bypass (CABG) surgery given its favorable long-term 90% patency at 10 years compared to saphenous vein grafts (SVG) [1, 2]. Left internal mammary artery (LIMA) side branches to the chest wall have been reported to occur in 10 to 20% of patients in preoperative and postoperative data [3]. Preferential blood flow through these unligated thoracic branches and subsequent coronary steal phenomena have been reported as potential causes of angina [4]. Successful ligation of these side branches surgically or through catheter embolization has been documented in the literature to effectively relieve anginal symptoms through mainly subjective measures [5, 6]. However, the hemodynamic significance of large thoracic side branches has been largely debated and is still controversial [7]. We report here a case of refractory angina in a patient with history of CABG surgery where we physiologically demonstrate coronary steal via a large unligated thoracic side branch by measuring coronary flow reserve before and after selective thoracic side branch balloon occlusion and successful treatment by coil embolization of the branch.

2. Case Report

A 50-year-old male with known history of coronary artery disease (CAD) and history of 2 vessel CABG 10 years previously presented to our facility with unstable angina. Over the preceding months, the patient experienced Canadian classification class III exertional angina despite maximal medical therapy with beta-blockers, calcium-channel blockers, and long acting nitrates. Given his worsening angina, a diagnostic catheterization was performed showing luminal irregularities in his circumflex artery (LCX), a 100% stenosis in his mid left anterior descending artery (LAD), and a 100% stenosis in his first diagonal artery. His right coronary artery (RCA) had a 95% stenosis in the posterolateral ventricular branch (PLV). His grafts showed a patent SVG to first diagonal and a small hypoplastic patent LIMA to LAD (Figure 1). There was no further progression of native coronary artery disease compared to prior cardiac catheterization expect for a large, laterally directed LIMA first intercostal thoracic side branch suggesting possible coronary steal and preferential blood flow through the intercostal branch. The large thoracic side branch was barely apparent on an angiogram done after his bypass surgery. The PLV branch was presumed to be the culprit

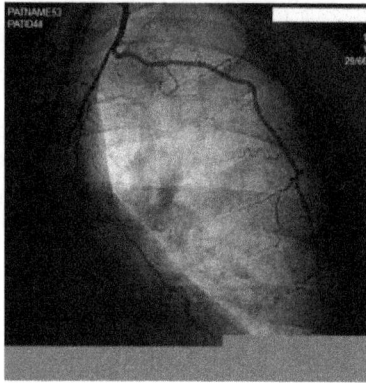

FIGURE 1: Patent hypoplastic LIMA with large thoracic side branch.

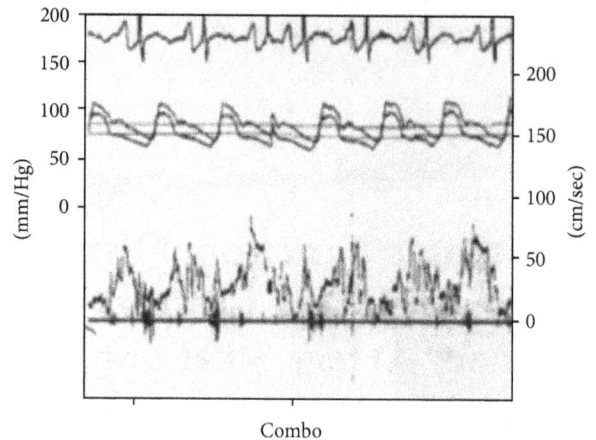

Combo

HR: 74
FFR-I.C.: 0.87
CFR: 3.4
HSR: 0.38
HMR: 2.9

FIGURE 2: Coronary flow reserve (CFR) tracing during intravenous adenosine infusion prior to balloon directed occlusion revealing a value of 3.4 after IV adenosine 140 mcg/kg/min.

lesion causing the patient's anginal symptoms and a 2.5 mm × 23 mm Promus drug eluting stent (Promus PREMIER™, Boston Scientific, Natick, MA) was deployed in the PLV with excellent angiographic results.

Despite coronary intervention, the patient continued to experience significant exertional angina. A cardiac positron emission tomography (PET) scan was performed demonstrating a 10–15% reversible anteroapical and anterolateral ischemic defect confirming suspicion of possible coronary steal from the LIMA thoracic side branch. In light of the PET result, the patient was brought back to the catheterization laboratory with coronary flow reserve (CFR) chosen to measure the functional significance of the thoracic branch.

The LIMA was engaged with a 6-French IMA guiding catheter (Cordis Corporation, Miami, FL). The coronary Doppler wire (FloWire, Volcano, San Diego, CA) was advanced into the mid-portion of LIMA distal to the first thoracic branch collateral. CFR after systemic intravenous (IV) adenosine injection (140 mcg/kg/min) was measured, and a baseline value of 3.4 was recorded (Figure 2). We then advanced, in parallel with the CFR wire, an exchange length Intuition wire (Medtronic, Minneapolis, MN) into the large first intercostal side branch over which a 2.0 × 20 mm Sprinter Legend balloon (Medtronic, Minneapolis, MN) was advanced. The balloon was inflated within the thoracic side branch inducing complete occlusion of flow (Figure 3). The CFR measurement was repeated with IV adenosine infusion (140 mcg/min/kg) during thoracic side branch occlusion revealing a value of 5.3. The discrepancy in CFR measurement from the time before and after side branch occlusion was consistent with significant coronary steal through this branch from the left internal mammary artery (Figure 4). The decision was made to proceed with embolization of the thoracic branch to restore primary graft flow to the LAD territory. The CFR wire was removed and the balloon was exchanged over the Intuition wire for a Tornado delivery catheter (Cook Medical, Bloomington, IN) deep into the thoracic side branch. Through the delivery catheter, four 3 × 2 mm Cook Miraflex microcoils (Miraflex™,

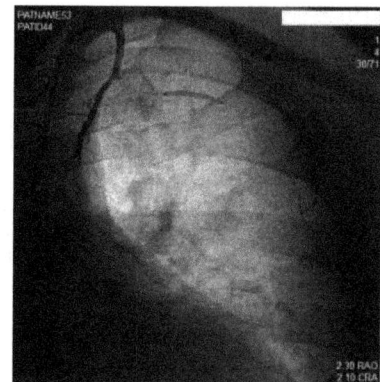

FIGURE 3: The LIMA was engaged with a 6-French IMA guide catheter. The Doppler wire was then advanced into the mid-portion of the LIMA distal to the first thoracic branch collateral with balloon occlusion of side branch.

Cook Medical, Bloomington, IN) were successfully delivered using a long 0.018″ Steelcore wire (Abbott Vascular, Santa Clara, CA) with successful closure of the side branch. Functional closure of the thoracic branch was tested by selective injection of contrast through the microdelivery catheter. Once complete embolization was documented, the microdelivery catheter was removed and final images of the LIMA demonstrated significant increase in flow and caliber of the vessel (Figure 5). At three-month follow-up, the patient reported sustained significant improvement in angina. Given his marked improvement, repeat cardiac PET to assess him for ischemia was not justified in our opinion and would have exposed him to unnecessary radiation.

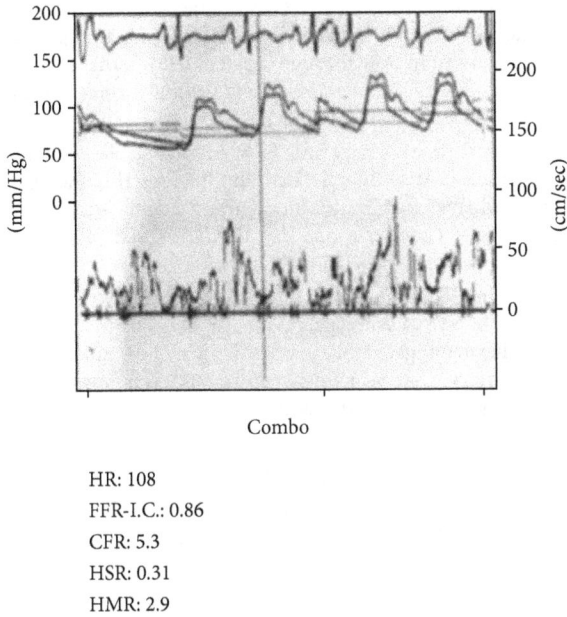

HR: 108
FFR-I.C.: 0.86
CFR: 5.3
HSR: 0.31
HMR: 2.9

FIGURE 4: Coronary flow reserve (CFR) tracing during 140 mcg/kg/min intravenous adenosine infusion following side branch balloon occlusion revealing a value of 5.3.

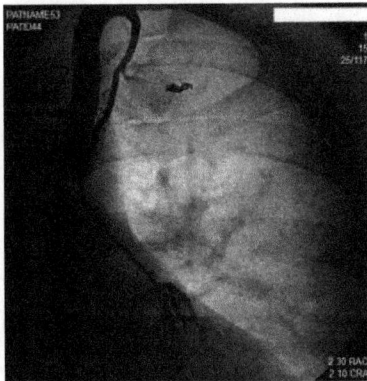

FIGURE 5: Angiogram of the LIMA showing successful microembolization of the thoracic side branch after placement of 4 microcoils with concomitant significant increase in LIMA size.

3. Discussion

LIMA is the conduit of choice for CABG surgery given its favorable long-term patency outcomes. Large unligated thoracic branches have been documented to occur in 10 to 20% of LIMA grafts. The clinical significance of these side branches has been largely debated and the decision to routinely ligate this branch at the time of CABG or later occlude the branch in the catheterization laboratory has remained controversial.

Previous reports supporting the concept of IMA thoracic side branch steal and interventions to occlude the thoracic side branch have postulated improvement in myocardial ischemia through predominantly subjective measures of symptomatic angina relief or through a few reports of resolution of myocardial ischemia on stress testing [8–11].

Opposing viewpoints have rejected the idea of utilizing subjective measurements as an endpoint to justify LIMA thoracic branch occlusion. In fact, Kern has suggested that LIMA side branch steal is defined as a systolic flow diversion and not a true coronary flow steal because the arterial flow to the chest wall is predominantly systolic opposed to coronary flow which is predominantly diastolic [12]. In addition, large unligated side branches have been described without any evidence of clinical symptom [13, 14] and studies that used intravascular Doppler techniques have mainly refuted this syndrome. Studies performed by Luise et al. [15], Abhyankar et al. [7], Guzon et al. [16], and Kern et al. [17] have failed to show any clinical and hemodynamic significance of IMA side branches on coronary pathophysiology under hyperemic conditions using adenosine with no change in coronary flow reserve. In addition, Gaudino et al. failed to show any significant change in LIMA coronary flow under conditions that produce both peripheral and coronary vasodilatation.

On the other hand, a study by Morocutti et al. was able to reproduce our findings. Using an intracoronary Doppler wire with IV adenosine, they demonstrated that a trial of balloon occlusion of a LIMA thoracic side branch increased flow through the LIMA (CFR of 1.6 to CFR of 3.3) confirming hemodynamically significant steal. They subsequently proceeded with successful microembolization in a similar fashion to our case [18].

The pathophysiology behind why IMA branch occlusion improves coronary flow in some and not in others is not fully known and needs to be further elucidated. Using intracoronary flow reserve and Doppler velocities, a trial occlusion of the LIMA side branch via balloon inflation can easily demonstrate whether flow downstream through the LIMA would increase after the intervention and would justify the risk of undergoing coil embolization or surgical ligation of the thoracic side branch. Ligation has been performed mainly by the means of coil embolization with one group deploying a vascular plug to obstruct flow into the side branch [19].

We highly recommend that the hemodynamic functional significance of an unligated thoracic side branch of the LIMA be confirmed using coronary flow reserve measurement after balloon occlusion of the side branch. This provides objective stratification of unligated side branches based on validated measures of coronary flow and can potentially improve the quality of life for patients suffering angina as a result of thoracic side branch coronary steal.

Conflict of Interests

The authors declare that there is no conflict of interests regarding the publication of this paper.

References

[1] R. N. Singh and J. A. Sosa, "Internal mammary artery—coronary artery anastomosis. Influence of the side branches on surgical result," *Journal of Thoracic and Cardiovascular Surgery*, vol. 82, no. 6, pp. 909–914, 1981.

[2] H. B. Barner, J. W. Standeven, and J. Reese, "Twelve-year experience with internal mammary artery for coronary artery bypass," *Journal of Thoracic and Cardiovascular Surgery*, vol. 90, no. 5, pp. 668–675, 1985.

[3] E. P. Bauer, M. C. Bino, L. K. von Segesser, A. Laske, and M. I. Turina, "Internal mammary artery anomalies," *Thoracic and Cardiovascular Surgeon*, vol. 38, no. 5, pp. 312–315, 1990.

[4] M. D. Eisenhauer, D. M. Mego, and P. A. Cambier, "Coronary steal by IMA bypass graft side-branches: a novel therapeutic use of a new detachable embolization coil," *Catheterization and Cardiovascular Diagnosis*, vol. 45, no. 3, pp. 301–306, 1998.

[5] G. J. Mishkel and R. Willinsky, "Combined PTCA and microcoil embolization of a left internal mammary artery graft," *Catheterization and Cardiovascular Diagnosis*, vol. 27, no. 2, pp. 141–146, 1992.

[6] C. Schmid, B. Heublein, S. Reichelt, and H. G. Borst, "Steal phenomenon caused by a parallel branch of the internal mammary artery," *The Annals of Thoracic Surgery*, vol. 50, no. 3, pp. 463–464, 1990.

[7] A. D. Abhyankar, A. S. Mitchell, and L. Bernstein, "Lack of evidence for improvement in internal mammary graft flow by occlusion of side branch," *Catheterization and Cardiovascular Diagnosis*, vol. 42, no. 3, pp. 291–293, 1997.

[8] E. Sbarouni, L. Corr, and A. Fenech, "Microcoil embolization of large intercostal branches of internal mammary artery grafts," *Catheterization and Cardiovascular Diagnosis*, vol. 31, no. 4, pp. 334–336, 1994.

[9] R. W. Ayres, C.-T. Lu, K. H. Benzuly, G. A. Hill, and J. D. Rossen, "Transcatheter embolization of an internal mammary artery bypass graft sidebranch causing coronary steal syndrome," *Catheterization and Cardiovascular Diagnosis*, vol. 31, no. 4, pp. 301–303, 1994.

[10] M. S. Firstenberg, G. Guy, C. Bush, and S. V. Raman, "Impaired myocardial perfusion from persistent mammary side branches: a role for functional imaging and embolization," *Cardiology Research and Practice*, vol. 2010, Article ID 203459, 2 pages, 2010.

[11] E. Chalvatzoulis, O. Ananiadou, A. Madesis, T. Christoforidis, V. Katsaridis, and G. Drossos, "Unligated left internal mammary artery side branch resulting in coronary artery steal syndrome," *Journal of Cardiac Surgery*, vol. 26, no. 5, pp. 487–490, 2011.

[12] M. J. Kern, "Mammary side branch steal: is this a real or even clinically important phenomenon?" *The Annals of Thoracic Surgery*, vol. 66, no. 6, pp. 1873–1875, 1998.

[13] T. Ivert, K. Huttunen, C. Landou, and V. O. Bjork, "Angiographic studies of internal mammary artery grafts 11 years after coronary artery bypass grafting," *Journal of Thoracic and Cardiovascular Surgery*, vol. 96, no. 1, pp. 1–12, 1988.

[14] D. R. Lakkireddy, T. J. Lanspa, N. J. Mehta, H. L. Korlakunta, and I. A. Khan, "Internal mammary artery steal syndrome secondary to an anomalous lateral branch," *International Journal of Cardiology*, vol. 101, no. 2, pp. 319–322, 2005.

[15] R. Luise, G. Teodori, G. Di Giammarco et al., "Persistence of mammary artery branches and blood supply to the left anterior descending artery," *Annals of Thoracic Surgery*, vol. 63, no. 6, pp. 1759–1764, 1997.

[16] O. J. J. Guzon, K. Klatte, A. Moyer, S. Khoukaz, and M. J. Kern, "Fallacy of thoracic side-branch steal from the internal mammary artery: analysis of left internal mammary artery coronary flow during thoracic side-branch occlusion with pharmacologic and exercise-induced hyperemia," *Catheterization and Cardiovascular Interventions*, vol. 61, no. 1, pp. 20–28, 2004.

[17] M. J. Kern, R. G. Bach, T. J. Donohue, E. A. Caracciolo, T. Wolford, and F. V. Aguirre, "Part XIII: role of large pectoralis branch artery in flow through a patent left internal mammary artery conduit," *Catheterization and Cardiovascular Diagnosis*, vol. 34, no. 3, pp. 240–244, 1995.

[18] G. Morocutti, D. Gasparini, L. Spedicato et al., "Functional evaluation of steal by unligated first intercostal branch before transcatheter embolization in recurrent angina after a LIMA-LAD graft," *Catheterization and Cardiovascular Interventions*, vol. 56, no. 3, pp. 373–376, 2002.

[19] H. Yorgun, U. Canpolat, E. B. Kaya, B. Çil, K. Aytemir, and A. Oto, "The use of Amplatzer Vascular Plug® to treat coronary steal due to unligated thoracic side branch of left internal mammary artery: four year follow-up results," *Cardiology Journal*, vol. 19, no. 2, pp. 197–200, 2012.

31

Spontaneous Coronary Dissection: "Live Flash" Optical Coherence Tomography Guided Angioplasty

Angela Pimenta Bento, Renato Gil dos Santos Pinto Fernandes, David Cintra Henriques Silva Neves, Lino Manuel Ribeiro Patrício, and José Eduardo Chambel de Aguiar

Hospital do Espirito Santo, Largo Senhor da Pobreza, 7000-811 Évora, Portugal

Correspondence should be addressed to David Cintra Henriques Silva Neves; dcneves25@hotmail.com

Academic Editor: Assad Movahed

Optical Coherence tomography (OCT) is a light-based imaging modality which shows tremendous potential in the setting of coronary imaging. Spontaneous coronary artery dissection (SCAD) is an infrequent cause of acute coronary syndrome (ACS). The diagnosis of SCAD is made mainly with invasive coronary angiography, although adjunctive imaging modalities such as computed tomography angiography, IVUS, and OCT may increase the diagnostic yield. The authors describe a clinical case of a young woman admitted with the diagnosis of ACS. The ACS was caused by SCAD detected in the coronary angiography and the angioplasty was guided by OCT. OCT use in the setting of SCAD has been already described and the true innovation in this case was this unique use of OCT. The guidance of angioplasty with live and short images was very useful as it allowed clearly identifying the position of the guidewires at any given moment without the use of prohibitive amounts of contrast.

1. Introduction

Optical Coherence tomography (OCT) is a light-based imaging modality which shows tremendous potential in the setting of coronary imaging. Compared to intravascular ultrasound (IVUS), OCT has a tenfold higher image resolution. It has the ability to characterize the structure and extent of coronary disease with unprecedented detail as the various components of atherosclerotic plaques have different properties. In daily practice OCT is useful in guiding complex interventions. Image acquisition has some particularities because blood must be displaced during OCT imaging. In fact OCT images are obtained and recorded as the coronary artery is flushed with contrast and the catheter-imaging tip is pulled back (usually at 20 mm/s). Spontaneous coronary artery dissection (SCAD) is an infrequent cause of acute coronary syndrome (ACS) typically affecting a younger, otherwise healthy population. The population-based incidence of SCAD is unknown. Retrospective registry studies have reported SCAD detection in 0.07% to 1.1% of all coronary angiograms performed.

Apparently there is a female preponderance and an association with peripartum or postpartum status. Other identified SCAD associations include connective tissue disorders, vasculitis, polycystic kidney disease, and exercise, suggesting an underlying vascular predisposition in some, although a unifying structural vessel wall abnormality has not yet been identified [1, 2]. The diagnosis of SCAD is made mainly with invasive coronary angiography, although adjunctive imaging modalities such as computed tomography angiography, IVUS, and OCT may increase the diagnostic yield [3]. OCT provides unique insights on the most relevant morphologic features of the condition including entry tear, intimomedial flap, double-lumen morphology, intramural hematoma, and associated thrombus [4]. The optimal treatment strategy for acute SCAD presentation remains undetermined and may vary according to the type and severity of presentation. Reports have demonstrated favorable outcomes with conservative management (with documented angiographic resolution), fibrinolysis, percutaneous coronary intervention (PCI), and coronary artery bypass grafting (CABG). Regardless of

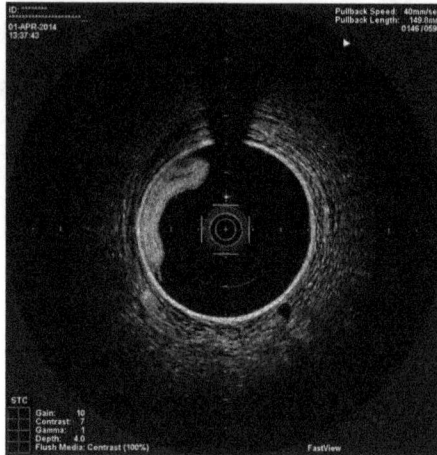

FIGURE 1: OCT image showing the guidewire in the false lumen as the true lumen is crushed against the vessel wall.

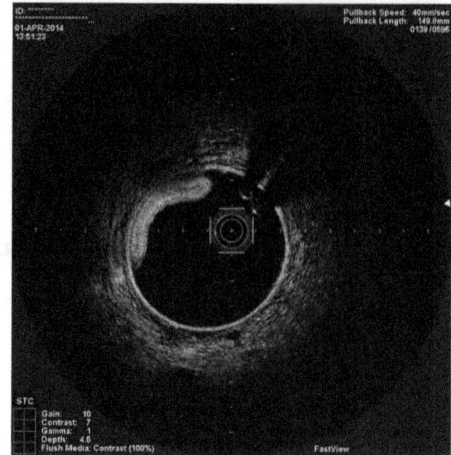

FIGURE 2: OCT image showing two guidewires in the false lumen.

initial treatment strategy, in-hospital and early outcomes have in general been reported to be favorable.

2. Case Report

A 41-year-old female with obesity and polycystic kidney disease is referred to the cath lab after an episode of chest pain with troponin elevation one week after primary PCI in the context of inferior acute myocardial infarction with ST elevation. Angiography at the time revealed a balanced-dominant circulation, with TIMI flow 3 in the right coronary artery (RCA) without stenotic lesions and a suboclusive lesion in a small posterolateral branch (PLB) from the circumflex artery which was considered to be the culprit lesion. Balloon angioplasty was performed with good final result and TIMI 3 flow.

In the present episode angiography showed persistent good result of the previous PCI, and total occlusion of the proximal RCA, that was suspected to be caused by spontaneous dissection because of the presence of haziness at the site of the occlusion and disappearance of several acute marginal branches as compared with the previous exam. We then decided to perform OCT (Terumo Lunawave® OFDI system) that clearly revealed the double-lumen morphology and also that the guidewire was in the false lumen (Figures 1 and 2). We then proceeded to angioplasty under OCT guidance. With live OCT images, without recording an actual pullback, we used small flushes of contrast until we were able to confirm that the guidewire was on the true lumen (Figures 3(a) and 3(b)). The OCT could also identify entry tear very clearly (Figure 4). Once the true lumen was secured, we proceeded to angioplasty with a drug-eluting stent sealing the entry tear in the proximal right coronary artery (Figure 5). There was final TIMI 3 flow, and the acute marginal branches were again visible, but there was a narrowing in the distal vessel where the false lumen was still visible but showing signs of thrombosis (Figure 6). To avoid making a full metal jacket, we decided to accept this result and perform

a control angiography one month later. After one uneventful month, follow-up angiography revealed persistence of a large dissection that extended to the distal vessel. There was an important compromise of the true lumen by the false lumen. Given the previous STEMI presentation and the negative angiographic evolution within a month, we carried out an OCT that confirmed the dissection and showed that the guidewire was now in the true lumen (Figures 7(a) and 7(b)). In this setting, we decided to seal the dissection with implantation of two more drug-eluting stents in the mid and distal RCA to guarantee the long-term patency of the vessel (Figure 8). There was residual dissection in the very distal segment, which was a small vessel.

3. Discussion

Diagnosis and management of SCAD is very challenging. However, an accurate and early diagnosis remains of paramount importance. There are few data concerning the utilization and value of OCT in this rare disease. In the case cited before, OCT was able to readily visualize the double-lumen morphology characteristic of this entity and to identify the entry tear and the circumferential nature and longitudinal extent of the disease. The compromise of the true lumen and the distribution of the false lumen were also clearly visualized. The low profile (catheter crossing profile: 2,6 Fr) and higher resolution (frame rate: 160 fps) of OCT were very useful in this case as they allowed obtaining high quality images of long segments of the artery. OCT is not, however, without potential harm. In a situation of a SCAD, it can further propagate the dissection and/or intimal tear, due to brisk intracoronary flow changes, so its use must take into account the potential benefit versus potential harm. Careful contrast injection speed is of paramount importance. In this case OCT was revealed to be particularly useful, since not only did it make it possible to correctly identify the dissection and intimal tear, it also made correct true lumen wiring possible, with live imaging during wire manipulation with a stationary OCT catheter. OCT usefulness in the setting

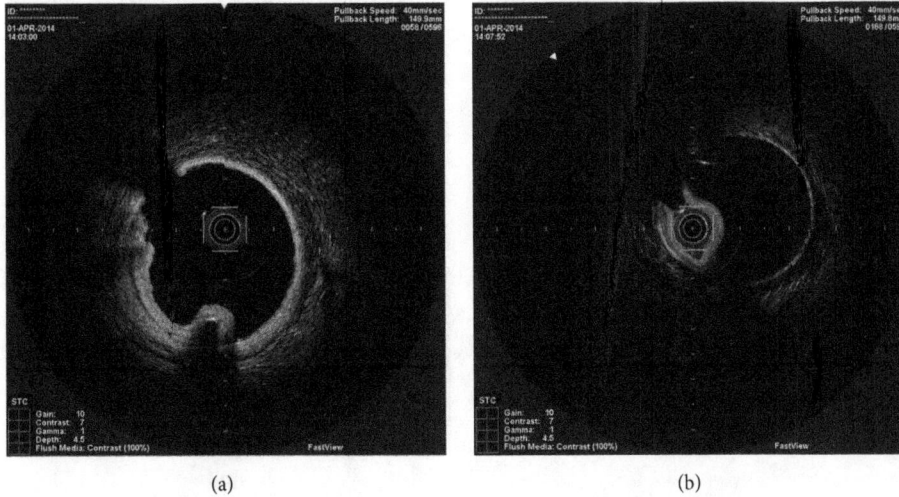

(a)

(b)

FIGURE 3: OCT image showing one guidewire in the false lumen and the other in the true lumen.

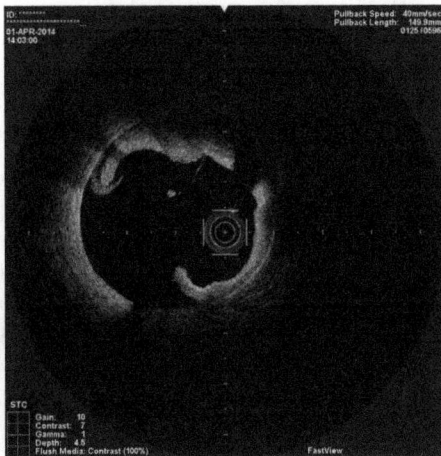

FIGURE 4: OCT image showing the entry tear of the spontaneous dissection.

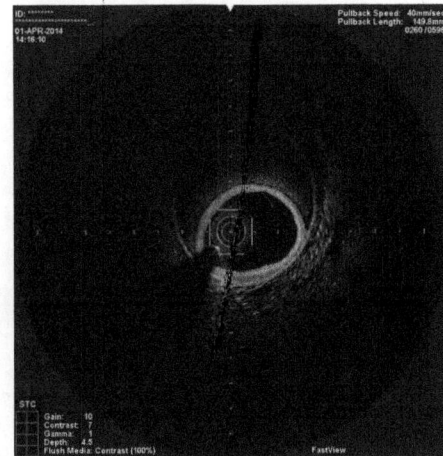

FIGURE 6: OCT image showing the guidewire in the true lumen and the false lumen with signs of thrombosis in process.

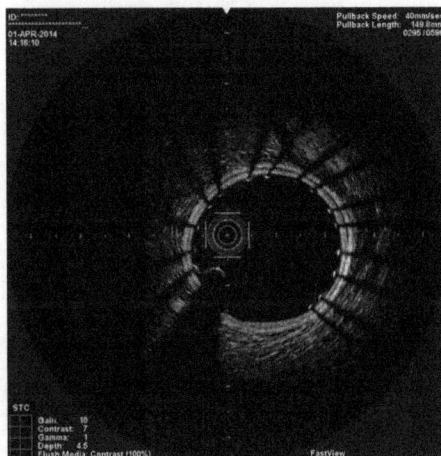

FIGURE 5: OCT performed after stent implantation showing good apposition.

of SCAD has already been reported, and the technique we describe in this case represents an innovation that may become even more interesting in the future, with OCT technical development. This technique opens a promising field for software development; for example, we think that it will be very useful to be able to also record images with a stationary OCT catheter and not only those obtained in the automated pullback with complete flush of the coronary artery. Another potential benefit of this technique (OCT) in SCAD setting is the possibility of doing 3D OCT online to improve the capability of identifying the entry tear. Regarding the angioplasty per se, we would have used bioresorbable scaffolds, were they available in our cath lab at the time of this procedure. In a more detailed analysis of the OCT images after the final procedure we realized that the entry tear was located behind the distal part of the previously implanted stent (Figure 7(b)). We now wonder if we could have sealed the dissection with just a balloon after dilatation.

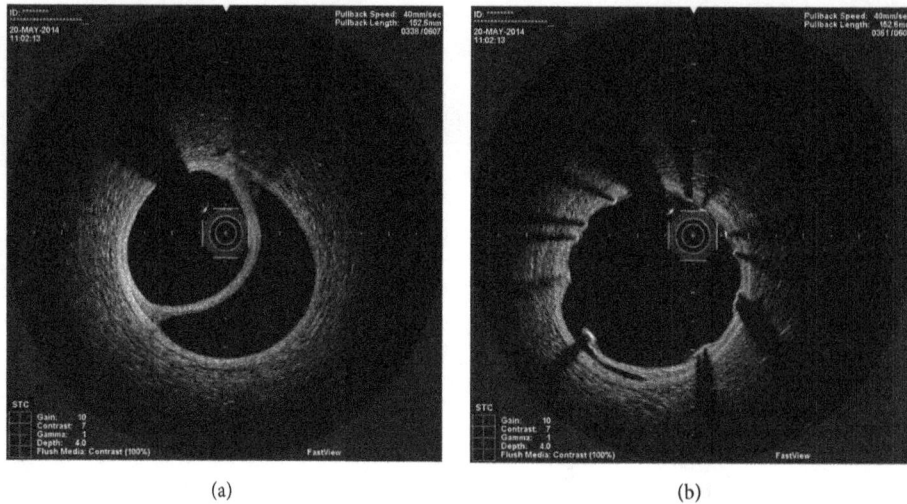

(a)   (b)

FIGURE 7: OCT performed one month after the stent angioplasty, showing the maintenance of the dissection. (a) shows clearly that the guide wire is in the true lumen.

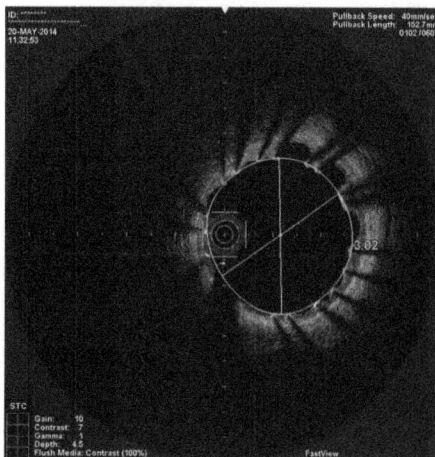

FIGURE 8: OCT performed after implantation of additional stents in medial and distal RCA and the balloon after dilatation.

4. Conclusion

Spontaneous coronary artery disease is an intriguing entity, in which a conservative approach seems to be the best option whenever possible, due to procedural complications. OCT can be decisive for correct diagnosis, planning, treatment, and optimization of PCI in SCAD.

Conflict of Interests

The authors declare that there is no conflict of interests regarding the publication of this paper.

References

[1] M. S. Tweet, S. N. Hayes, S. R. Pitta et al., "Clinical features, management, and prognosis of spontaneous coronary artery dissection," *Circulation*, vol. 126, no. 5, pp. 579–588, 2012.

[2] A. Yip and J. Saw, "Spontaneous coronary artery dissection—a review," *Cardiovascular Diagnosis and Therapy*, vol. 5, no. 1, pp. 37–48, 2015.

[3] F. Alfonso, M. Paulo, V. Lennie et al., "Spontaneous coronary artery dissection: long-term follow-up of a large series of patients prospectively managed with a 'conservative' therapeutic strategy," *JACC: Cardiovascular Interventions*, vol. 5, no. 10, pp. 1062–1070, 2012.

[4] C. Franco, L. Eng, and J. Saw, "Optical coherence tomography in the diagnosis and management of spontaneous coronary artery dissection," *Interventional Cardiology Clinics*, vol. 4, no. 3, pp. 309–320, 2015.

32

Pneumopericarditis: A Case of Acute Chest Pain with ST Segment Elevation

Erwin E. Argueta,[1] **Menfil A. Orellana-Barrios,**[1] **Teerapat Nantsupawat,**[2] **Alvaro Rosales,**[2] **and Scott Shurmur**[2]

[1]*Department of Internal Medicine, Texas Tech University, Lubbock, TX 79430, USA*
[2]*Department of Cardiovascular Medicine, Texas Tech University, Lubbock, TX 79430, USA*

Correspondence should be addressed to Menfil A. Orellana-Barrios; menfil@gmail.com

Academic Editor: Takatoshi Kasai

Pneumopericarditis describes a clinical scenario where fluid and air are found within the pericardial space. Although infrequent, pneumopericarditis should be considered in patients presenting with acute chest pain as a differential diagnosis. This is relevant in patients with history of upper gastrointestinal (GI) surgery, as this may lead to a fistula communicating the GI tract and the pericardium. We report a 42-year-old man with history of numerous surgical interventions related to a Nissen fundoplication that presented with acute chest pain and inferior lead ST segment elevations. Emergent coronary angiography was negative for coronary vascular disease but fluoroscopy revealed air in the pericardial space. Subsequent radiographic studies helped confirm air in the pericardial space with a fistulous communication to the stomach. Ultimate treatment for this defect was surgical closure.

1. Introduction

Pneumopericarditis involves a pericarditis clinical presentation, where fluid and air are found within the pericardial space. There are many reported cases of patients with a pneumopericardium, with only a few developing a classical pericarditis syndrome. This last condition has been described most frequently secondary to cardiovascular surgery, trauma, and gastrointestinal (GI) cancer. It may also result from abdominal surgery related complications, where the GI tract forms a fistula to the pericardial space. The latter is also known as a gastropericardial or esophagopericardial fistula depending on the organ involved. The pneumopericarditis clinical presentation varies from acute chest pain and hemodynamic compromise to a subacute and even chronic pericarditis picture. We present a patient with acute pneumopericarditis that had history of a Nissen fundoplication 14 years before with multiple postoperative complications requiring several interventions.

2. Case Presentation

A 42-year-old man, active smoker, presented to the emergency room complaining of anterior left side chest pain that started approximately three hours before arrival. He woke up around 3:00 am with sudden onset severe crushing chest pain that was constant. It was associated with shortness of breath and diaphoresis. His medical history was significant for gastroesophageal reflux, hypertension, major depression, and chronic left shoulder pain diagnosed as impingement syndrome. Family history was noncontributory. He had an extensive past surgical history, which included a laparoscopic Nissen fundoplication at age 25 due to severe gastroesophageal reflux disease and associated esophagitis. Several months after this procedure, he required two open revisions of the Nissen procedure. The first was due to a hiatal hernia, and the second was due to a diaphragmatic rupture requiring diaphragm repair with prosthetic material. The patient developed a subdiaphragmatic abscess at age 30 that required antibiotics and diaphragmatic surgery where the prosthetic

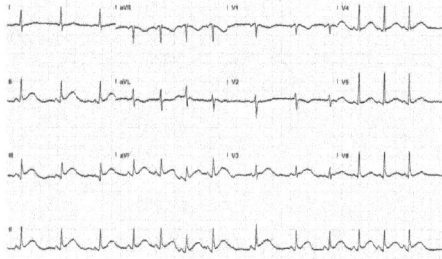

Figure 1: Admission EKG. ST segment elevations are noted in leads II, III, and aVF.

material was removed. In addition, at age 35 years, he had a spinal cord stimulator inserted, as treatment for chronic left shoulder and epigastric pain associated with persistent nausea and dry heaves. Three months prior to his current visit he had a diagnostic arthroscopy due to persistent left shoulder pain.

On physical exam, he was pale and in distress. Vital sings included an oral temperature of 97.6°F, blood pressure of 116/66 mmHg, heart rate of 45 beats per minute, respiratory rate of 18 breaths per minute, and oxygen saturation of 94% on room air. No rub or murmur was auscultated on initial cardiac examination. Lungs were clear to auscultation. The electrocardiogram (EKG) was significant for ST segment elevations in leads II, III, and aVF (Figure 1). TIMI risk score was 2 (based on chest pain and EKG changes). The patient was immediately taken for coronary angiography, which showed no coronary artery obstruction. However, a halo around the cardiac silhouette suggestive of air was noted (Figure 2). Laboratory results came back during the procedure and were significant for a white blood cell count of 15.42 K/μL (88.5% neutrophils), creatinine of 1.4 mg/dL, and glucose of 172 mg/dL. Troponin T was negative and the rest of the laboratory values were noncontributory.

A chest X-ray obtained after the angiogram also showed this halo around the left cardiac border suggesting a pneumopericardium (Figure 3). A chest computer tomography confirmed the diagnosis (Figure 4). During the following 12 hours while additional diagnostic workup was performed, the patient developed signs consistent with acute pericarditis. This included a mill wheel type murmur and diffuse ST segment elevations on the EKG (Figure 5). No pulsus paradoxus was detected. A transthoracic echocardiogram performed had technically limited images but was suggestive of a preserved ejection fraction and a pericardial effusion. A Gastrografin esophagogram suggested a pericardial fistula located at the level of the greater curvature of the cardia (Figure 6). After diagnostic workup, the patient was started on empiric antibiotic coverage with meropenem and was taken to the operating room. There he had a pericardial window and upper gastrointestinal endoscopy. About 300 mL of serosanguineous fluid was drained from the pericardial space. During endoscopy, an ulcer was noted at the level of the cardia with no obvious communication to the pericardium. Due to the high suspicion of a communication between these two structures, final treatment consisted in application of

a fibrin sealant to the ulcer. Drains were also left in the pericardium and removed later. A pericardial biopsy was consistent with fibrinopurulent pericarditis and a biopsy obtained from the gastric ulcer was negative for *H. pylori* and malignancy. The patient tolerated the surgery well and no organisms were recovered from the cultures obtained from the pericardial fluid.

3. Discussion

There have been numerous pneumopericardium case reports secondary to various etiologies, with fistula formation occurring in up to 30% of cases [1, 2]. From this last group, those that arise from the GI tract are associated with gastroesophageal trauma and/or surgery. They can occur after trauma or during the first year after surgery or years after [3, 4]. These fistulae occur secondary to complications from esophagectomy with gastric tube repair, gastric bypass surgery, and slipped Nissen fundoplications. They are found less frequently secondary to spontaneous gastric ulcer disease or gastrointestinal cancer [5–8]. There has also been an association between subphrenic abscesses with repeated gastroesophageal surgeries and fistula development [9]. Out of the patients with pneumopericardium secondary to fistula formation, the minority will develop an acute pericarditis clinical picture.

The common symptoms described by patients with pneumopericardium are chest pain and dyspnea. Left shoulder pain, or referred pain, may also be present and arises from diaphragmatic and/or pericardial irritation [10–12]. Of note, in some cases shoulder pain is chronic and persistent. On physical examination a classic mill wheel murmur, or "bruit de moulin," can be present, which is a metallic tinkling rub found in patients with pneumopericardium [1]. Diagnosis is based on imaging studies which include upright chest X-rays, echocardiography, and chest computed tomography. GI imaging studies, like contrast esophagography, may show a fistula to the pericardium. Electrocardiographic findings can vary from those consistent with pericarditis to those with localized ST segment elevations. For example, much like in the case presented, these electrocardiographic findings have led to angiography and thrombolysis (Table 1) [2, 8, 9, 13, 14]. Treatment includes conservative management, described in few cases, and surgical intervention with fistula correction. Cases with conservative management have a worse prognosis, with the mortality being as high as 85% [8, 15]. A case has been described where the fistula was unrepaired and the patient had recurrent disease five years later [16].

In our case, the patient may have had chronic diaphragmatic irritation leading to his chronic left shoulder pain. It is difficult to say over what period of time he started to have pericardial irritation with a fistula formation. A possible explanation for the absence of clinical signs of tamponade is that the fistula could have a bidirectional flow thereby impeding higher pressure buildup in the pericardial space over time. In this sense, a possible acute decompensation with increase in symptoms may have been due to changes in the fistula flow or gastric content/pressure leading to his acute symptoms and hospital visit. This would also be

TABLE 1: Pneumopericardium case reports where EKG ST segment elevations were found during initial presentation.

Author	Gender	Age	Risk factor	Chest X-ray[*]	ST elevation[†]	Intervention
Kato et al. [8]	M	65	Esophagectomy	Yes	V5-V6	None
Bruhl et al. [2]	M	63	Spontaneous	No	I, II, aVL, V3–V6	Angiogram
Ruano Poblador et al. [15]	M	56	Billroth I gastrectomy	Yes	Lower, lateral	None
Gagné et al. [13]	F	43	Roux-y-gastric bypass	Yes	I, II, aVL	Angiogram
Sihvo et al. [9]	M	54	Nissen Fundoplication	No	Inferior	Thrombolysis
Grandhi et al. [14]	M	29	Diaphragmatic hernia repair	Yes	V1, V2	None

[*]Chest X-rays usually obtained when there were other exam findings such as fever.
[†]Per case report description.

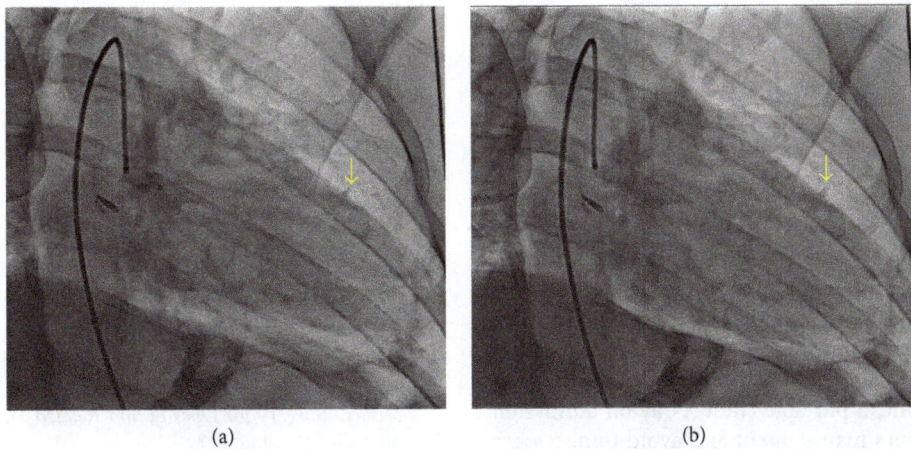

(a)   (b)

FIGURE 2: Left ventriculogram. Air around the cardiac borders noted in systole (a) and diastole (b).

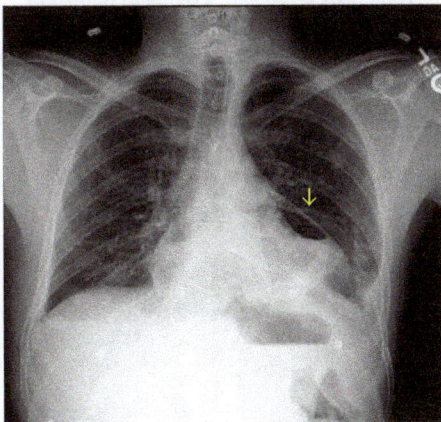

FIGURE 3: PA chest X-ray. A halo is visible around the left cardiac border.

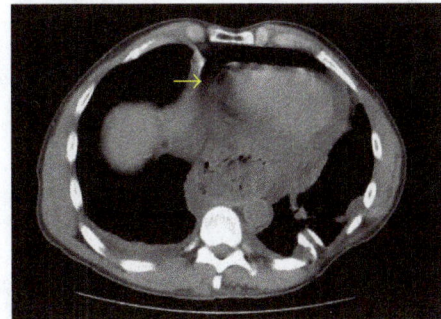

FIGURE 4: Chest computed tomography. There is an air fluid level in the pericardial space.

supported by his clinical course while in the hospital. We present electrocardiographic changes that were present after admission in Figure 5. Other cases where EKG changes were not suggestive of pericarditis are shown in Table 1. In patients with risk factors for developing gastropericardial fistulas, chest pain, and ST segment elevations we consider that a chest X-ray performed during the initial assessment should be considered.

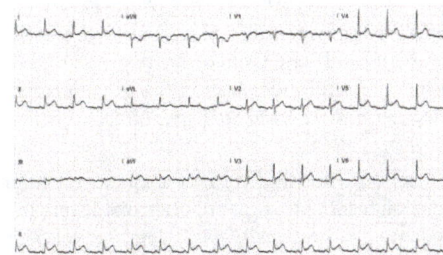

FIGURE 5: EKG 24 hrs after admission. Diffuse ST segment elevation and slight PR segment depression.

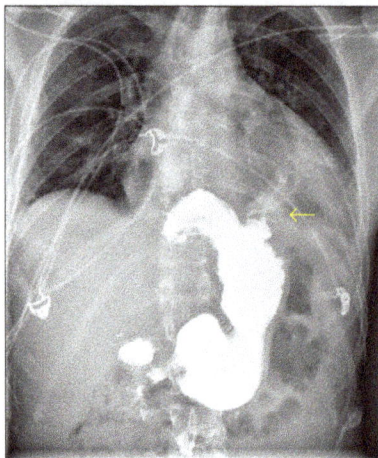

FIGURE 6: Contrast esophagogram. There is evidence that suggests a fistula located at the level of the cardia.

In conclusion, pneumopericarditis should be considered as a differential diagnosis for acute chest pain in the patient with extensive gastroesophageal surgery. A key clinical finding such as chronic left shoulder pain and history of multiple GI interventions should heighten the suspicion for a possible gastropericardial fistula. In addition, associated EKG findings should be evaluated with caution in this clinical setting. In cases such as this one, a portable chest X-ray on admission may change a patient's management and avoid unnecessary interventions.

Conflict of Interests

All authors have no conflict of interests to disclose.

References

[1] L. Brander, D. Ramsay, D. Dreier, M. Peter, and R. Graeni, "Continuous left hemidiaphragm sign revisited: a case of spontaneous pneumopericardium and literature review," *Heart*, vol. 88, no. 4, article e5, 2002.

[2] S. R. Bruhl, K. Lanka, and W. R. Colyer Jr., "Pneumopericardial tamponade resulting from a spontaneous gastropericardial fistula," *Catheterization and Cardiovascular Interventions*, vol. 73, no. 5, pp. 666–668, 2009.

[3] S. Murthy, J. Looney, and M. T. Jaklitsch, "Gastropericardial fistula after laparoscopic surgery for reflux disease," *The New England Journal of Medicine*, vol. 346, no. 5, pp. 328–332, 2002.

[4] F. Farjah, C. B. Komanapalli, I. Shen, and M. S. Sukumar, "Gastropericardial fistula and *Candida kruzei* pericarditis following laparoscopic nissen fundoplication (gastropericardial fistula)," *Thoracic and Cardiovascular Surgeon*, vol. 53, no. 6, pp. 365–367, 2005.

[5] J. J. Reicher and R. Mindelzun, "Case report: benign gastric ulcer erosion leading to a gastropericardial fistula in a patient with no known risk factors," *Clinical Imaging*, vol. 38, no. 4, pp. 547–549, 2014.

[6] F. A. Marasca, G. R. T. Alves, R. C. Pires, T. C. Dallasta, R. V. De Andrade Silva, and J. R. Missel Corrêa, "Gastropericardial fistula," *Annals of Thoracic Surgery*, vol. 95, no. 6, article e161, 2013.

[7] D. Rodriguez and M. T. Heller, "Pneumopericardium due to gastropericardial fistula: a delayed, rare complication of gastric bypass surgery," *Emergency Radiology*, vol. 20, no. 4, pp. 333–335, 2013.

[8] T. Kato, T. Mori, and K. Niibori, "A case of gastropericardial fistula of a gastric tube after esophagectomy: a case report and review," *World Journal of Emergency Surgery*, vol. 5, no. 1, article 20, 2010.

[9] E. I. T. Sihvo, J. V. Räsänen, M. Hynninen, T. K. Rantanen, and J. A. Salo, "Gastropericardial fistula, purulent pericarditis, and cardiac tamponade after laparoscopic nissen fundoplication," *Annals of Thoracic Surgery*, vol. 81, no. 1, pp. 356–358, 2006.

[10] W. J. Kim, E. J. Choi, Y.-W. Oh, K. T. Kim, and C. W. Kim, "Gastropericardial fistula-induced pyopneumopericardium after esophagectomy with esophagogastrectomy," *Annals of Thoracic Surgery*, vol. 91, no. 1, pp. e10–e11, 2011.

[11] S. Park, J.-H. Kim, Y. C. Lee, and J. B. Chung, "*Gastropericardial fistula* as a complication in a refractory gastric ulcer after esophagogastrostomy with gastric pull-up," *Yonsei Medical Journal*, vol. 51, no. 2, pp. 270–272, 2010.

[12] D. Pop, N. Venissac, L. Rami, and J. Mouroux, "Gastropericardial fistula after laparoscopic surgery for gastroesophageal reflux disease," *Journal of Thoracic and Cardiovascular Surgery*, vol. 133, no. 6, pp. 1676–1677, 2007.

[13] D. J. Gagné, P. K. Papasavas, T. Birdas, J. Lamb, and P. F. Caushaj, "Gastropericardial fistula after Roux-en-Y gastric bypass: a case report," *Surgery for Obesity and Related Diseases*, vol. 2, no. 5, pp. 533–535, 2006.

[14] T. M. Grandhi, D. Rawlings, and C. G. Morran, "Gastropericardial fistula: a case report and review of literature," *Emergency Medicine Journal*, vol. 21, no. 5, pp. 644–645, 2004.

[15] A. Ruano Poblador, A. M. Gay Fernández, M. T. García Martínez et al., "Pneumopericardium caused by gastropericardial fistula," *Revista Espanola de Enfermedades Digestivas*, vol. 99, no. 3, pp. 168–171, 2007.

[16] E. L. Servais, B. M. Stiles, J. A. Spector, N. K. Altorki, and J. L. Port, "Gastropericardial fistula: a late complication of esophageal reconstruction," *Annals of Thoracic Surgery*, vol. 93, no. 5, pp. 1729–1731, 2012.

33

Early Cardiac Tamponade in a Patient with Postsurgical Hypothyroidism

Archana Sinha,[1] **Sri Lakshmi Hyndavi Yeruva,**[2] **Rajan Kumar,**[1] **and Bryan H. Curry**[3]

[1]*Division of Cardiology, Saint Luke's University Health Network, Bethlehem, PA 18015, USA*
[2]*Division of Hematology and Oncology, Howard University Hospital, 2041 Georgia Avenue NW, Washington, DC 20060, USA*
[3]*Division of Cardiology, Howard University Hospital, 2041 Georgia Avenue NW, Washington, DC 20060, USA*

Correspondence should be addressed to Archana Sinha; sinha.archana7@gmail.com

Academic Editor: Gerard Devlin

Pericardial effusion is a common cardiac manifestation of hypothyroidism, but effusion resulting in cardiac tamponade is extremely rare. We present a case of a 56-year-old African American woman with slurred speech and altered mental status that was initially suspected to have stroke. Her chest X-ray revealed cardiomegaly and subsequent echocardiogram showed a large pericardial effusion with echocardiographic evidence of cardiac tamponade. Clinically, patient did not have pulsus paradoxus or hypotension. Further questioning revealed a history of total surgical thyroidectomy and noncompliance with thyroid replacement therapy. Pericardiocentesis was performed promptly and thyroxine replacement therapy was started. Thereafter, her mental status improved significantly. The management of pericardial effusion associated with hypothyroidism varies depending on size of effusion and hemodynamic stability of the patient. The management strategy ranges from conservative management with close monitoring and thyroxine replacement to pericardiocentesis or creation of a pericardial window.

1. Introduction

Pericardial effusion may be caused by acute pericarditis, tumor, uremia, hypothyroidism, trauma, cardiac surgery, or other inflammatory conditions. Pericardial effusion is a known complication of hypothyroidism with the incidence ranging from 3–6% in mild cases of hypothyroidism to 30%–80% in severe hypothyroidism [1]. Cardiac tamponade secondary to hypothyroidism is rare as the fluid accumulates slowly, allowing for pericardial sac distension [2]. Even a small pericardial effusion can cause clinically significant tamponade, if it accumulates rapidly. It is important to suspect tamponade when patients have hemodynamic compromise regardless of the amount of pericardial effusion present. We report here a case of early cardiac tamponade, due to untreated postsurgical hypothyroidism.

2. Case Report

A 56-year-old African American woman with past medical history of hypothyroidism, hypertension, dyslipidemia, seizures, schizophrenia, and mood disorders was brought to emergency room by her estranged son for slurred speech and altered mental status. On further questioning, patient revealed a history of total surgical thyroidectomy done about ten years ago and admitted noncompliance with all her medications including thyroid replacement therapy for the last 4 years. She did not report any symptoms of constipation, cold intolerance, or weight gain. Her family history was unknown, social history was negative for any substance abuse, and she stayed alone.

Her vitals on presentation were temperature of 98°F, blood pressure of 167/90 mmHg, pulse rate of 91 beats per min, and respiratory rate of 18 per min. Her physical exam showed dry skin, brittle hair, jugular venous distention, pulsus paradoxus < 10 mm of Hg, distant and muffled heart sounds, and delayed relaxation of ankle jerk. She also had slow slurred speech and slow mentation. In the emergency room, CT scan and MRI of head were negative for acute stroke. Her anteroposterior chest radiograph revealed massive cardiomegaly (Figure 1(a)). 12-lead Electrocardiography

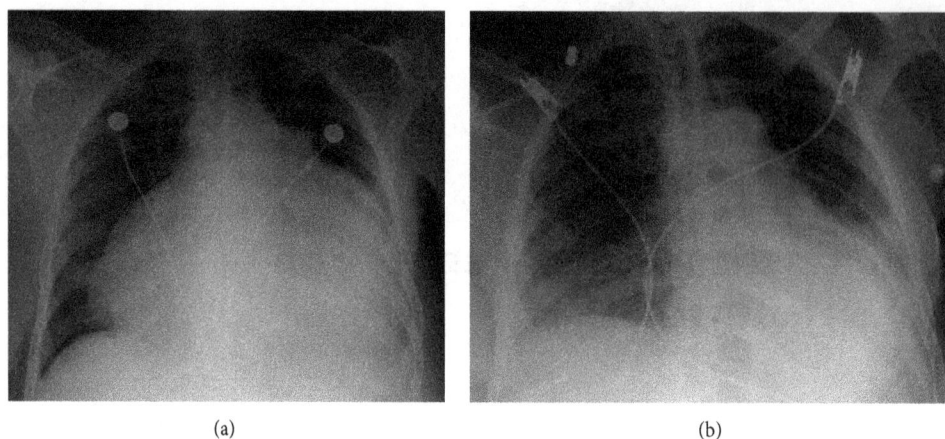

(a)   (b)

FIGURE 1: CXR. (a) Classical "water bottle" shaped cardiomegaly due to pericardial fluid. (b) Resolution of cardiomegaly after pericardial fluid drainage.

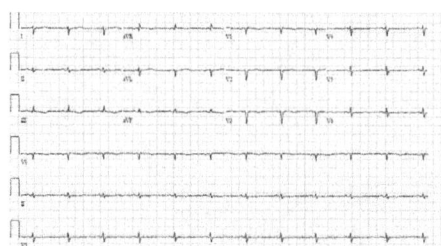

FIGURE 2: EKG. Low voltage QRS complexes.

TABLE 1: Pericardial fluid analysis.

Pericardial fluid	Our patient	Normal
Appearance	Hazy	Clear
Color	Golden yellow	Pale yellow
Glucose	80 mg/dL	106–159 mg/dL
LDH	150 mg/dL	276–517 mg/dL
Total protein	5.5 g/dL	2.8–4.8 g/dL
WBC	51	0–5
Polymorphs	73	None
RBC	101	0–20
Mesothelial cells	Few	None
Adenosine deaminase	4.7	<9.2
Specific gravity	1.035	—
Cholesterol	68 mg/dL	<55 mg/dL

(EKG) revealed low voltage QRS complexes in all leads (Figure 2). A transthoracic echocardiogram was performed which showed ejection fraction of 55–60% and large (>3 cm) pericardial effusion with evidence of diastolic collapse of the right heart chambers (Figures 3(a) and 3(b)) and a significant respiratory variation of mitral and tricuspid inflow velocities. Cardiology consult was placed for further management.

Her blood chemistry panel was normal except for abnormal thyroid profile reflecting severe hypothyroidism with thyroid stimulating hormone of 89.33 mIU/L, total thyroxine (T4) of 5.15 nmol/L, and total triiodothyronine (T3) of 0.46 nmol/L. Her erythrocyte sedimentation rate (ESR) was 104 mm/Hg. She was started on levothyroxine 75 mcg, with plan to up-titrate it to optimal dose depending on clinical tolerability.

Transthoracic echocardiogram guided pericardiocentesis via the subxiphoid approach was performed. Samples of the hazy, yellow pericardial fluid were sent for biochemistry, cytology, microscopy, and sensitivity testing. Therapeutic pericardiocentesis was performed and pericardial drain was left in place. Patient's hemodynamic status was continuously monitored, during and after the pericardiocentesis. Lim et al. have shown association of fatal postprocedural "pericardial decompression syndrome" with pericardiocentesis [3]. Three liters of hazy, yellowish/"gold paint" pericardial fluid was drained (Figure 4).

The patient's vital signs remained stable and a repeat chest X ray (Figure 1(b)) and echocardiogram revealed that the pericardial effusion had decreased considerably in size. Pericardial fluid analysis was performed (Table 1). Pericardial fluid bacterial and fungal cultures were negative. Her creatinine phosphokinase was 527 U/L and troponin I was negative. Her ANA titre was positive at 1 : 1280 with centromere pattern. ANA titer can be false positive in 5% of tested women and elderly and can also be high in patients with thyroid disease. Rheumatoid factor, ds DNA, SM, RNP, and nucleosomal chromatin antibody were all negative. We ruled out all other possible etiologies of pericardial effusion. Hypothyroidism was the only abnormality that could explain the large pericardial effusion and subsequent early tamponade in our patient. She was started on thyroxine supplementation, which improved her mental status and speech considerably. She was discharged with outpatient follow-up with endocrinology and cardiology.

3. Discussion

The British physician C. Parry in 1785 was the first to report the deleterious effect of excess thyroid hormone on heart,

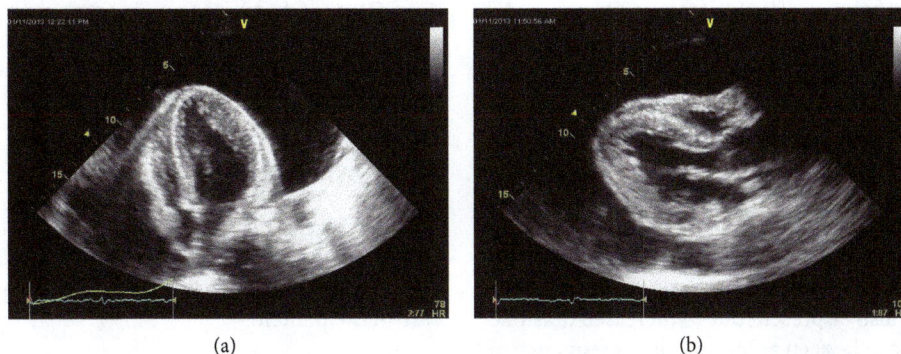

(a)   (b)

FIGURE 3: Echocardiogram. (a) Apical four-chamber view showing "swinging heart" and large pericardial effusion, (b) parasternal long axis view showing right ventricular diastolic collapse.

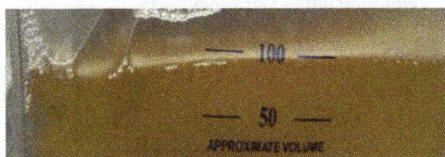

FIGURE 4: "Gold paint effusion" of hypothyroidism.

who described heart enlargement as a consequence of hyperthyroidism [4]. H. Zondeck showed that hypothyroidism could cause cardiac enlargement (pericardial effusion) along with decrease pulsations and low electrocardiographic voltage, which was subsequently called "myxedema heart."

Cardiovascular abnormalities are common in those with abnormal thyroid functions and changes include abnormal cardiac contractility, heart rate, and peripheral vascular resistance [5]. Pericardial effusion can be a common finding in hypothyroidism but an effusion large enough to cause cardiac tamponade is rare with only few reports in English literature [6–11].

The rare occurrence of cardiac tamponade can be attributed to the pericardial distensibility and the slow accumulation of fluid, allowing significant fluid accumulation without hemodynamic compromise. Even though heart failure is unusual in hypothyroidism, it should be differentiated from tamponade because of similar presentations [12]. The volume of pericardial effusion is directly related to the duration and severity of the hypothyroidism but there has been no correlation with thyroid stimulating hormone levels and the existence or severity of the effusions. The factors responsible for development of pericardial effusion in hypothyroidism include increased capillary permeability with efflux of proteins rich fluid and glycosaminoglycans into the pericardial sac decreased lymphatic drainage and high retention of salt and water [13].

The diagnosis of hypothyroidism as the cause of cardiac tamponade in emergent situations at times can be difficult because of its slow onset, nonspecific signs, and symptoms [14].

Pericardial effusions associated with hypothyroidism have an insidious onset and initially present without significant hemodynamic changes; if left untreated, development of effusion into cardiac tamponade can be explained in a sequential manner. Initially there is moderate to large pericardial effusions without tamponade, followed by echocardiographic tamponade without paradoxical pulse and finally when pericardial pressure remains continuously above the intracavitary pressure, overt hemodynamic collapse develops [15]. Our patient had echocardiographic evidence of tamponade but lacked clinical signs of tamponade. This scenario might be present very early in the tamponade physiology. Even though the pericardial pressure transiently exceeds the intracavity pressure, cardiac output may still be maintained owing to the very slow rate of pericardial fluid accumulation.

The usual presenting clinical triad of cardiac tamponade which includes hypotension, distant heart sounds, and jugular vein engorgement, popularly referred to as Beck's triad, may be present or absent. On the contrary, our patient was noted to be hypertensive, which could be explained by profound vasoconstriction, as a result of sympathetic overactivity. Previous studies have shown that subacute to chronic tamponade may present with hypertension in approximately one-third of patients, especially in those with preexisting hypertension and renal failure [16]. The absence of sinus tachycardia in patients diagnosed with cardiac tamponade should arouse strong suspicion of hypothyroidism [17]. Bradycardia can also be seen in cardiac tamponade as a consequence of hypothyroidism. It has been suggested that it can be due to decreased sympathetic activity, but indirect measurements of sympathetic activity have showed it to be elevated. There is some evidence of blunted sympathetic excitatory and tachycardic response to hypotension, and depressed arterial baroreflex, with elevated dependence on the resting sympathetic tone that could explain the presence of bradycardia [18]. Wang et al. studied hypothyroid pericardial effusion and recommended that if heart rate is approximately 80 beats per minute in hypothyroid patients with echocardiographic signs of tamponade, clinical tamponade is evident and possibly warrants emergent drainage [15].

The EKG findings include decreased voltage with electrical alternans, T wave flattening which has been mentioned to be associated with myxedema heart disease [15]. QT prolongation has also been observed in patients with hypothyroidism and tamponade likely secondary to the hypothyroidism. The presence of sinus bradycardia, low QRS voltage, diffuse flat T waves, and long QT has positive predictive value for hypothyroidism [19]. Echocardiogram (M or 2D mode) is the preferred investigation for diagnosis of cardiac tamponade. The findings suggestive of cardiac tamponade on echocardiography include pericardial effusion, diastolic right atrial and right ventricular collapse, inferior vena cava dilation, and loss of respiratory variations and respiratory increase of interventricular dependence. Left ventricle "pseudohypertrophy" can also be present due to increased diastolic wall thickness. This can be seen as an overall consequence of hypothyroidism. Hypothyroidism gives rise to arterial wall stiffness and induces hypertension, which if not treated can produce LV concentric hypertrophy [20, 21].

The management of cardiac tamponade is guided by the hemodynamic status of the patient. Early tamponade with only mild hemodynamic compromise may be treated conservatively. Thyroxine replacement is the mainstay of treatment along with fluid restriction and close observation. In patients with severe hemodynamic compromise needle pericardiocentesis or surgical drainage with creation of a pericardial window is employed. In such individuals, quick removal of pericardial fluid is imperative because there is direct relationship between volume of pericardial fluid and pericardial pressure. Removal of as little as 50 mL of pericardial fluid can produce appreciable hemodynamic and symptomatic improvement. Conscious effort should be made to avoid measures that can decrease venous filling pressures and can negatively affect cardiac output [22]. Echocardiogram guided pericardiocentesis is well tolerated by patients and can be quickly performed even in unstable patients. The success rate is close to 97% and the preferred route of approach is the subxiphoid region [23]. The recurrence of effusion after pericardiocentesis has been observed in the past and this should be anticipated while draining effusion caused by hypothyroidism [24].

4. Conclusion

Our patient did not present with typical symptoms of clinical tamponade and severe hypothyroidism posing clinical dilemma. A high index of suspicion must be maintained for timely diagnosis of cardiac tamponade due to severe hypothyroidism, followed by prompt intervention. All the patients diagnosed with cardiac tamponade without sinus tachycardia or with bradycardia should be worked up for hypothyroidism. The management of cardiac tamponade caused by hypothyroidism is different from other causes of tamponade, cases with mild hemodynamic compromise can be managed conservatively with thyroxine replacement, and those with severe hemodynamic compromise need needle pericardiocentesis or surgical drainage.

Consent

Patient's consent was obtained for the publication.

Conflict of Interests

The authors declare that there is no conflict of interests regarding the publication of this paper.

Acknowledgments

The authors extend their acknowledgement to all the patients who allow them to be part of their lives. They sincerely thank Dr. J. Diggs for his constant support and guidance in taking care of the patient.

References

[1] G. Datillo, S. Crosca, S. Tarvella, F. Marte, and S. Patanè, "Pericardial effusion associated with subclinical hypothyroidism," *International Journal of Cardiology*, vol. 153, no. 3, pp. e47–e50, 2011.

[2] A. Butala, S. Chaudhari, and A. Sacerdote, "Cardiac tamponade as a presenting manifestation of severe hypothyroidism," *BMJ Case Reports*, 2013.

[3] A. S. A. L. Lim, E. Paz-Pacheco, M. Reyes, and F. Punzalan, "Pericardial decompression syndrome in a patient with hypothyroidism presenting as massive pericardial effusion: a case report and review of related literature," *BMJ Case Reports*, vol. 2011, 2011.

[4] A. A. Khaleeli and N. Memon, "Factors affecting resolution of pericardial effusions in primary hypothyroidism: a clinical, biochemical and echocardiographic study," *Postgraduate Medical Journal*, vol. 58, no. 682, pp. 473–476, 1982.

[5] I. Klein and S. Danzi, "Thyroid disease and the heart," *Circulation*, vol. 116, no. 15, pp. 1725–1735, 2007.

[6] R. Cohen, P. Loarte, S. Opris, and B. Mirrer, "Cardiac tamponade as the initial manifestation of severe hypothyroidism: a case report," *World Journal of Cardiovascular Diseases*, vol. 2, no. 4, pp. 321–325, 2012.

[7] N. S. H. D. S. Setty, K. S. Sadananda, M. C. Nanjappa, S. Patra, H. Basappa, and S. Krishnappa, "Massive pericardial effusion and cardiac tamponade due to cholesterol pericarditis in a case of subclinical hypothyroidism: a rare event," *Journal of the American College of Cardiology*, vol. 63, no. 14, p. 1451, 2014.

[8] R. Bajaj, R. Mehrzad, K. Singh, and J. P. Gupta, "Cardiac tamponade in hypothyroidism," *BMJ Case Reports*, 2014.

[9] A. Motabar, R. Anousheh, R. Shaker, and R. G. Pai, "A rare case of amiodarone-induced hypothyroidism presenting with cardiac tamponade," *The International Journal of Angiology*, vol. 20, no. 3, pp. 177–180, 2011.

[10] M. Ekka, I. Ali, P. Aggarwal, and N. Jamshed, "Cardiac tamponade as initial presenting feature of primary hypothyroidism in the ED," *The American Journal of Emergency Medicine*, vol. 32, no. 6, pp. 683.e1–683.e3, 2014.

[11] H. Yamaguchi, M. Inoshita, A. Shirakami, S. Hashimoto, C. Ichimiya, and T. Shigekiyo, "A case of severe hypothyroidism causing cardiac tamponade associated with lithium intoxication," *Journal of Cardiology Cases*, vol. 8, no. 1, pp. e42–e45, 2013.

[12] A. Rachid, L. C. Caum, A. P. Trentini, C. A. Fischer, D. A. J. Antonelli, and R. P. Hagemann, "Pericardial effusion with cardiac tamponade as a form of presentation of primary hypothyroidism," *Arquivos Brasileiros de Cardiologia*, vol. 78, no. 6, pp. 580–585, 2002.

[13] U. M. Kabadi and S. P. Kumar, "Pericardial effusion in primary hypothyroidism," *American Heart Journal*, vol. 120, no. 6, part 1, pp. 1393–1395, 1990.

[14] Y.-J. Chen, S.-K. Hou, C.-K. How et al., "Diagnosis of unrecognized primary overt hypothyroidism in the ED," *The American Journal of Emergency Medicine*, vol. 28, no. 8, pp. 866–870, 2010.

[15] J.-L. Wang, M.-J. Hsieh, C.-H. Lee et al., "Hypothyroid cardiac tamponade: clinical features, electrocardiography, pericardial fluid and management," *The American Journal of the Medical Sciences*, vol. 340, no. 4, pp. 276–281, 2010.

[16] E. Argulian, E. Herzog, D. G. Halpern, and F. H. Messerli, "Paradoxical hypertension with cardiac tamponade," *The American Journal of Cardiology*, vol. 110, no. 7, pp. 1066–1069, 2012.

[17] Y. Valibey, A. N. Calik, S. Satilimis, and H. Iliksu, "First and only manifestation of Hashimoto's disease: pericardial tamponade," *Turk Kardiyoloji Dernegi Arsivi*, vol. 40, no. 5, pp. 454–457, 2012.

[18] C. M. Foley, R. M. McAllister, and E. M. Hasser, "Thyroid status influences baroreflex function and autonomic contributions to arterial pressure and heart rate," *The American Journal of Physiology—Heart and Circulatory Physiology*, vol. 280, no. 5, pp. H2061–H2068, 2001.

[19] D. L. Glancy and W. L. Wang, "Electrocardiogram in a 55-year-old woman with an endocrine disorder," *Proceedings (Baylor University. Medical Center)*, vol. 20, no. 1, pp. 81–82, 2007.

[20] B. Maisch, P. M. Seferović, A. D. Ristić et al., "Guidelines on the diagnosis and management of pericardial diseases executive summary; The Task force on the diagnosis and management of pericardial diseases of the European society of cardiology," *European Heart Journal*, vol. 25, no. 7, pp. 587–610, 2004.

[21] S. Fazio, E. A. Palmieri, G. Lombardi, and B. Biondi, "Effects of thyroid hormone on the cardiovascular system," *Recent Progress in Hormone Research*, vol. 59, pp. 31–50, 2004.

[22] R. N. Alsever and M. R. Stjernholm, "Cardiac tamponade in myxedema," *The American Journal of the Medical Sciences*, vol. 269, no. 1, pp. 117–121, 1975.

[23] H. A. Gumrukcuoglu, D. Odabasi, S. Akdag, and H. Ekim, "Management of cardiac tamponade: a comperative study between echo-guided pericardiocentesis and surgery-a report of 100 patients," *Cardiology Research and Practice*, vol. 2011, Article ID 197838, 7 pages, 2011.

[24] A. K. Karu, W. I. Khalife, R. Houser, and J. VanderWoude, "Impending cardiac tamponade as a primary presentation of hypothyroidism: case report and review of literature," *Endocrine Practice*, vol. 11, no. 4, pp. 265–271, 2005.

34

Rapid Switch from Intra-Aortic Balloon Pumping to Percutaneous Cardiopulmonary Support Using Perclose ProGlide

Kenichi Sakakura, Yusuke Adachi, Yousuke Taniguchi, Hiroshi Wada, Shin-ichi Momomura, and Hideo Fujita

Division of Cardiovascular Medicine, Saitama Medical Center, Jichi Medical University, 1-847 Amanuma, Omiya, Saitama 330-8503, Japan

Correspondence should be addressed to Kenichi Sakakura; ksakakura@jichi.ac.jp

Academic Editor: Magnus Baumhäkel

We present a case of a patient who needed rapid switch from intra-aortic balloon pumping (IABP) to percutaneous cardiopulmonary support (PCPS)/venoarterial extracorporeal membrane oxygenation. It is difficult to switch from IABP to PCPS, because 0.035-inch guidewires cannot pass the IABP guidewire lumen (0.025-inch compatible), and the IABP sheath needs to be removed together with the IABP catheter. First, a 0.025-inch guidewire was inserted into the IABP wire lumen, and then the IABP catheter together with the 8 Fr IABP sheath was removed, leaving the 0.025-inch guidewire in place. We used the Perclose ProGlide for safe and rapid exchange of the 0.025-inch guidewire for a 0.035-inch guidewire. This allowed insertion of a PCPS cannula and the prompt initiation of PCPS.

1. Introduction

Intra-aortic balloon pumping (IABP) plays a crucial role during cardiogenic shock. However, some catastrophic situations require the use of more aggressive support such as percutaneous cardiopulmonary support (PCPS)/venoarterial extracorporeal membrane oxygenation. It is not difficult to add a PCPS cannula as long as another femoral artery is available. However, it is difficult to exchange an IABP catheter for a PCPS cannula in the same femoral artery, because a 0.035-inch guidewire cannot pass the IABP guidewire lumen (0.025-inch size). Therefore, the IABP catheter together with the 8 Fr IABP sheath needs to be removed over a 0.025-inch guidewire, and then the 0.025-inch guidewire needs to be exchanged for a 0.035-inch guidewire to introduce a PCPS cannula. It is very difficult to exchange a 0.025-inch guidewire for a 0.035-inch guidewire safely without a sheath. Also, an 8 Fr sheath compatible with a 0.025-inch guidewire is usually not available. We present a case of a patient who needed rapid switch from IABP to PCPS. We used the Perclose ProGlide

(Abbott Vascular, Abbott Park, IL, USA) for safe and rapid switch from a 0.025-inch guidewire to a 0.035-inch guidewire.

2. Case Report

A 78-year-old man who had chest discomfort on exertion was referred to our medical center for coronary artery disease. He had diabetes mellitus, hypertension, and dyslipidemia as coronary risk factors; stress scintigraphy at the previous hospital revealed inferior ischemia. Coronary angiography revealed three tandem stenoses in the right coronary artery (RCA) (Figures 1(a) and 1(b)). Since the patient had been treated with dual antiplatelet therapy (aspirin and clopidogrel), we performed ad hoc percutaneous coronary intervention (PCI) of the RCA. A 7 Fr, AL1.0ST SH guiding catheter (Mach 1, Boston Scientific, Natick, MA, USA) was inserted via the right femoral artery. Three everolimus-eluting stents (3.0 × 18 mm, 3.0 × 38 mm, and 3.5 × 38 mm) were successfully deployed (Figure 2). The initial activated coagulation time (ACT) was 333 seconds, while the final ACT was 239 seconds.

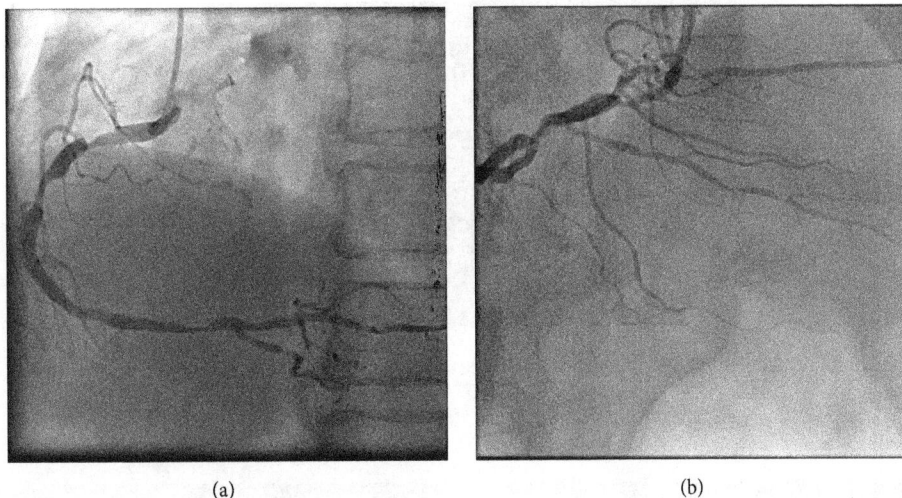

(a)

(b)

FIGURE 1: (a) Left anterior oblique view of the right coronary artery. There are three tandem stenoses. (b) Cranial view of the right coronary artery. There are several stenoses in the posterior descending branch and atrioventricular branch.

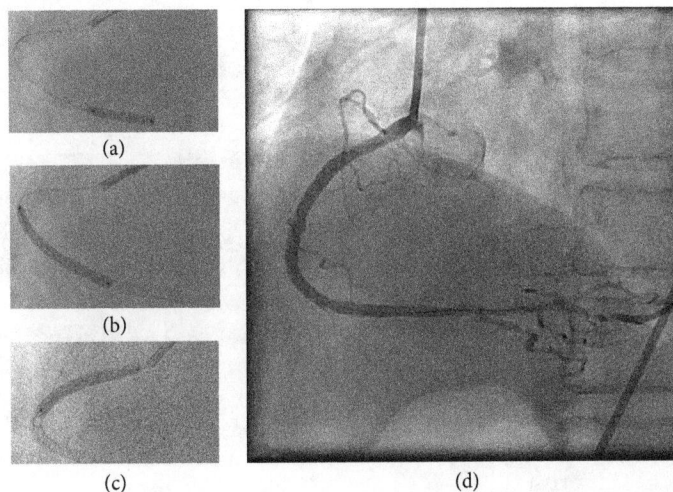

(a)

(b)

(c)

(d)

FIGURE 2: (a) A 3.0 × 18 mm everolimus-eluting stent was deployed in the distal segment of the right coronary artery. (b) A 3.0 × 38 mm everolimus-eluting stent was deployed in the middle segment of the right coronary artery. (c) A 3.5 × 38 mm everolimus-eluting stent was deployed in the proximal segment of the right coronary artery.

Protamine sulfate (10 mg) was injected intravenously, and then the 7 Fr sheath was removed from the right femoral artery. After achieving hemostasis by manual compression, the patient was moved from the catheter laboratory to a general ward.

One hour later, the patient returned to the catheter laboratory in shock. Although the patient was conscious, his systolic blood pressure was <50 mmHg. Furthermore, the electrocardiogram showed ST-segment elevation in leads II, III, and aVF. Therefore, we suspected that he had cardiogenic shock due to acute stent thrombosis. We inserted an 8 Fr IABP catheter (TOKAI 8 Fr IABP 40 cc L, TOKAI Medical Products, Kasugai, Japan) via the left femoral artery. At the same time, we noticed swelling of the right lower abdomen. We realized that he also had hypovolemic shock due to retroperitoneal or abdominal bleeding. We compressed the right lower abdomen manually, and normal saline and 5% albumin were rapidly injected to restore intravascular volume. Despite these measures, the patient remained in shock, and the ST elevation was sustained (Figure 3). Since we recognized that he had hypovolemic as well as cardiogenic shock, we decided to use PCPS as a life-saving intervention. Since we could not use the right femoral artery, we had to exchange the IABP catheter for a PCPS cannula via the left femoral artery. First, we inserted a 0.025-inch guidewire (220 cm) into the IABP catheter lumen and then removed the IABP catheter together with the 8 Fr IABP sheath and left the 0.025-inch guidewire in place. We then inserted a Perclose ProGlide via the 0.025-inch guidewire, removed the 0.025-inch guidewire, and left the Perclose ProGlide in place. We next inserted a 0.035-inch guidewire from the exit port of the Perclose ProGlide, removed the Perclose

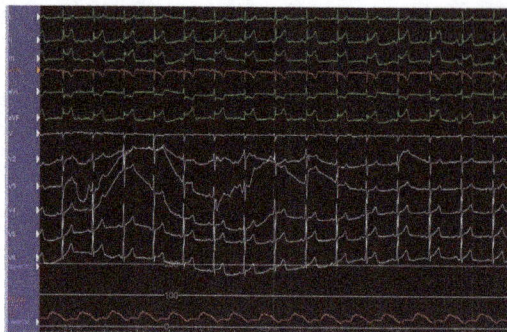

FIGURE 3: The electrocardiogram showed ST-segment elevation in leads II, III, and aVF. Aortic blood pressure with intra-aortic balloon pumping was <50 mmHg.

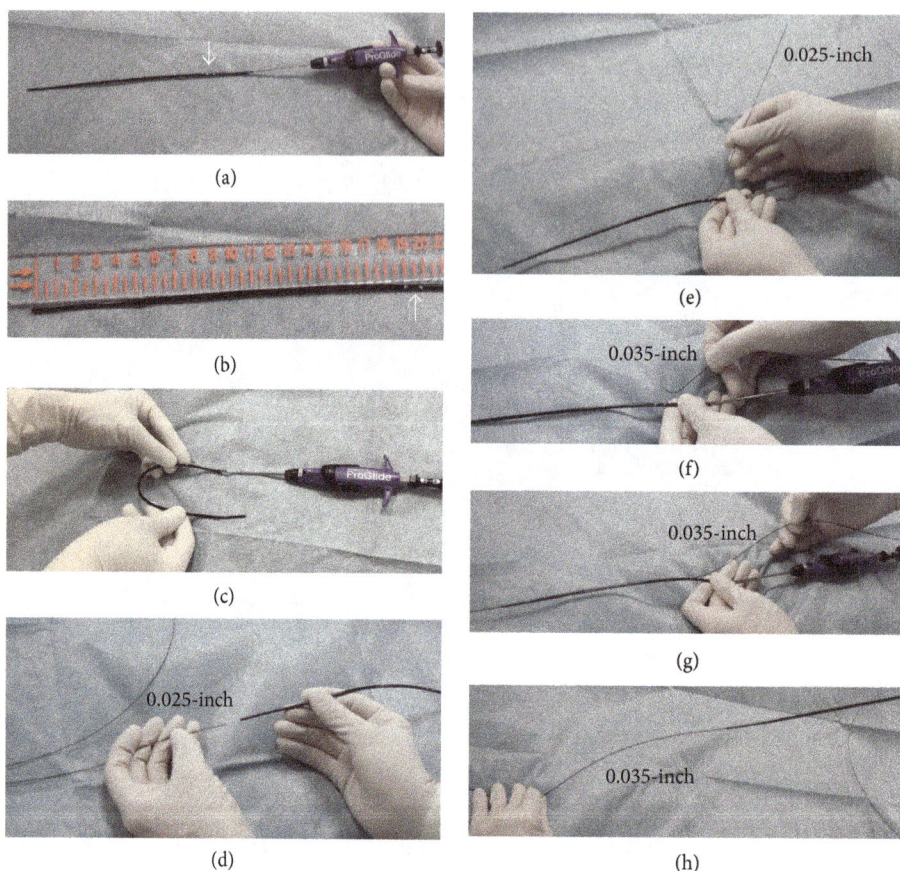

(a)

(b)

(c)

(d)

(e)

(f)

(g)

(h)

FIGURE 4: The ex vivo procedure for guidewire exchange. (a) Perclose ProGlide (Abbott vascular, Abbott Park, Illinois, USA). A white arrow shows the position of the exit port. (b) The length between the tip and exit port (white arrow) of the Perclose ProGlide is approximately 19.5 cm. (c) The rubber part of the Perclose ProGlide is flexible. (d) A 0.025-inch guidewire is inserted via the tip of the Perclose ProGlide. (e) A 0.025-inch guidewire is pulled out from the exit port of the Perclose ProGlide. (f) A 0.035-inch guidewire is inserted via the exit port of the Perclose ProGlide. (g) A 0.035-inch guidewire is advanced and pulled out from the tip of the Perclose ProGlide. (h) The Perclose ProGlide is pulled out, and the 0.035-inch guidewire is left in place. This completes the switch from a 0.025-inch guidewire to a 0.035-inch guidewire.

ProGlide, and left the 0.035-inch guidewire in place (these procedures are illustrated ex vivo in Figure 4). Since the PCPS cannula was smoothly inserted via the 0.035-inch guidewire, we started PCPS promptly. Following PCPS support, his blood pressure recovered and the ST elevation spontaneously resolved. We performed coronary angiography to check the patency of the deployed stents via the right brachial artery and confirmed that all stents were patent (Figure 5). Since there were several stenoses in the distal segments of the RCA, ischemia in the RCA territory might have been induced by insufficient coronary perfusion due to hypovolemia [1].

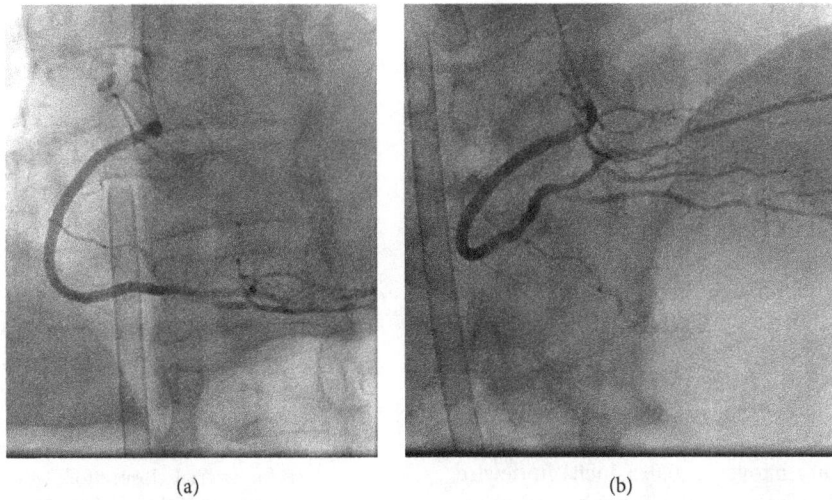

(a)   (b)

FIGURE 5: (a) Left anterior oblique view of the right coronary artery following insertion of the percutaneous cardiopulmonary support (PCPS) cannula. (b) Cranial view of the right coronary artery following PCPS cannula insertion.

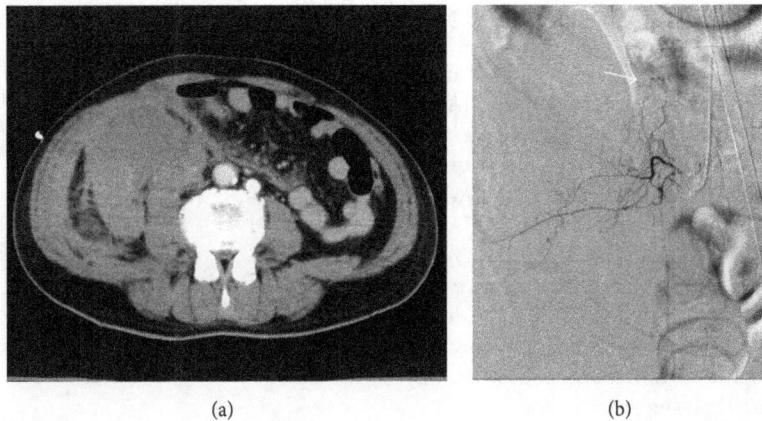

(a)   (b)

FIGURE 6: (a) Computed tomography of the abdomen revealed a large hematoma in the right abdomen. (b) Selective angiography revealed bleeding (arrow) from the right lumbar artery.

We performed abdominal computed tomography and abdominal angiography to find the source of the hemorrhage. Radiologists confirmed hemorrhage of the right lumber artery (Figure 6) and performed transcatheter arterial embolization. Since this patient was on dual antiplatelet therapy and there was substantial anticoagulation due to heparin for PCI (initial ACT, 333 seconds), spontaneous lumber artery hemorrhage was the most likely diagnosis [2, 3]. Furthermore, since we used the modified J-type guidewire (SUWANEXCEL guidewire, AuBEX, Tokyo, Japan) under fluoroscopic guidance, it is unlikely that the guidewire perforated the lumber artery. The patient was ambulatory and discharged on day 16 following PCI.

3. Discussion

The Perclose ProGlide, which is usually used for femoral artery closure after PCI [4], was very useful in our case for switch from a 0.025-inch guidewire to a 0.035-inch guidewire.

Generally, switch from a 0.025-inch guidewire to a 0.035-inch guidewire is very easy if there is a sheath. However, since the IABP catheter is usually removed together with the 8 Fr IABP sheath, it is not easy to switch from a 0.025-inch guidewire to a 0.035-inch guidewire. Furthermore, it is very difficult to puncture the same femoral artery again if guidewire exchange fails, because of the large hole (8 Fr) that must be compressed manually. Since there is no commercially available 8 Fr sheath compatible with a 0.025-inch guidewire, we had to find a method of guidewire exchange.

Although we could not puncture the contralateral femoral artery due to hematoma, it is better to insert a PCPS cannula from the contralateral femoral artery without removal of the IABP, especially in patients with severely reduced ejection fraction [5]. However, it may be difficult to puncture the femoral artery correctly for insertion of a PCPS cannula in patients with cardiogenic shock. Our method does not need an additional puncture, which may reduce the total procedure time in patients with cardiogenic shock. Furthermore, the combination of transfemoral PCI with transfemoral IABP is common during high-risk PCI such as unprotected left main stenting [6]. We would need to stop transfemoral PCI to secure the femoral artery for PCPS, if we could not exchange an IABP catheter for a PCPS cannula.

The Perclose ProGlide has several advantages for guidewire exchange. First, the length from the tip hole to the exit port is enough long (approximately 19.5 cm) (Figure 4(b)) to ensure that the tip of device is beyond the femoral artery (it is likely in the common iliac artery), even when the patient's subcutaneous tissue is thick (obesity). Second, the tip of device is soft and flexible (Figure 4(c)), which allows the device to enter the femoral artery along with a 0.025-inch guidewire. It is usually difficult and dangerous to insert 0.035-inch guidewire compatible devices such as a conventional 8 Fr sheath over a 0.025-inch guidewire, because of the mismatch between the insufficient backup force of the 0.025-inch guidewire and the stiffness of 0.035-inch guidewire compatible devices. Finally, a Perclose ProGlide is a 6–8 Fr compatible device. Therefore, continuous bleeding from the puncture site is less likely when a Perclose ProGlide is inserted following the removal of an IABP 8 Fr sheath.

Although the Perclose ProGlide for guidewire exchange is one of the available solutions for switching from IABP to PCPS, other options are available. For example, a specific IABP catheter (MAQUET, Fairfield, NJ, USA) can be removed separately from the 8 Fr IABP sheath, thus allowing a 0.035-inch guidewire to be inserted directly via the IABP sheath. With this system, the use of a Perclose ProGlide for guidewire exchange would not be necessary; however, preparation for switching from IABP to PCPS should be done in advance in each catheter laboratory, because failure to exchange could be catastrophic in an emergency situation. This is the first case report that suggests the novel utility of a Perclose ProGlide for guidewire exchange in a life-threatening situation.

Abbreviations

IABP: Intra-aortic balloon pumping
PCPS: Percutaneous cardiopulmonary support
RCA: Right coronary artery
PCI: Percutaneous coronary intervention
ACT: Activated coagulation time.

Conflict of Interests

Dr. Kenichi Sakakura received speaking honoraria from Abbott Vascular, Boston Scientific, Daiichi-Sankyo, Terumo, Sanofi, and Medtronic Cardiovascular. The Division of Cardiovascular Medicine (Saitama Medical Center, Jichi Medical University) received a research grant from Abbott Vascular.

Acknowledgment

The authors thank Dr. Kohei Hamamoto for the diagnosis and treatment of lumbar artery hemorrhage.

References

[1] M. D. Seeberger, M. K. Cahalan, K. Rouine-Rapp et al., "Acute hypovolemia may cause segmental wall motion abnormalities in the absence of myocardial ischemia," *Anesthesia and Analgesia*, vol. 85, no. 6, pp. 1252–1257, 1997.

[2] S. Surani, B. Estement, S. Manchandan, S. Sudhakaran, and J. Varon, "Spontaneous extraperitoneal lumbar artery hemorrhage," *Journal of Emergency Medicine*, vol. 40, no. 6, pp. e111–e114, 2011.

[3] J.-M. Isokangas and J. M. Perälä, "Endovascular embolization of spontaneous retroperitoneal hemorrhage secondary to anticoagulant treatment," *CardioVascular and Interventional Radiology*, vol. 27, no. 6, pp. 607–611, 2004.

[4] J. L. Martin, A. Pratsos, E. Magargee et al., "A randomized trial comparing compression, perclose proglide and angioseal VIP for arterial closure following percutaneous coronary intervention: the CAP trial," *Catheterization and Cardiovascular Interventions*, vol. 71, no. 1, pp. 1–5, 2008.

[5] A. Gass, C. Palaniswamy, W. S. Aronow et al., "Peripheral venoarterial extracorporeal membrane oxygenation in combination with intra-aortic balloon counterpulsation in patients with cardiovascular compromise," *Cardiology*, vol. 129, no. 3, pp. 137–143, 2014.

[6] C. Briguori, F. Airoldi, A. Chieffo et al., "Elective versus provisional intraaortic balloon pumping in unprotected left main stenting," *American Heart Journal*, vol. 152, no. 3, pp. 565–572, 2006.

35

Small Bowel Obstruction Masquerading as Acute ST Elevation Myocardial Infarction

Manan Parikh,[1] **Martin Miguel Amor,**[1] **Isha Verma,**[1] **Jeffrey Osofsky,**[2] **and Madhu Paladugu**[1]

[1]*Department of Internal Medicine, Monmouth Medical Center, 300 2nd Avenue, Long Branch, NJ 07740, USA*
[2]*Department of Cardiology, Monmouth Medical Center, 300 2nd Avenue, Long Branch, NJ 07740, USA*

Correspondence should be addressed to Manan Parikh; manan_cnv@yahoo.com

Academic Editor: Man-Hong Jim

ST segment elevation on EKG remains among the most important presentations of acute myocardial infarction. Due to the urgency of intervention for this finding, other clinical scenarios causing ST elevations on EKG may sometimes go unaddressed and can lead to fatal complications. We present a case of an 86-year-old male presenting with small bowel obstruction leading to EKG findings of ST segment elevation in the absence of critical coronary obstruction. The EKG finding resolved after the improvement of small bowel obstruction reflecting the reversible cause of the changes.

1. Introduction

ST segment elevation on EKG remains among the most important presentations of acute myocardial infarction, requiring immediate diagnosis and management to prevent permanent damage to the myocardium and reduce mortality. Due to the urgency of intervention for this finding, other clinical scenarios causing ST elevations on EKG may sometimes go unaddressed and can lead to fatal complications. Herein, we present an unusual case of an 86-year-old male with ST segment elevations on EKG, which while initially thought to be cardiac were later found to be due to small bowel obstruction.

2. Case Report

An 86-year-old male presented to the ED with a chief complaint of vomiting and epigastric pain of 24-hour duration. He had a past medical history significant for paroxysmal atrial fibrillation, hypertension, chronic kidney disease, anemia of chronic disease, Barrett's esophagus, esophageal rupture, and pneumomediastinum requiring surgical repair. Ten years

prior to this ED visit, the patient had undergone an emergency esophageal rupture repair with prolonged postsurgical course requiring jejunostomy and tracheostomy but had subsequently recovered from it. He had a nuclear stress test 10 months prior to this visit with no signs of inducible ischemia. He started experiencing epigastric abdominal pain as well as nausea 24 hours prior to presentation. In the following hours, he had three episodes of vomiting and one bowel movement. There was no note of any hematemesis, hematochezia, or melena. Upon arrival at the ED, his vital signs were stable with blood pressure of 166/70 mmHg, pulse rate of 83, respiratory rate of 14, and temperature of 98.2 F. His initial hemoglobin was 11.0 mg/dL. He also had elevated amylase and lipase levels of 198 IU/L and 76 IU/L, respectively, which increased to 474 IU/L and 527 IU/L the next morning. Abdominal obstructive series revealed scant small bowel gas without clear evidence of obstruction. Ultrasound of the abdomen showed a large gallstone in common bile duct with no gall bladder wall thickening or pericholecystic fluid. An EKG obtained at this time showed sinus rhythm with no ST segment elevation (Figure 1). He was admitted as a case of acute pancreatitis. On the succeeding hospital day, he was noted to have severe epigastric pain and another EKG

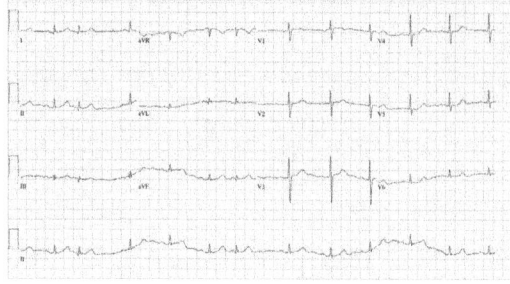

FIGURE 1: 12-lead EKG on admission showing normal sinus rhythm.

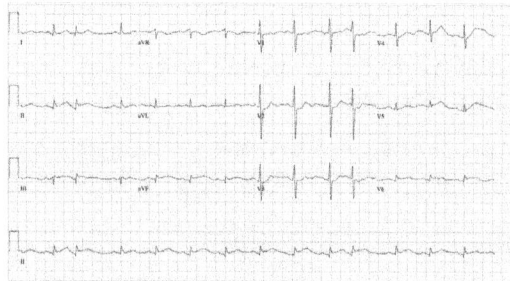

FIGURE 2: 12-lead EKG showing ST segment elevations in leads II, III, and aVF with reciprocal changes in anterior precordial leads, consistent with acute inferior wall ST segment elevation myocardial infarction (STEMI).

was obtained. The EKG (Figure 2) showed ST segment elevations in inferior leads with reciprocal changes in anterior precordial leads consistent with acute inferior wall ST segment elevation myocardial infarction (STEMI). Troponin was noted to be 0.04. Emergent cardiac catheterization revealed 70% stenosis of the right coronary artery (RCA), as well as diffuse calcific disease of posterolateral branches, with 40% left anterior descending artery stenosis. None of the vessels showed plaque rupture or acute thrombus. Serial monitoring of troponin levels yielded normal results. In light of the patient's ongoing gastrointestinal complaints, intervention for the noncritical RCA lesion was deferred. The patient subsequently underwent an abdominal CT scan and was found to have small bowel obstruction, with transition point in the jejunum with a markedly dilated stomach containing foci of air (Figure 3). He also had a dilated gall bladder with gallstones, but the pancreas was normal in appearance. Small bowel obstruction and gastric distention were conservatively treated with nasogastric tube placement over the next 2 days. As the patient's gastric distention improved, the inferior wall ST segment elevations in his EKG also resolved, as was noted on serial EKGs (Figure 4). The patient subsequently underwent laparoscopic cholecystectomy without complications. He was eventually discharged home with stable follow-up.

3. Discussion

Despite the variety of diagnostic tests available, the EKG remains the primary diagnostic tool to diagnose acute myocardial infarction. Hence, it is important to know about conditions which can present with ST elevations on EKG.

Other than myocardial infarction, common cardiac conditions causing ST elevations on EKG include myocarditis [1, 2], early repolarization, ventricular hypertrophy, and aneurysms [3]. Other noncardiac conditions, which may present with ST elevations on EKG, include cholecystitis [4], esophageal perforation [5], pancreatitis [6], and stomach distention [7]. These are usually misdiagnosed as acute myocardial infarction resulting in emergent angiography and unwanted thrombolytic therapy for early reperfusion. The ST segment elevations seen on EKG in these noncardiac conditions may be explained by disease processes involving the intrathoracic cavity, producing a shift in the main QRS axis of the heart as a result of displacement of the intrathoracic contents. Specifically, these EKG changes occur secondary to displacement of the heart in the anterior-posterior plane, or due to the thickness of the contents between the chest wall and heart [8].

In our patient, distention of the stomach and esophagus secondary to small bowel obstruction possibly caused changes in the relative position of the heart to the other thoracic organs. This presented on EKG in the form of ST elevations in leads II, III, and aVF, which was mistaken for acute inferior wall myocardial infarction. Subsequently, the patient was taken for immediate angiography, but no critical lesion was found. Appropriate intervention to relieve small bowel obstruction resulted in improvement of the symptoms and resolution of the EKG changes.

In conclusion, while the EKG remains an indispensable tool to diagnose acute myocardial infarction, it is important to rule out other cardiac conditions presenting with ST elevations on EKG before pursuing aggressive interventions. It is equally important to be cognizant of noncardiac conditions presenting with ST segment elevations on EKG, to guide

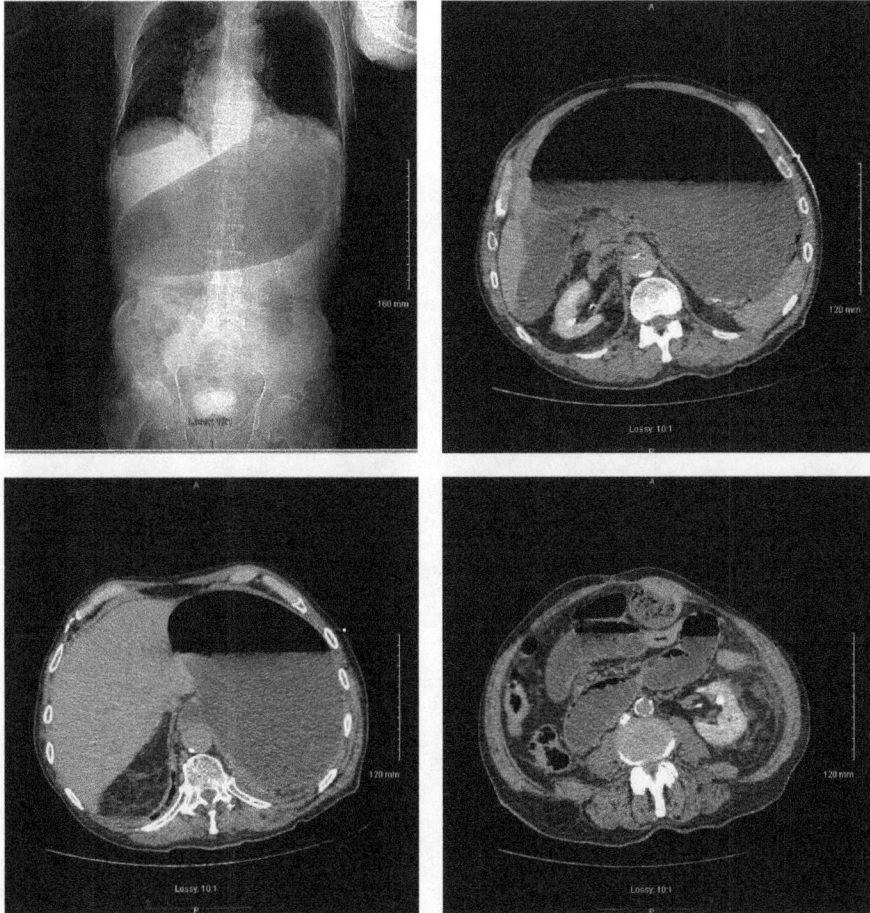

FIGURE 3: CT scan of the abdomen showing small bowel obstruction, with transition point in the jejunum with a markedly dilated stomach containing foci of air. Also a dilated gall bladder with gallstones and normal-appearing pancreas is noted.

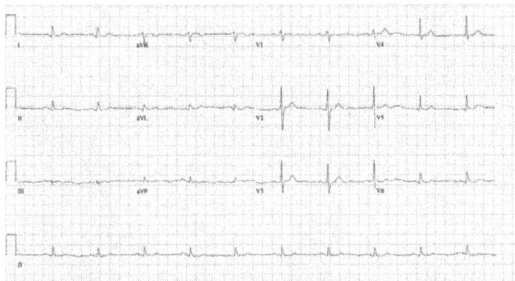

FIGURE 4: 12-lead EKG showing normal sinus rhythm, with resolution of the previously seen ST segment elevations in the inferior wall leads (II, III, and aVF).

us in choosing the most appropriate intervention. With this case report, we intend to add small bowel obstruction to the growing list of noncardiac conditions presenting as ST elevations on EKG.

Disclosure

All the authors report no financial disclosure.

Conflict of Interests

The authors declare that there is no conflict of interests regarding the publication of this paper.

References

[1] G. W. Dec Jr., H. Waldman, J. Southern, J. T. Fallon, A. M. Hutter Jr., and I. Palacios, "Viral myocarditis mimicking acute myocardial infarction," *Journal of the American College of Cardiology*, vol. 20, no. 1, pp. 85–89, 1992.

[2] C. Chrysohoou, E. Tsiamis, S. Brili, J. Barbetseas, and C. Stefanadis, "Acute myocarditis from coxsackie infection, mimicking subendocardial ischaemia," *Hellenic Journal of Cardiology*, vol. 50, no. 2, pp. 147–150, 2009.

[3] K. Wang, R. W. Asinger, and H. J. Marriott, "ST-segment elevation in conditions other than acute myocardial infarction," *The New England Journal of Medicine*, vol. 349, no. 22, pp. 2128–2135, 2003.

[4] E. T. Ryan, P. H. Pak, and R. W. DeSanctis, "Myocardial infarction mimicked by acute cholecystitis," *Annals of Internal Medicine*, vol. 116, no. 3, pp. 218–220, 1992.

[5] M. Mosseri, R. Eliakim, and P. Mogle, "Perforation of the esophagus electrocardiographically mimicking myocardial infarction," *Israel Journal of Medical Sciences*, vol. 22, no. 6, pp. 451–454, 1986.

[6] J. Patel, A. Movahed, and W. C. Reeves, "Electrocardiographic and segmental wall motion abnormalities in pancreatitis mimicking myocardial infarction," *Clinical Cardiology*, vol. 17, no. 9, pp. 505–509, 1994.

[7] S. Asada, T. Kawasaki, T. Taniguchi, T. Kamitani, S. Kawasaki, and H. Sugihara, "A case of ST-segment elevation provoked by distended stomach conduit," *International Journal of Cardiology*, vol. 109, no. 3, pp. 411–413, 2006.

[8] J. R. Diamond and N. M. Estes, "ECG changes associated with iatrogenic left pneumothorax simulating anterior myocardial infarction," *American Heart Journal*, vol. 103, no. 2, pp. 303–305, 1982.

36

Endovascular Therapy Is Effective for Leriche Syndrome with Deep Vein Thrombosis

Tasuku Higashihara, Nobuo Shiode, Tomoharu Kawase, Hiromichi Tamekiyo, Masaya Otsuka, Tomokazu Okimoto, and Yasuhiko Hayashi

Cardiovascular Center, Division of Cardiology, Akane Foundation, Tsuchiya General Hospital, 3-30 Nakajima-cho, Naka-ku, Hiroshima 730-8655, Japan

Correspondence should be addressed to Nobuo Shiode; nobucode.0317@kfd.biglobe.ne.jp

Academic Editor: Man-Hong Jim

A 65-year-old man presented to our hospital due to intermittent claudication and swelling in his left leg. He had Leriche syndrome and deep vein thrombosis. We performed endovascular therapy (EVT) for Leriche syndrome, and a temporary filter was inserted in the inferior vena cava. He received anticoagulation therapy for deep vein thrombosis. The stenotic lesion in the terminal aorta was stented with an excellent postprocedural angiographic result and dramatic clinical improvement after EVT. This case suggests that EVT can be a treatment for Leriche syndrome.

1. Introduction

Leriche syndrome is a chronic obstruction of the aortic bifurcation, extending to both the infrarenal aorta and the common iliac arteries, and is classically associated with a triad of symptoms comprising intermittent claudication, absent or diminished peripheral pulses, and erectile dysfunction in men [1]. The disease manifested as Leriche syndrome is nowadays categorized as a type D aortoiliac lesion by the Trans-Atlantic Inter-Society Consensus for the Management of Peripheral Arterial Disease (TASC II) [2]. May-Thurner syndrome is an iliac vein compression syndrome in which anatomic compression of the left common iliac vein by the overlying right common iliac artery occurs, therefore, resulting in development of left lower extremity deep vein thrombosis (DVT) [3].

Here we report a case of Leriche syndrome with DVT resembling May-Thurner syndrome that we treated with endovascular therapy (EVT).

2. Case Report

A 65-year-old male presented to our hospital due to intermittent claudication of both legs and swelling in his left leg.

The claudication had started 4 weeks earlier and was ongoing at the time of presentation, and the pain had worsened. His left lower limb had become swollen 2 weeks before admission. On admission, the pulsation of his bilateral femoral, popliteal, and anterior tibial arteries was weak. The ankle-brachial index (ABI) was significantly low bilaterally.

Ultrasonography showed that there were massive thrombi in the veins extending from the left external iliac vein to the left popliteal vein (Figure 1). At the same time, there was no discernible arterial blood flow from the infrarenal abdominal aorta to both the common iliac arteries. Further, the inside echo of the occlusion site was low, so the occlusion seemed to be due to a thrombus. Pulmonary thromboembolism was ruled out by echocardiographic examination. The echocardiography showed normal left ventricular function (left ventricular ejection fraction 73%), mild left ventricular hypertrophy, and no tricuspid regurgitation. We considered that if pulmonary thromboembolism had occurred, the grade was not severe. In the computed tomography (CT) findings, the terminal aorta was occluded with thrombus and there was a venous thrombus in his left iliac vein that appeared in the proximal site that was compressed by the left common iliac artery (Figure 2). The patient was diagnosed with Leriche syndrome accompanied with DVT. His thyroid function

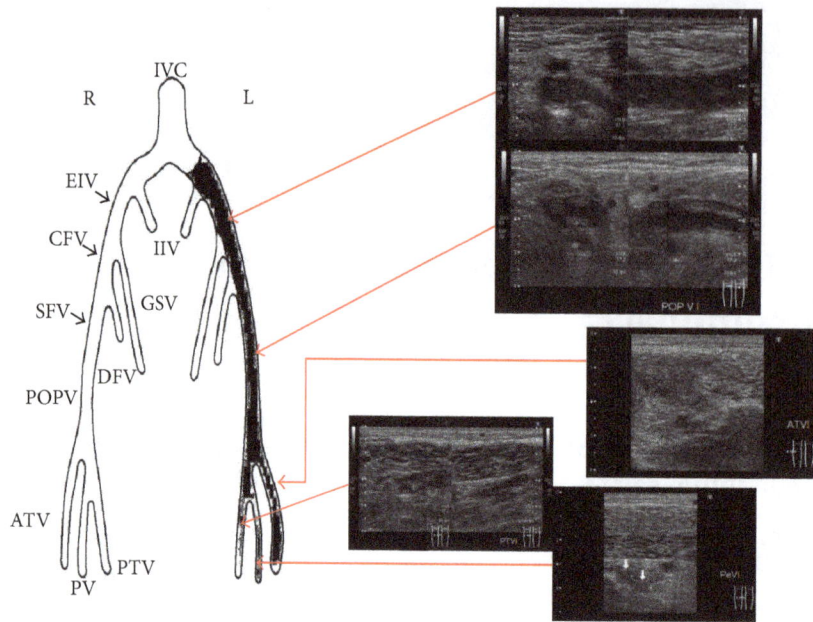

FIGURE 1: Ultrasonography showed the left iliac vein was occluded with a thrombus.

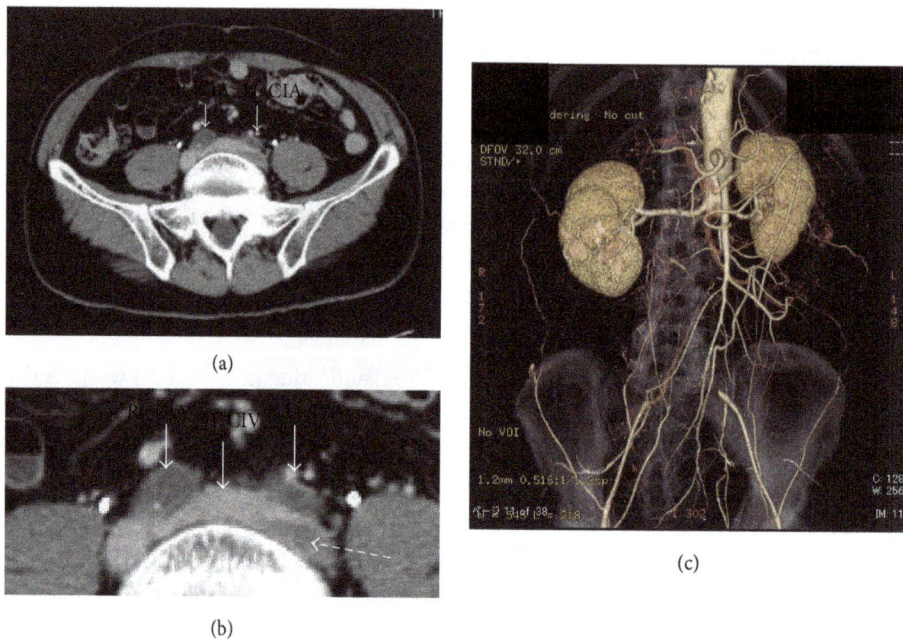

FIGURE 2: (a) The left common iliac vein (Lt. CIV) was compressed by the left common iliac artery (Lt. CIA) resulting in formation of a venous thrombus at this point. (b) The thrombus was observed in left common iliac vein (dotted arrow). (c) CT showed that the terminal aorta was occluded from the level of renal artery to the bilateral common iliac arteries.

tests were normal and his hypercoagulable workup including serum protein C, protein S, anti-cardiolipin antibodies, and lupus anticoagulant antibody was found to be negative.

On day 1, a temporary inferior vena cava (IVC) filter was inserted to prevent pulmonary embolism. Oral warfarin administration and intravenous heparin infusion were started for DVT. Oral cilostazol (200 mg/day) was started for ischemia of the lower extremities. Coronary angiography

(CAG) and aortography were done to plan the treatment strategy. There was 75% stenosis in the middle of the left circumflex coronary artery; however, he had no chest symptom, so we decided to continue observation with oral medication.

We planned the treatment strategy as follows. CT showed that the terminal aorta was occluded with thrombus. The high density area was observed in low density area (Figure 3). It seemed that thrombus was comparatively fresh. The patient

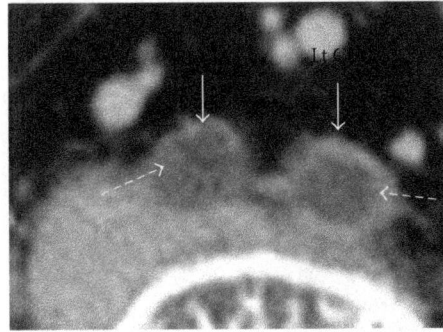

FIGURE 3: CT showed that the bilateral common iliac arteries were occluded with thrombus. The high density area was observed in low density area (dotted arrows).

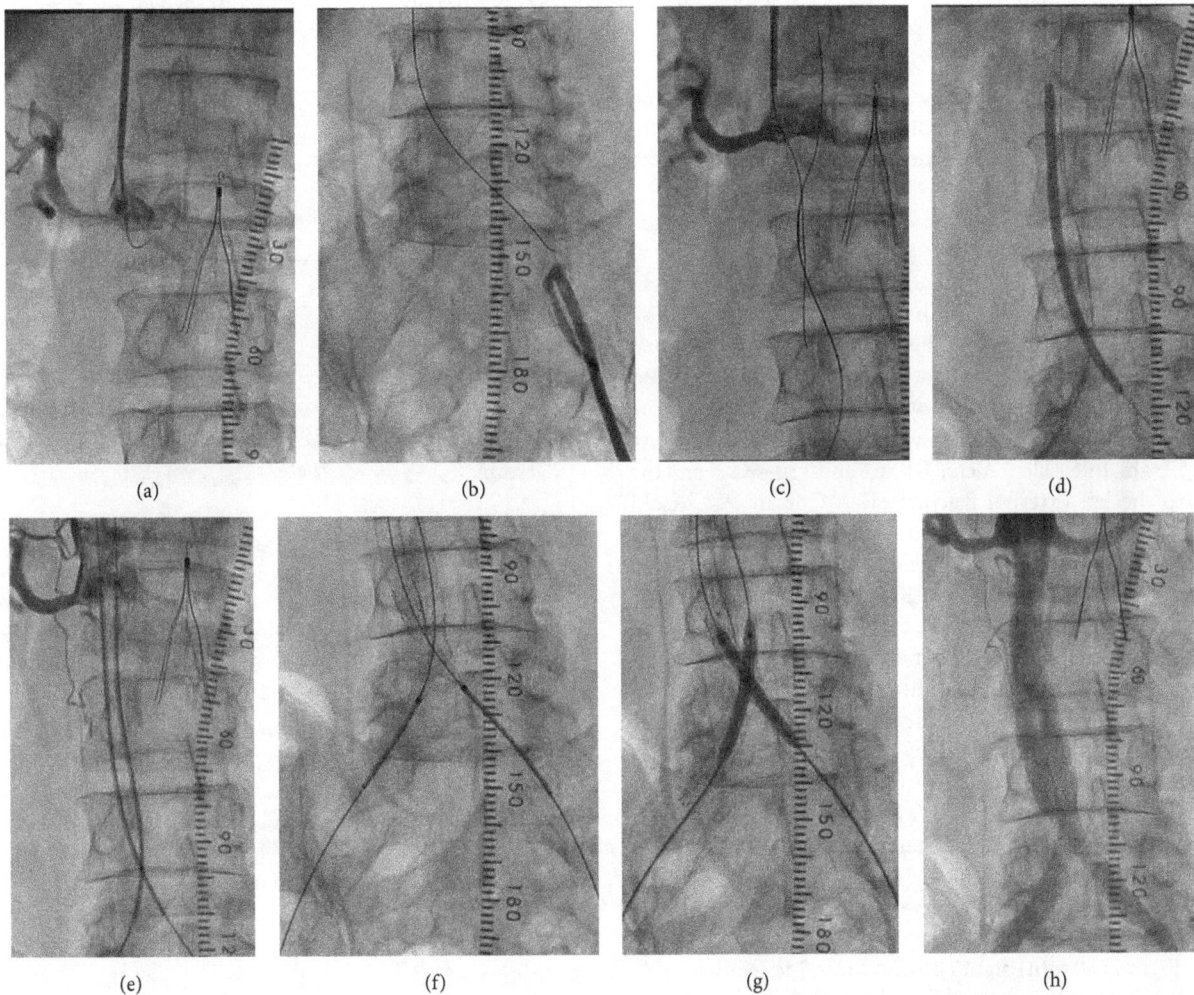

(a)

(b)

(c)

(d)

(e)

(f)

(g)

(h)

FIGURE 4: (a) The proximal fibrous cap of the occlusion site of terminal aorta was penetrated by using a multipurpose catheter and a 0.035-inch Radifocus guidewire. (b) Treasure XS12 was crossed from the aorta to the left external iliac artery. (c) Another Treasure XS12 was advanced from the right femoral artery to the aorta. (d) The occluded segments of the bilateral iliac arteries were predilated with either of the two 4.0 mm balloons. (e, f) An Epic 10 mm (98 mm) and a 10 mm (80 mm) stent were inserted from the right common iliac artery and advanced to the aorta. Also, an Epic 10 mm (98 mm) and a 10 mm (60 mm) stent were inserted in the left iliac artery from the left common iliac artery and advanced to the aorta. (g) The postdilatation of the bilateral stents was performed simultaneously with two 5.0 mm balloons. (h) The final angiogram.

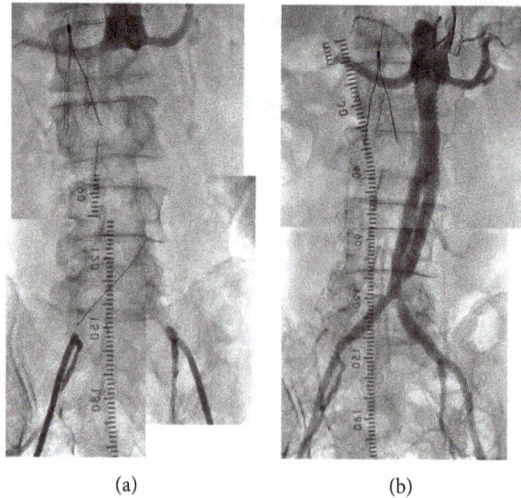

(a)   (b)

FIGURE 5: (a) Aortography showed that the terminal aorta was occluded from the level of the renal artery to the bilateral common iliac arteries. (b) After EVT, aortography showed that the bilateral common iliac arterial flow was restored. EVT: endovascular therapy.

had received abdominal surgery for intestinal obstruction about 20 years before, so the adhesion of abdominal organs was suspected. Therefore, we decided to perform EVT for Leriche syndrome.

Following local anesthesia, a 90 cm 6F sheath was inserted from the right brachial artery and advanced to the distal abdominal aorta. The 6F sheath was placed in the right femoral artery and a 7F sheath was placed in the left FA. The proximal fibrous cap of the occlusion site of terminal aorta was penetrated by using a multipurpose catheter and a 0.035-inch Radifocus guidewire (GW) (Terumo Corp., Japan). Then the Radifocus GW was exchanged for a Treasure XS12 (Asahi Intec Co., Aichi, Japan) and crossed from the aorta to the left external iliac artery. A Corsair PV (Asahi Intec Co., Aichi, Japan) was crossed from the left femoral artery to the aorta by the Rendez-Vous Technique, and we exchanged the GW for a Runthrough Ph guidewire (Terumo Corp., Japan). Next, we crossed the Corsair PV and Treasure XS12 from the right femoral artery to the aorta and exchanged the GW for the Runthrough Ph. The intraluminal position of the GW was confirmed by the intravascular ultrasound. After the two wires were successfully passed through, the thrombi were aspirated using a Thrombuster II for 8F aspiration catheter (Kaneka Medix Corp., Japan) and next with a 6F guide catheter Heartrail BL3.5 (Terumo Corp., Japan). The occluded segments of the bilateral iliac arteries were predilated simultaneously with either of the two 4.0 mm balloons. After that, an Epic 10 mm (98 mm) and a 10 mm (80 mm) stent (Boston Scientific, Natick, MA, USA) were inserted from the right common iliac artery and advanced to the aorta. Also, an Epic 10 mm (98 mm) and a 10 mm (60 mm) stent were inserted in the left iliac artery from the left common iliac artery and advanced to the aorta, and postdilatation of the bilateral stents was performed simultaneously with two 5.0 mm balloons. The final angiogram showed no thromboembolism in the distal arteries (Figures 4 and 5).

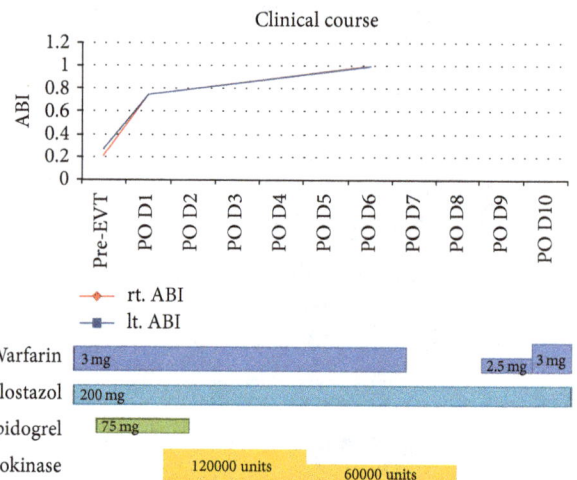

FIGURE 6: Clinical course after endovascular therapy. ABI: ankle-brachial index, EVT: endovascular therapy, and POD: postoperative day.

The clinical course after the EVT is showed in Figure 6. The ABI dramatically improved (right 0.21 to 0.97 and left 0.27 to 0.98). On day 12 after EVT, the ultrasonography revealed that the venous thrombi in his left leg had decreased (Figure 7). On day 17 after EVT, the IVC filter was removed and the patient was discharged on the 28th hospital day (20th day after EVT).

3. Discussion

In general, surgical treatment has been recommended as a revascularization therapy for Leriche syndrome [2]. Recently the devices for EVT have improved and EVT is becoming more widely used. However, the clinical outcome of EVT for Leriche syndrome remains unclear. A retrospective cohort study demonstrated that EVT for Leriche syndrome had a favorable outcome [4, 5].

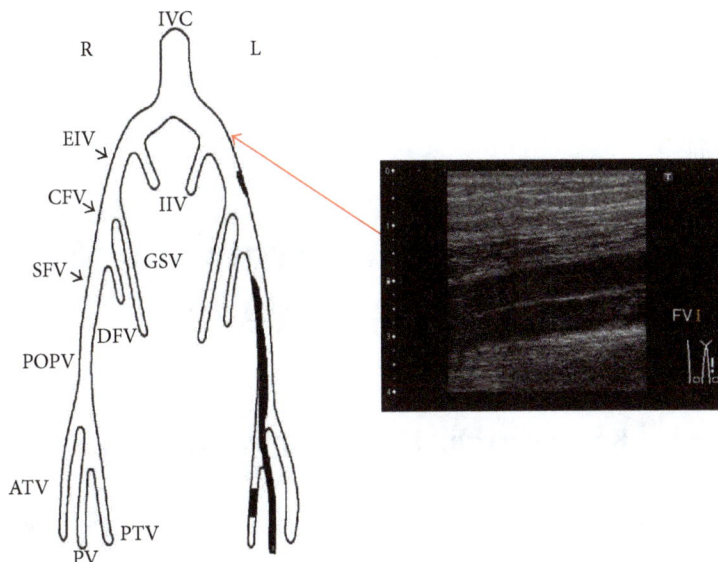

FIGURE 7: After anticoagulant therapy and EVT, the venous thrombi in the left leg decreased as seen in the ultrasonography of leg veins.

There are a few case reports of simultaneous occurrence of DVT and Leriche syndrome [6]. From clinical course of this case, we speculated that Leriche syndrome had occurred firstly; after that, the left common iliac vein had been compressed by the left common iliac artery continuously and finally DVT had occurred. May-Thurner syndrome is an iliac vein compression syndrome in which compression of the left common iliac vein occurs by the overlying right common iliac artery [3]. In this case the left common iliac vein was compressed with the "left" common iliac artery. So this case was not exactly May-Thurner syndrome.

In this case, the tissue at the occlusion site in the terminal aorta seemed to be soft tissue from the CT findings, so we speculated that the occlusion was not so old. Furthermore, the patient had received abdominal surgery for intestinal obstruction about 20 years before. At that time the long hospital stay had been needed due to wound complications. And there was possibility of the adhesion of the abdominal organ. The adhesiolysis during reoperation was associated with an increase of sepsis incidence, intra-abdominal complications and wound infection, and longer hospital stay [7]. Therefore, we decided to treat Leriche syndrome with EVT. In this case, the terminal aorta was occluded with a massive thrombus. In such a case, distal embolization is one of the adverse complications. To prevent distal embolization, thrombus aspiration was done and dilatation after stenting was performed with small-size balloons. Fortunately, distal embolization did not occur in this case; however, it is important to take care of distal embolization. The clinical course of this case was excellent. So we concluded that EVT can be considered as a treatment option for Leriche syndrome.

4. Conclusion

We reported a case of Leriche syndrome accompanied with DVT treated with EVT for Leriche syndrome and the clinical course was excellent. EVT may be a treatment option for Leriche syndrome.

Conflict of Interests

The authors declare that there is no conflict of interests regarding the publication of this paper.

References

[1] R. Leriche and A. Morel, " The syndrome of thrombotic obliteration of the aortic bifurcation," *Annals of Surgery*, vol. 127, no. 2, pp. 193–206, 1948.

[2] L. Norgren, W. R. Hiatt, J. A. Dormandy, M. R. Nehler, K. A. Harris, and F. G. R. Fowkes, "Inter-society consensus for the management of peripheral arterial disease (TASC II)," *Journal of Vascular Surgery*, vol. 45, no. 1, supplement, pp. S5–S67, 2007.

[3] N. F. Brazeau, H. B. Harvey, E. G. Pinto, A. Deipolyi, R. L. Hesketh, and R. Oklu, "May-Thurner syndrome: diagnosis and management," *Vasa*, vol. 42, no. 2, pp. 96–105, 2013.

[4] H. Krankenberg, M. Schlüter, C. Schwencke et al., "Endovascular reconstruction of the aortic bifurcation in patients with Leriche syndrome," *Clinical Research in Cardiology*, vol. 98, no. 10, pp. 657–664, 2009.

[5] T. Dohi, O. Iida, M. Uematsu, K. Ikeoka, S. Okamoto, and S. Nagata, *Endovascular Therapy for Leriche Syndrome: Initial and Midterm Results*, vol. 1, CVIT, 2009, (Japanese).

[6] Y. Gouëffic, T. Piffeteau, and P. Patra, "Acute leriche syndrome due to paradoxical embolism," *European Journal of Vascular and Endovascular Surgery*, vol. 33, no. 2, pp. 220–222, 2007.

[7] R. P. G. T. Broek, C. Strik, Y. Issa, R. P. Bleichrodt, and H. van Goor, "Adhesiolysis-related morbidity in abdominal surgery," *Annals of Surgery*, vol. 258, no. 1, pp. 98–106, 2013.

37

Raghib Syndrome Presenting as a Cryptogenic Stroke: Role of Cardiac MRI in Accurate Diagnosis

Vistasp J. Daruwalla,[1] Keyur Parekh,[2] Hassan Tahir,[1] Jeremy D. Collins,[2] and James Carr[2]

[1]*Conemaugh Memorial Hospital/Temple University, USA*
[2]*Department of Cardiovascular Radiology, Northwestern University Feinberg School of Medicine, USA*

Correspondence should be addressed to Vistasp J. Daruwalla; vdaruwal@conemaugh.org

Academic Editor: Gianluca Pontone

Raghib Syndrome is a rare developmental complex, which consists of persistence of the left superior vena cava (PLSVC) along with coronary sinus ostial atresia and atrial septal defect. This Raghib complex anomaly has also been associated with other congenital malformations including ventricular septal defects, enlargement of the tricuspid annulus, and pulmonary stenosis. Our case demonstrates an isolated PLSVC draining into the left atrium along with coronary sinus atresia in a young patient presenting with cryptogenic stroke without the atrial septal defect. Majority of the cases reported in the literature were found to have the lesion during the postmortem evaluation or were characterized at angiography and/or echocardiography. We stress the importance of modern day imaging like the computed tomography (CT) angiography and cardiac MRI in diagnosis and surgical management of such rare lesions leading to cryptogenic strokes.

1. Introduction

Persistence of the left superior vena cava (PLSVC) is seen in 0.3%–0.5% of normal subjects [1, 2] and in up to 2.1%–4.3% of patients with congenital heart disease [3]. Coronary sinus ostial atresia with a PLSVC is usually associated with an anomalous connection between the coronary sinus ostium and the left atrium [4, 5]. Atresia of the coronary sinus ostium without this anomalous communication is rare since first described in 1738 [6]. Raghib syndrome is a rare developmental complex, which consists of PLSVC draining in the left atrium, coronary sinus ostial atresia, and atrial septal defect in the posteroinferior angle of the atrial septum. Okumori et al. stated that the atrial septal defect was true and this specific type of atrial septal defect associated with an absent coronary sinus [7]. Cases of an intact atrial septum and with PLSVC into left atrium were noted [8].

Due to the association with cardiac level right to left shunts, Raghib Syndrome has a significant risk of paradoxical embolization and is associated with varied degrees of reduced arterial blood oxygen saturation. Most of the cases reported in the literature were detected during postmortem evaluation or were characterized at angiography and/or echocardiography. We report a case of isolated PLSVC draining into the left atrium along with coronary sinus atresia in a young patient presenting with cryptogenic stroke evaluated with transthoracic echocardiography, computed tomography (CT), angiography and Cardiac MRI.

2. Case Presentation

The patient is a 31-year-old African-American, left handed female who was recently diagnosed with hypertension. She presented with left handed clumsiness, most notably in her left index finger and thumb, she also complains of an episode of slurred speech and left sided facial numbness that lasted for about 30 minutes to 1 hour. The patient was initially seen in a local hospital nearby and was reported to have an abnormal EKG with T wave inversions in leads v2–v4 and left ventricular hypertrophy but the patient refused admission and was admitted to our institution 10 days later. Her symptoms had improved two days after the attack but she

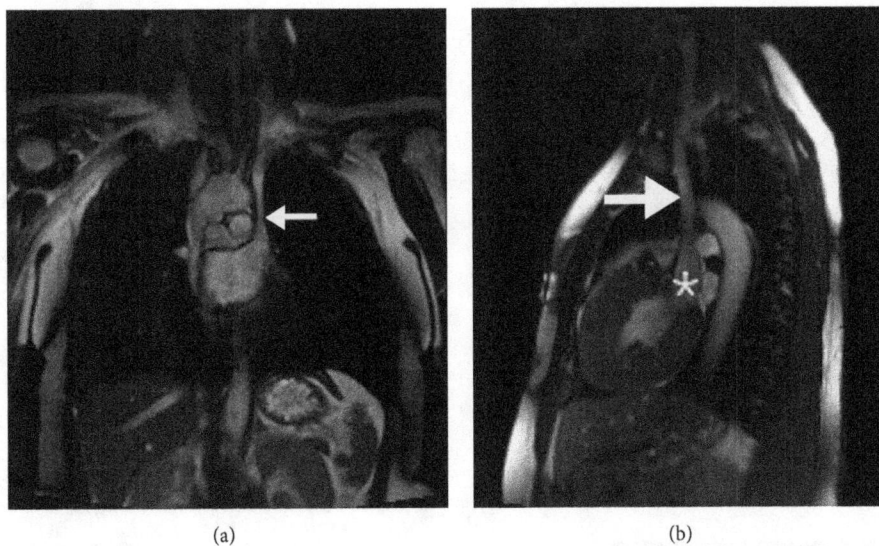

FIGURE 1: Coronal and sagittal T2 weighted images show a persistent left superior vena cava (arrow) draining in to the left atrial appendage (star).

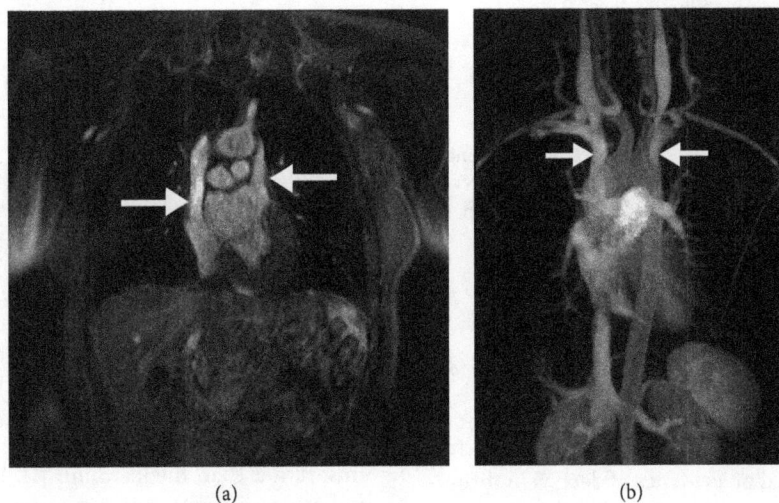

FIGURE 2: Static and three-dimensional MR angiography confirms the presence of right and left superior vena cava (arrows) draining in to the corresponding atrial chambers leading to a right-to-left shunt.

still had difficulty with fine motor task like typing. During her stay she maintained a saturation of 95-96%.

Her neurological work-up included an MRI of the brain, which demonstrated a subacute infarct within the right precentral gyrus, involving the region of the hand knob correlating with her left hand weakness (Figure 5).

Transthoracic echocardiography revealed moderate left ventricular hypertrophy without regional wall motion abnormalities. The left atrium was mildly dilated. There was an increased mitral valve E point, ventricular septal separation; the visually estimated ejection fraction was 45–50%. There was no evidence of right to left shunting by agitated saline bubble contrast study performed in the right arm.

Her chest radiography demonstrated abnormal soft tissue densities along the right paratracheal region extending to the right main stem bronchus and along the right cardiomediastinal margin of unclear etiology which was further evaluated with a CT scan. CT imaging demonstrated persistence of the left superior vena cava draining into the left atrium without visualization of a coronary sinus. Cardiac venous drainage is seen directly into the inferior vena cava via the great cardiac vein. Subtle high attenuation contrast extends deep into the interventricular septum. While this may be a myocardial cleft in the same setting of possible left ventricular hypertrophy, the alternate possibility of a sinusoidal VSD is raised as a potential component of Raghib Syndrome. The mass seen in

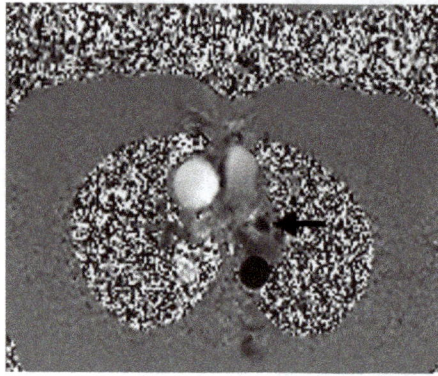

FIGURE 3: Axial 2D phase contrast images in the upper chest show caudally directed flow in the left superior vena cava (arrow).

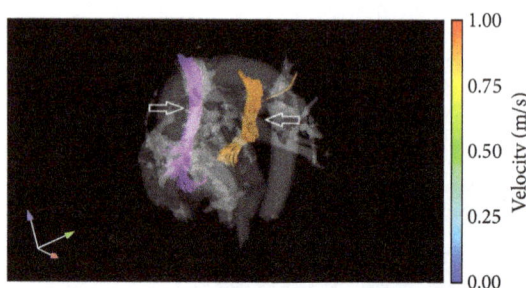

FIGURE 4: Whole heart 4D flow image demonstrating differential flow into the atria. Flow from the right superior vena cava (SVC) to the right atrium and left superior vena cava to the left atrium.

the chest radiograph along the cardiomediastinal margin was correlated to be a 5.4 cm pericardial cyst, and a 1 mm right middle lobe nodule was also noted.

For cryptogenic stroke, the patient underwent upper and lower extremity Doppler ultrasound as well as cardiac MRI. Doppler ultrasound showed no evidence of deep vein thrombosis. Cardiac MR demonstrated concentric hypertrophic cardiomyopathy, with relative sparing of the apical chamber. Left ventricular systolic function was moderately reduced with a calculated ejection fraction of 36%. The persistent left superior vena cava drained into the left atrium resulting in a right to left shunt with a $Qp/Qs = 0.694$ (Figure 1).

The patient's clinical diagnosis was Raghib syndrome with paradoxical embolization causing stroke. Although PLSVC serves as a right to left shunt, our patient during her stay has maintained oxygen saturation of above 90%. The right to left shunt caused by PLSVC is usually small and does not lead to significant oxygen desaturation. Transcatheter treatment is performed in patients with unroofed coronary sinus or an ASD and also seen in a reported case of LSVC which had a bridging with the RSVC by left brachiocephalic vein, such a treatment option was not considered in our patient as she did not have any of the above. She was discharged on aspirin, metoprolol, and a Holter monitor was placed prior to discharge. She will continue to follow up with the hospital for further evaluation 6 months later with a cardiac MRI.

3. Discussion

Raghib Syndrome is a rare cardiac anomaly that was originally described by Raghib et al. in 1965 as a developmental complex consisting of termination of the left superior vena cava in the left atrium, absence of the coronary sinus, and an atrial septal defect commonly located at the posterior-inferior angle of the atrial septum [9]. This complex was considered unique to Raghib Syndrome; however, cases with a normal atrial septum have been reported where the orifice of the unroofed coronary sinus functions as the interatrial communication [10]. Our patient demonstrated an isolated persistent left superior vena cava draining into the left atrium along with an absence of the coronary sinus (Figure 6) and absence of ASD (Figure 7). She also has hypertrophic cardiomyopathy leading to ventricular dysfunction; association of this condition with Raghib syndrome has not been reported before.

Embryologically, persistence of the left superior vena cava (PLSVC) occurs due to failure of involution of the left horn of the embryonic sinus venosus and is one the most common venous anomalies of the chest. Drainage of the PLSVC into the left atrium due to congenital defects which prevent the rotation of the sinoatrial region; this in turn causes the left and the right cardinal veins to lie at the same level rather than the usual inferior location of the right cardinal vein, thus blocking the development of the coronary sinus. As a result a PLSVC draining into left atrium is commonly associated with coronary sinus ostial atresia [7]. LSVC may serve as a collateral channel secondary to coronary sinus atresia. This anatomic configuration is vital to recognize at open heart surgery so that the cardiac venous return can be identified and preserved. Retrograde administration of cardioplegia is also relatively contraindicated. The coronary sinus catheter balloon may not be able to occlude the dilated coronary sinus, resulting in failure to ensure retrograde flow of cardioplegia to the myocardium. Also, cardioplegia delivered would largely be distributed to the left internal jugular and left subclavian veins, rather than myocardium [11, 12]. Careful mapping of the coronary venous anatomy and dissection of the coronary sinus are necessary before reanastomoses of the PLSVC into the right atrium is attempted [11].

Precise anatomical detailing and multiresolution image building capacity of cardiac CT scan is of high yield in such cases especially in the plane of the atrioventricular groove in a short axis view. The shunt between the left atrium and the coronary sinus can be easily detected on a cardiac CT scan by insertion of contrast in the left arm vein and noting its presence in the left atrium [13]. MRI on the other hand with its phase contrast cine images may demonstrate turbulent flow from left atrium to coronary sinus, thus providing a distinctive advantage in detecting left to right shunt and estimating the ratio of pulmonary to systemic flow (Figure 3). The 3D images of cardiac CT scan and MRI not only facilitate in diagnosing the anomaly but also play an important role in planning surgical interventions like closure of PLSVC with coils or coronary sinus stent placement (Figure 2) [14, 15]. A novel cardiac MRI 4D flow technique, still under research phase, displays differential flow into the atria (Figure 4).

(a)

(b)

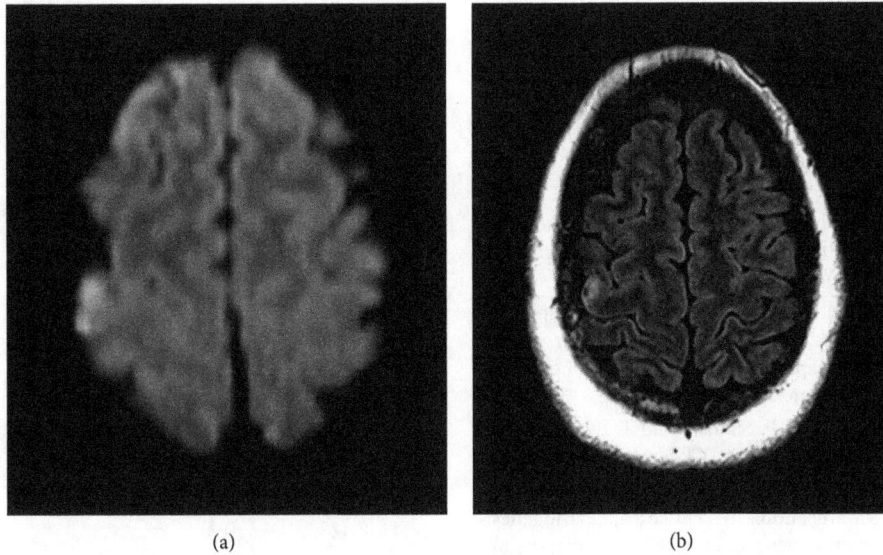

FIGURE 5: Restricted diffusion on DWI with increase T2 signal on FLAIR and postcontrast enhancement in right frontal lobe is consistent with subacute infarct within the right precentral gyrus.

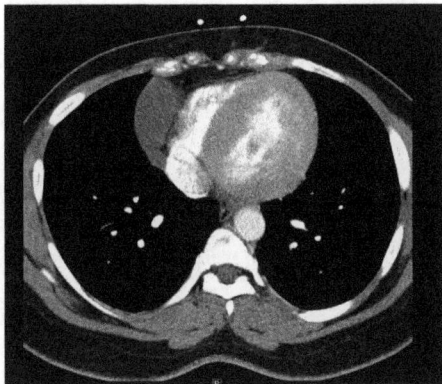

FIGURE 6: Coronary sinus atresia: absence of coronary sinus at the expected location on axial contrast CT chest image.

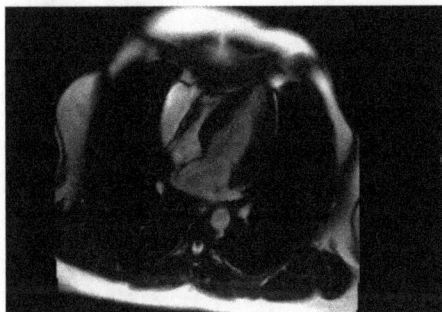

FIGURE 7: Four chamber steady-state free precession imaging shows intact interatrial septum. No ASD noted.

Overall cardiac Ct scan and MRI provide an unparalleled edge in visualization of such rare developmental anomalies and assist in prevention of paradoxical cerebral embolization and abscess formation [16].

4. Conclusion

Raghib Syndrome is considered to be a benign anomaly yet is associated with paradoxical embolization, diminished arterial oxygen saturation, and has implications for cardiac surgery as well as considerations for the location of intravenous access. Cardiac MRI and cardiac CT are useful imaging modalities in the evaluation of anomalies of the systemic venous return, enabling quantification of the flow disturbance and characterization of the anatomy.

Conflict of Interests

The authors declare that there is no conflict of interests regarding the publication of this paper.

References

[1] M. Biffi, G. Boriani, L. Frabetti, G. Bronzetti, and A. Branzi, "Left superior vena cava persistence in patients undergoing pacemaker or cardioverter-defibrillator implantation: a 10-year experience," *Chest*, vol. 120, no. 1, pp. 139–144, 2001.

[2] J. K. Perloff, "Congenital anomalies of vena caval connection," in *The Clinical Recognition of Congenital Heart Disease*, pp. 703–714, WB Saunders, Philadelphia, Pa, USA, 4th edition, 1994.

[3] J. C. Horrow and N. Lingaraju, "Unexpected persistent left superior vena cava: diagnostic clues during monitoring," *Journal of Cardiothoracic Anesthesia*, vol. 3, no. 5, pp. 611–615, 1989.

[4] E. Mantini, C. M. Grondin, C. W. Lillehei, and J. E. Edwards, "Congenital anomalies involving the coronary sinus," *Circulation*, vol. 33, no. 2, pp. 317–327, 1966.

[5] M. R. de Leval, D. G. Ritter, D. C. McGoon, and G. K. Danielson, "Anomalous systemic venous connection: surgical

considerations," *Mayo Clinic Proceedings*, vol. 50, no. 10, pp. 599–610, 1975.

[6] Le Cat, *Histoire de l'Acad Royale des Sciences*, Le Cat, Paris, France, 1738.

[7] M. Okumori, M. Hyuga, S. Ogata, T. Akamatsu, S. Otomi, and S. Ota, "Raghib's syndrome: a report of two cases," *Japanese Journal of Surgery*, vol. 12, no. 5, pp. 356–361, 1982.

[8] D. A. Goor and C. W. Lillehei, *Congenital Malformations of the Heart: Embryology, Anatomy, and Operative Considerations*, Grune & Stratton, New York, NY, USA, 1975.

[9] G. Raghib, H. D. Ruttenberg, R. C. Anderson, K. Amplatz, P. Adams, and J. E. Edwards, "Termination of left superior vena cava in left atrium, atrial septal defect, and absence of coronary sinus," *Circulation*, vol. 31, pp. 906–918, 1965.

[10] H. D. Allen, D. J. Driscoll, R. E. Shaddy, and T. F. Feltes, *Moss and Adam's Heart Disease in Infants, Children and Adolescent*, Lippincott Williams & Wilkins, 2012.

[11] E. N. Nsah, G. W. Moore, and G. M. Hutchins, "Pathogenesis of persistent left superior vena cava with a coronary sinus connection," *Pediatric Pathology*, vol. 11, no. 2, pp. 261–269, 1991.

[12] J. Paval and S. Nayak, "A persistent left superior vena cava," *Singapore Medical Journal*, vol. 48, no. 3, pp. e90–e93, 2007.

[13] G. Brancaccio, F. Miraldi, F. Ventriglia, G. Michielon, R. M. di Donato, and M. de Santis, "Multidetector-row helical computed tomography imaging of unroofed coronary sinus," *International Journal of Cardiology*, vol. 91, no. 2-3, pp. 251–253, 2003.

[14] J. K. Hahm, Y. W. Park, J. K. Lee et al., "Magnetic resonance imaging of unroofed coronary sinus: three cases," *Pediatric Cardiology*, vol. 21, no. 4, pp. 382–387, 2000.

[15] Y. H. Choe, I.-S. Kang, S. W. Park, and H. J. Lee, "MR imaging of congenital heart disease in adolescents and adults," *Korean Journal of Radiology*, vol. 2, no. 3, pp. 121–131, 2001.

[16] E. M. Kim, P. B. Moore, S. P. Singh, and S. G. Lloyd, "Cardio-vascular magnetic resonance imaging of the Raghib complex," *Journal of the American College of Cardiology*, vol. 57, no. 8, article e15, 2011.

38

Severe Hyperthyroidism Presenting with Acute ST Segment Elevation Myocardial Infarction

Dayan Zhou, Zongjie Qu, Hao Wang, Zhe Wang, and Qiang Xu

Department of Cardiology, Fifth People's Hospital of Chongqing, Renji Road No. 24, Nanan District, Chongqing 400062, China

Correspondence should be addressed to Qiang Xu; 24725373@qq.com

Academic Editor: Kjell Nikus

Introduction. Acute myocardial infarction is life-threatening. A cardiac troponin rise accompanied by typical symptoms, ST elevation or depression is diagnostic of acute myocardial infarction. Here, we report an unusual case of a female who was admitted with chest pain. However, she did not present with a typical profile of an acute myocardial infarction patient. *Case Presentation.* A 66-year-old Han nationality female presented with chest pain. The electrocardiogram (ECG) revealed arched ST segment elevations and troponin was elevated. However, the coronary angiography showed a normal coronary arterial system. Thyroid function tests showed that this patient had severe hyperthyroidism. *Conclusion.* Our case highlights the possibility that hyperthyroidism may cause a large area of myocardium injury and ECG ST segment elevation. We suggest routine thyroid function testing in patients with chest pain.

1. Introduction

A patient is diagnosed with acute myocardial infarction if a typical rise and gradual fall (troponin) or a more rapid rise and fall (creatine kinase-MB, CK-MB) of biochemical markers of myocardial necrosis are seen with at least one of the following: (a) ischemic symptoms; (b) development of pathologic Q waves on the electrocardiogram (ECG); or (c) ECG changes indicative of ischemia (ST segment elevation or depression) [1]. When myocardial necrosis occurs, troponin rises before CK/CK-MB. Here, we report an unusual case of a 66-year-old female who was admitted with chest pain. The ECG revealed ST segment elevations and troponin was elevated. However, she did not present with a typical profile of an acute myocardial infarction patient.

2. Case Presentation

A 66-year-old Han nationality female, who had experienced a cerebral infarction 1 year previously and showed lingering muscle weakness in the right limbs, was admitted with chest pain and palpitations for 2 days. There was no significant family history of cardiac disease, and she had two healthy children. She did not have any risk factors, such as hypertension, diabetes, hyperlipidemia, or smoking.

Physical examination at the intensive care unit showed that her body weight was normal. Her temperature was 37.2°C, blood pressure was 105/65 mmHg, heart rate was about 131 beats per minute, and respiratory rate was about 24 breaths per minute. Heart sounds were normal. A small amount of rales could be heard at the bottom of both lungs.

On admission, the ECG showed sinus tachycardia, 2 to 3 mm ST segment elevations in II, III, and aVF, and 2 to 9 mm ST segment elevations in V2 to V6 (Figure 1). A diagnosis of acute myocardial infarction was made, and the patient was immediately started on standard medication (aspirin, clopidogrel, atorvastatin, low-molecular-weight heparin, and metoprolol). An emergency coronary angiogram was not arranged; this is done only when patients have had chest pain within 12 hours. However this patient had chest pain for 2 days.

Laboratory workup revealed the following results: troponin I levels were markedly raised (7.959 μg/L); myocardial enzymes (CK 299.0 IU/L, CK-MB 26.6 IU/L) and NT pro-Brain Natriuretic Peptide (NT-proBNP, 18497.0 pg/mL) were elevated; blood gas, glucose, liver function, and renal function were in normal ranges; initial laboratory tests revealed

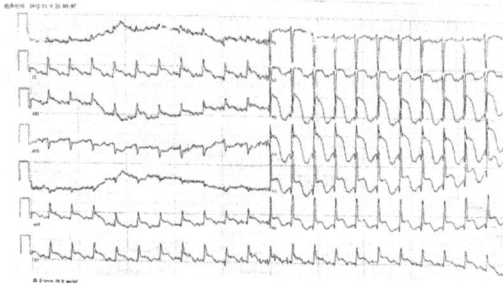

FIGURE 1: ECG upon arrival at hospital.

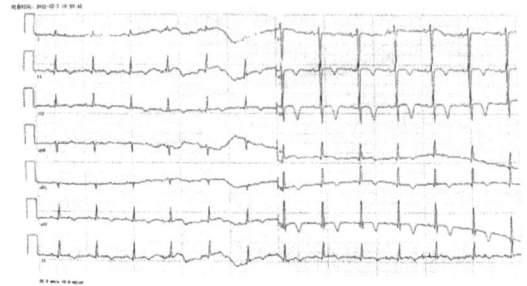

FIGURE 3: ECG 2 weeks after discharge from hospital.

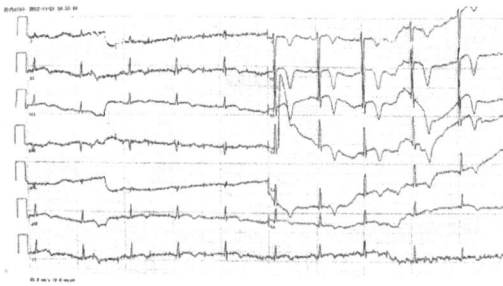

FIGURE 2: ECG 11 days after admission.

normal electrolytes; and plasma lipids showed surprisingly low concentrations (total cholesterol 2.8 mmol/L, triglycerides 0.83 mmol/L, LDL-cholesterol 1.75 mmol/L, and HDL-cholesterol 0.87 mmol/L).

However, the patient had persistent tachycardia (about 110–120 beats/minute) after drug treatment. Therefore, thyroid function tests were requested; these revealed hyperthyroidism (free T3 48.71 pmol/L (reference range 2.8–7.1), T3 8.59 nmol/L (1.3–3.1), free T4 > 100 pmol/L (12–22), T4 > 320 nmol/L (66–181), and thyroid-stimulating hormone < 0.005 μIU/mL (0.27–4.2)). An acute myocardial infarction complicated by hyperthyroidism and threatened hyperthyroidism crisis could not be ruled out. She was therefore referred for an endocrine consultation and started on propylthiouracil.

After 11 days of such a complicated condition, the patient's condition had stabilized. Blood pressure was 115/65 mm Hg and the heart rate was 95 beats per minute. ECG showed sinus rhythm and negative T waves on anterior and inferior derivations and no abnormal Q waves over the anterior and inferior leads (Figure 2). Echocardiography one week after admission showed normal left ventricle systolic function with the left ventricular ejection fraction of 65%. A thyroid ultrasound scan showed no focal lesions. Percutaneous angiography was also performed. Coronary angiography showed a normal coronary arterial system, a normal supply of blood to the heart, and no blockages.

The patient was successfully discharged after 2 weeks of treatment. A follow-up ECG showed no pathological Q waves over the anterior and inferior leads (Figure 3). She remained euthyroid on propylthiouracil, which was discontinued after 18 months. She denied any anginal symptoms.

Patient's ECG upon arrival at the hospital shows the following: sinus tachycardia, 2 to 3 mm ST segment elevations in II, III, and aVF, and 2 to 9 mm ST segment elevations in V2 to V6.

Patient's ECG 11 days after admission shows the following: sinus rhythm, T waves inversion on anterior and inferior leads, and no Q waves on anterior and inferior leads.

Patient's ECG 2 weeks after discharge from hospital shows the following: sinus rhythm, negative T waves on anterior and inferior derivations, and no Q waves.

3. Discussion

Myocardial infarction can occur with thyrotoxicosis [2, 3]. There is evidence that thyrotoxicosis is directly associated with the presence of a prothrombotic state [4]. Some long-term follow-up studies have revealed increased mortality from cardiovascular and cerebrovascular disease in persons with a history of overt hyperthyroidism [5], as well as in those with subclinical hyperthyroidism [6]. In another study, an elevated FT3 concentration was associated with a 2.6-fold greater likelihood of coronary events [7]. In the absence of fixed coronary artery disease or coronary artery spasm, thyrotoxicosis is rarely associated with acute myocardial infarction. Therefore, acute myocardial infarction and hyperthyroidism (especially thyrotoxic storm) are a difficult and dangerous combination. Although acute myocardial infarction and hyperthyroidism are curable when diagnosed early, they can be fatal if left undiagnosed or treated incorrectly.

The cause of myocardial ischemia and infarction in thyrotoxic patients with normal coronary arteries is unclear. It may be a result of in situ coronary thrombosis or a direct metabolic effect of thyroid hormone on the myocardium, or it may be secondary to supraventricular tachycardia or atrial fibrillation [8]. In addition, coronary vasospasm might be another factor contributing to the development of acute myocardial infarction. There are some reports of severe coronary artery spasm leading to myocardial infarction in young subjects with thyrotoxicosis, but without classical cardiovascular disease risk factors [3, 8, 9].

According to the typical ST segment elevation on the ECG, the chest pain, and the elevated myocardial enzymology, there was no doubt about the initial diagnosis of acute myocardial infarction in our patient. However, coronary angiography showed a normal coronary arterial system without any stenotic lesions. Admission ECG showed 2 to 3 mm ST segment elevations in II, III, and aVF and 2 to 9 mm ST segment elevations in V2 to V6, while long-term follow-up ECG showed no abnormal Q waves over the anterior and inferior leads. Therefore, the diagnosis of acute myocardial infarction had to be reconsidered. A thrombophilic tendency or severe spasm may be considered in our patient. According to the Third Universal Definition of Myocardial Infarction, our patient may have a type 2 myocardial infarction [10]. But we did not perform ergonovine or acetylcholine provocation test during coronary angiography. This was a limitation which could not differentiate vasospasm from causal disease. Thyroid function tests showed that this patient had severe hyperthyroidism, causing a large area of injury to the myocardium and leading to decreased cardiac function. Since it is known that thyroid hormones increase the demand for oxygen, the rapid elevation of oxygen utilization caused by thyrotoxicosis is likely responsible for this patient's myocardium injury. At the first physical examination rale sounds were heard and NT-proBNP levels were clearly elevated, indicating reduced left ventricular function. However, ventriculography or echocardiography was not performed in the acute phase. Transient systolic dysfunction of left ventricle, ST elevation, elevated troponin T and inverted T wave with no Q wave seem to be consistent with Takotsubo cardiomyopathy. Takotsubo cardiomyopathy is characterized by transient left ventricular dysfunction with chest symptoms, elevated cardiac enzymes, and ECG changes such as ST segment elevation and/or T-wave inversion without coronary artery occlusion [11]. The association of Takotsubo syndrome and hyperthyroidism has been reported before [12–14]. Therefore Takotsubo cardiomyopathy may be considered in our patient. However, such typical ST segment elevation in a patient with severe hyperthyroidism is rare and easy to misdiagnose.

4. Conclusion

Our case highlights the possibility that hyperthyroidism may cause a large area of myocardium injury and ECG ST segment elevation. We suggest routine thyroid function testing in patients with chest pain.

Consent

Written informed consent was obtained from the patient for publication of this case report and accompanying images.

Disclaimer

The contents of this paper are solely the responsibility of the authors and do not necessarily represent the official views of the supporting offices.

Conflict of Interests

The authors declare that they have no conflict of interests.

Authors' Contribution

Dayan Zhou, Zongjie Qu, and Qiang Xu contributed in acquisition of data; Hao Wang and Zhe Wang did literature search; Dayan Zhou did drafting of the paper. All authors read and approved the final paper.

Acknowledgment

The authors thank Professor TC He for language modification of the paper.

References

[1] J. S. Alpert, K. Thygesen, E. Antman, and J. P. Bassand, "Myocardial infarction redefined—a consensus document of the Joint European Society of Cardiology/American College of Cardiology Committee for the redefinition of myocardial infarction," *Journal of the American College of Cardiology*, vol. 36, no. 3, pp. 959–969, 2000.

[2] K. C. Lewandowski, T. Rechciński, M. Krzemińska-Pakuła, and A. Lewiński, "Acute myocardial infarction as the first presentation of thyrotoxicosis in a 31-year old woman—case report," *Thyroid Research*, vol. 3, no. 1, article 1, 2010.

[3] J. Al Jaber, S. Haque, H. Noor, B. Ibrahim, and J. Al Suwaidi, "Thyrotoxicosis and coronary artery spasm: case report and review of the literature," *Angiology*, vol. 61, no. 8, pp. 807–812, 2010.

[4] M. K. Horne III, K. K. Singh, K. G. Rosenfeld et al., "Is thyroid hormone suppression therapy prothrombotic?" *Journal of Clinical Endocrinology and Metabolism*, vol. 89, no. 9, pp. 4469–4473, 2004.

[5] J. A. Franklyn, P. Maisonneuve, M. C. Sheppard, J. Betteridge, and P. Boyle, "Mortality after the treatment of hyperthyroidism with radioactive iodine," *The New England Journal of Medicine*, vol. 338, no. 11, pp. 712–718, 1998.

[6] J. V. Parle, P. Maisonneuve, M. C. Sheppard, P. Boyle, and J. A. Franklyn, "Prediction of all-cause and cardiovascular mortality in elderly people from one low serum thyrotropin result: a 10-year cohort study," *The Lancet*, vol. 358, no. 9285, pp. 861–865, 2001.

[7] A. Peters, M. Ehlers, B. Blank et al., "Excess triiodothyronine as a risk factor of coronary events," *Archives of Internal Medicine*, vol. 160, no. 13, pp. 1993–1999, 2000.

[8] N. D. Masani, D. B. Northridge, and R. J. C. Hall, "Severe coronary vasospasm associated with hyperthyroidism causing myocardial infarction," *British Heart Journal*, vol. 74, no. 6, pp. 700–701, 1995.

[9] Z. Grąbczewska, T. Białoszyński, and J. Kubica, "Acute myocardial infarction in a patient with iatrogenic thyrotoxicosis—a case report," *Kardiologia Polska*, vol. 65, no. 3, pp. 280–282, 2007.

[10] K. Thygesen, J. S. Alpert, A. S. Jaffe, M. L. Simoons, B. R. Chaitman, and H. D. White, "Third universal definition of myocardial infarction," *Circulation*, vol. 126, no. 16, pp. 2020–2035, 2012.

[11] T. M. Pilgrim and T. R. Wyss, "Takotsubo cardiomyopathy or transient left ventricular apical ballooning syndrome: a systematic review," *International Journal of Cardiology*, vol. 124, no. 3, pp. 283–292, 2008.

[12] S. Omar, E. Ali, H. Mazek, T. Mahmoud, S. Soontrapa, and J. Suarez, "Takotsubo cardiomyopathy associated with hyperthyroidism treated with thyroidectomy," *Proceedings (Baylor University. Medical Center)*, vol. 28, no. 2, pp. 194–195, 2015.

[13] M. Eliades, D. El-Maouche, C. Choudhary, B. Zinsmeister, and K. D. Burman, "Takotsubo cardiomyopathy associated with

thyrotoxicosis: a case report and review of the literature," *Thyroid*, vol. 24, no. 2, pp. 383–389, 2014.

[14] D. C. Hutchings, D. Adlam, V. Ferreira, T. D. Karamitsos, and K. M. Channon, "Takotsubo cardiomyopathy in association with endogenous and exogenous thyrotoxicosis," *QJM*, vol. 104, no. 5, pp. 433–435, 2011.

39

Superdominant Right Coronary Artery with Absence of Left Circumflex and Anomalous Origin of the Left Anterior Descending Coronary from the Right Sinus: An Unheard Coronary Anomaly Circulation

Marcos Danillo Peixoto Oliveira, Fernando Roberto de Fazzio, José Mariani Junior, Carlos M. Campos, Luiz Junya Kajita, Expedito E. Ribeiro, and Pedro Alves Lemos

Department of Interventional Cardiology, Heart Institute(InCor) of the University of São Paulo, Avenida Dr. Enéas de Carvalho Aguiar 44, 05403-900 São Paulo, SP, Brazil

Correspondence should be addressed to Expedito E. Ribeiro; expribeiro@incor.usp.br

Academic Editor: Monvadi Barbara Srichai

Coronary artery anomalies are congenital changes in their origin, course, and/or structure. Most of them are discovered as incidental findings during coronary angiographic studies or at autopsies. We present herein the case of a 70-year-old man with symptomatic severe aortic valvar stenosis whose preoperative coronary angiogram revealed a so far unreported coronary anomaly circulation pattern.

1. Introduction

Coronary artery anomalies (CAA) are a diverse group of congenital disorders, and the pathophysiological mechanisms and manifestations are highly variable. Several controversies remain in terms of incidence, classification, screening, heredity, and treatment [1–3]. The absence of the left circumflex (LCX) artery with a superdominant right coronary artery (RCA) is very rare, and the concomitant anomalous origin of the left anterior descending (LAD) artery turns this association into an unheard, up to now, CAA presentation.

2. Case Report

A 70-year-old man, active and Caucasian, presented with a three-month history of exertional angina, one episode of syncope after a normal effort, and dyspnea in usual daily activities. There were no previous episodes of myocardial infarction, stroke, coronary artery disease, or personal or familiar histories of sudden cardiac death. The resting electrocardiogram (ECG) showed sinus rhythm and left atrial and ventricular overload. A rest transthoracic echocardiogram revealed preserved left ventricular ejection fraction (0.58, Simpson) and severe aortic valvar stenosis, defined by an orifice area of $0.7 \, cm^2$ and a transvalvular medium gradient of 50 mmHg. The surgical aortic valve replacement (SAVR) was proposed to him and a preoperative coronary angiogram was, then, requested. The RCA showed a superdominant pattern, with various posterior descending branches, extending beyond the *crux cordis* and circling the atrioventricular groove almost completely, following the expected path of the absent circumflex artery (Figures 1 and 2). A nonselective injection of contrast media into the left coronary sinus revealed no emergent arteries (Figure 2). The left coronary artery, instead, arose from the right coronary sinus, near to the RCA ostium, and reached the anterior intraventricular course of the left anterior descending artery, after passing in front of the pulmonary trunk (Figure 3). There was massive calcification into the aortic valve topography. The systolic transvalvular gradient was 100 mmHg, without intraventricular gradient. The patient is, at the time of this report, waiting the call for the proposed SAVR, in the same functional

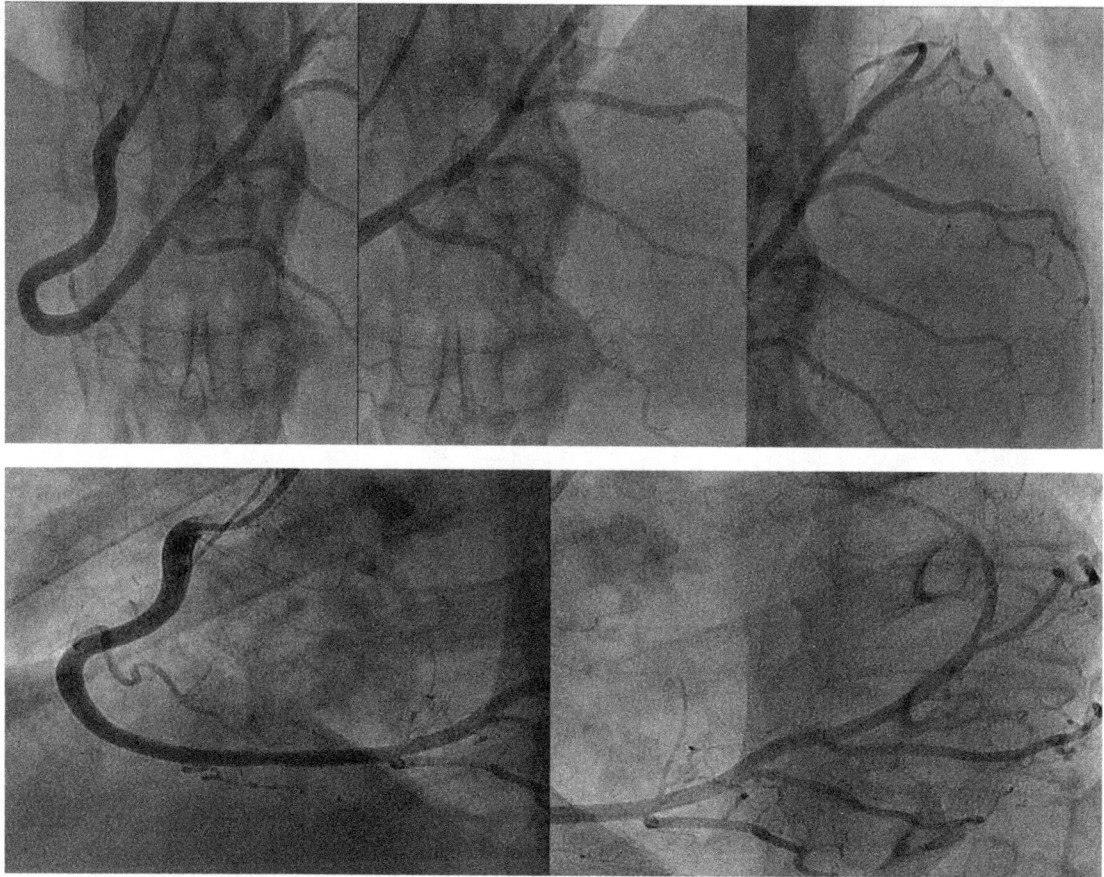

FIGURE 1: Reconstruction, by subsequent images, of the superdominant RCA, with various posterior descending branches, extending beyond the *crux cordis* and circling the atrioventricular groove, following the expected path of the absent circumflex artery. Superior panel: cranial left anterior oblique view. Inferior panel: left anterior oblique view. RCA: right coronary artery.

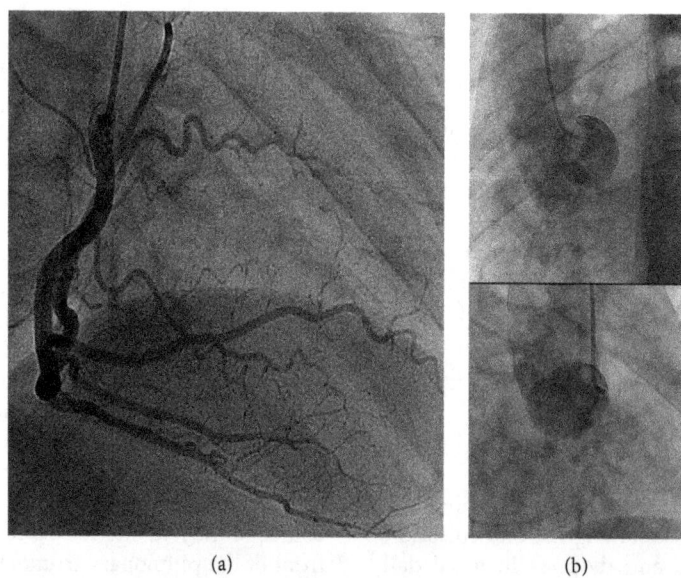

(a)   (b)

FIGURE 2: (a) The superdominant RCA in right anterior oblique view. (b) Nonselective injections of contrast media into the left coronary sinus showing no emergent arteries.

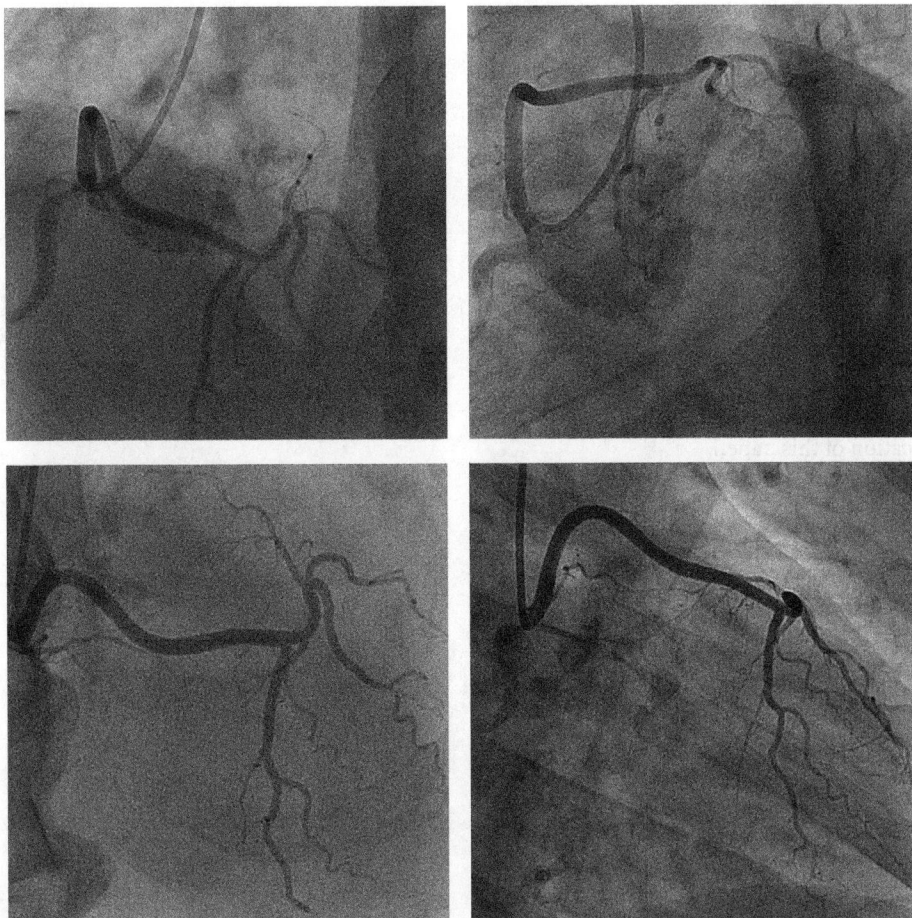

FIGURE 3: The LCA arising from the right coronary sinus, near to the RCA ostium, and reaching the anterior intraventricular course of the LAD. LCA: left coronary artery; RCA: right coronary artery; LAD: left anterior descending.

status, without readmissions or major adverse cardiac or cerebrovascular events.

3. Discussion

CAA are congenital changes in their origin, course, and/or structure. Several controversies remain in terms of incidence, classification, screening, heredity, and treatment. Despite being mostly asymptomatic, clinical presentation in adults may result from myocardial ischemia, manifesting as angina, syncope, arrhythmias, and even sudden death. In young athletes, apparently healthy, they are the second most frequent cause of sudden death [3].

Most CAA are discovered as incidental findings during coronary angiographic study or at autopsy with incidence rate of 0.64% to 1.3% reported in the literature [4].

Yamanaka and Hobbs described 126.595 patients undergoing cardiac catheterization from 1960 to 1988 [5]. Separate origins of the LAD and LCX arteries from the left sinus of Valsalva were the most common anomaly, occurring in about 0.41% of the patients studied [4]. Absence of the LCX artery is a very rare congenital anomaly of the coronary circulation in which the artery fails to develop in the left atrioventricular

groove, with a few cases reported in the literature [4, 6], and a frequency of only 0.003% according to those authors [5]. In this condition, the inferior, lateral, and posterior walls of the left ventricle are supplied by a superdominant RCA and, sometimes, by a large diagonal branch [4, 5].

If the LCX artery cannot be visualized during angiography, either an ostial total occlusion or congenital agenesis should be suspected. Anomalous origin of the LCX is diagnosed when it is not visualized during left coronary injection in the absence of proximal occlusion, but, instead, it arises separately from the right sinus of Valsalva or as an extension of the RCA [4].

After an extensive review in the pertinent literature, we did not find any report of the herein described association of absence of LCX with superdominant RCA and anomalous origin of the LAD from the right coronary sinus.

In our case, despite the presence of degenerative severe aortic valvar stenosis, no significant lesions were noted in any of the coronary arteries, so the symptoms recently reported by the patient were really due to the progression of the valvar dysfunction.

All interventional cardiologists and cardiac surgeons should be familiar with these anatomic variants since accurate recognition of the course and distribution of the coronary vessels is crucial for proper revascularization strategies in the presence of coronary artery disease [7].

4. Conclusion

To the best of our knowledge, this is the first report of this so far unheard coronary anomaly circulation, characterized by the absence of LCX with superdominant RCA and anomalous origin of the LAD from the right sinus of Valsalva.

Conflict of Interests

The authors declare that there is no conflict of interests regarding the publication of this paper.

References

[1] P. Angelini, "Coronary artery anomalies: an entity in search of an identity," *Circulation*, vol. 115, no. 10, pp. 1296–1305, 2007.

[2] M. D. P. Oliveira, P. H. M. C. de Melo, A. E. Filho, L. J. Kajita, E. E. Ribeiro, and P. A. Lemos, "Type 4 dual left anterior descending artery: a very rare coronary anomaly circulation," *Case Reports in Cardiology*, vol. 2015, Article ID 580543, 3 pages, 2015.

[3] C. Almeida, R. Dourado, C. Machado et al., "Anomalias das artérias coronárias," *Portuguese Journal of Cardiology*, vol. 31, no. 7-8, pp. 477–484, 2012.

[4] F. A. Ali, S. A. Khan, J. M. Tai, S. H. Fatimi, and S. H. Dhakam, "Congenital absence of left circumflex artery with a dominant right coronary artery," *BMJ Case Reports*, 2009.

[5] O. Yamanaka and R. E. Hobbs, "Coronary artery anomalies in 126,595 patients undergoing coronary arteriography," *Catheterization and Cardiovascular Diagnosis*, vol. 21, no. 1, pp. 28–40, 1990.

[6] A. Quijada-Fumero, R. Pimienta-González, and M. Rodriguez-Esteban, "Absence of left circumflex with superdominant right coronary artery," *BMJ Case Reports*, 2014.

[7] M. Maheshwari and S. R. Mittal, "Superdominant right coronary artery with double posterior descending artery," *Heart Views*, vol. 16, no. 1, pp. 19–20, 2015.

40

Fibromuscular Dysplasia Leading to Spontaneous Coronary Artery Dissection with Sudden Cardiac Arrest

Ata Bajwa, Udit Bhatnagar, Amit Sharma, Hani El-Halawany, and Randall C. Thompson

Saint Luke's Mid America Heart Institute, University of Missouri-Kansas City School of Medicine, Kansas City, MO, USA

Correspondence should be addressed to Ata Bajwa; bajwaa@umkc.edu

Academic Editor: Markus Ferrari

A 30-year-old previously healthy female, who was six-week postpartum, experienced sudden collapse and tonic-clonic seizure. Emergency medicine services arrived at the scene and the patient was found to be in ventricular fibrillation. Advanced cardiovascular life support (ACLS) was initiated with return of spontaneous circulation. Afterwards, her initial EKG showed atrial fibrillation with rapid ventricular rate, ST elevation in leads II, III, and aVF, and ST depression in V2–V4. She was transferred to a tertiary care hospital where emergent angiogram was performed revealing obstruction of blood flow in the proximal and mid right coronary artery (RCA). A hazy and irregularly contoured appearance of the RCA was consistent with diagnosis of fibromuscular dysplasia. Subsequently, intravascular ultrasonogram (IVUS) was performed which confirmed the diagnosis of RCA dissection. Successful revascularization of the RCA was performed using two bare mental stents. After a complicated course in hospital, she was discharged in stable condition and did very well overall.

1. Introduction

Fibromuscular dysplasia has been frequently cited to have close association with spontaneous coronary artery dissection (SCAD) which is an increasingly recognized cause of acute coronary syndrome, especially in young women. Prompt diagnosis and treatment can improve survival in patients with SCAD which otherwise may prove fatal.

2. Case

A 30-year-old Caucasian female presented after a sudden collapse followed by seizure activity that was witnessed by her husband. It was reported that she had woken up early in the morning and noticed abnormal sensations in both arms before collapsing. She had no significant past medical history and had spontaneous vaginal delivery of a healthy term infant, six weeks prior. On arriving at the scene, emergency medicine services found her in ventricular fibrillation. She was successfully defibrillated and taken to a nearby critical care hospital. Her initial EKG showed atrial fibrillation with rapid ventricular rate, ST segment elevation in the inferior leads, and ST depression in the anterior precordial leads.

The ST elevation resolved spontaneously on subsequent EKGs, but ST depression persisted. She could not be airlifted because of inclement weather and, after few hours delay, was transferred to a tertiary care hospital via ambulance. Therapeutic hypothermia was initiated at the outlying hospital prior to transfer and was continued per protocol at our facility. Her serum troponin rose to 17.5 ng/mL. After her transfer, coronary angiogram was performed emergently.

Coronary angiography, as evident in Figure 1, showed 70% stenosis in the proximal and mid right coronary artery (RCA). The lesion was irregularly contoured and hazy and became more severe after intracoronary nitroglycerin was administered, progressing to 99% occlusion with TIMI II flow (Figure 2). Worsening of stenosis following nitroglycerin administration was considered to be inconsistent with coronary vasospasm. The angiographic appearance, young age of the patient, and lack of traditional risk factors for atherosclerotic disease were all consistent with a diagnosis of fibromuscular dysplasia. Coronary intravascular ultrasound (IVUS) was performed following angiography and showed dissection as well as thrombus in right coronary artery. The left main, left anterior descending, and circumflex coronary artery segments were angiographically normal.

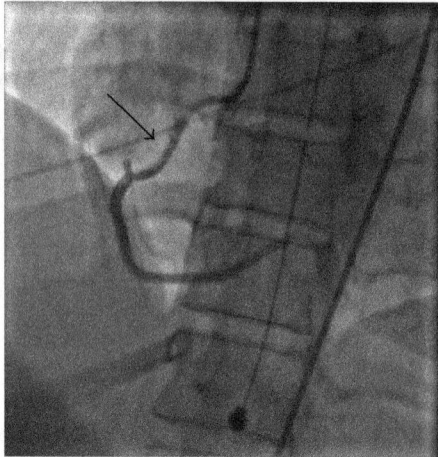

FIGURE 1: Coronary angiogram was performed within few hours after onset of symptoms and it showed 70% stenosis in proximal RCA flow. The lesion was irregularly contoured and hazy, which was consistent with fibromuscular dysplasia leading to spontaneous coronary artery dissection.

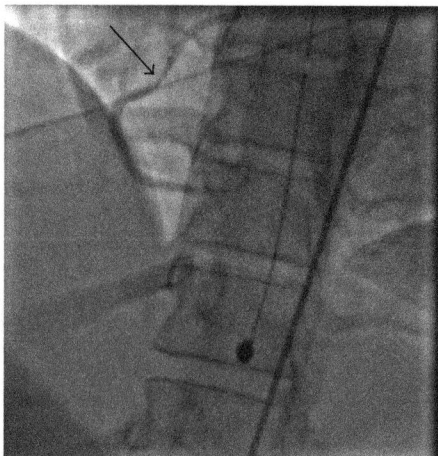

FIGURE 2: Stenosis seen in RCA became progressively worse after IC NTG and progressed to 99% occlusion. IVUS was performed and demonstrated coronary artery dissection.

The patient had originally presented after suffering cardiac arrest and she remained persistently hypotensive after being transferred to our facility. Because of the severe and worsening nature of the stenosis and the patient's hemodynamic instability, it was decided that IVUS directed coronary stent implantation would be appropriate. 3.5 mm × 30 mm and 3.5 × 15 mm integrity bare metal stent (Medtronic Corp) were implanted into the proximal right coronary artery and dilated to 14 atm. TIMI 3 flow was seen in RCA after the procedure (Figure 3). Optimal poststent implantation and expansion were confirmed with IVUS. Bare metal stents were chosen instead of drug eluting ones primarily because the patient had a very low predicted rate of restenosis based on our decision support algorithm. The low predicted rate was largely driven by the large caliber of the right coronary artery and the individual patient characteristics. The patient was comatose at the time of the procedure and limited

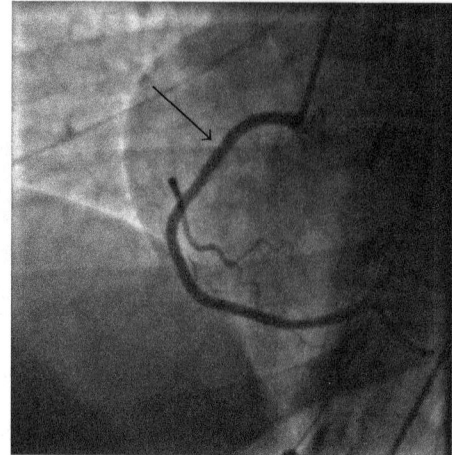

FIGURE 3: Emergent PCI was performed with placement of bare metal stents in proximal and mid RCA leading to restoration of the normal coronary blood flow (TIMI 3 flow).

medical history was available and there was some concern about bleeding risk with prolonged dual platelet therapy which would be necessary if drug eluting stents were used. She was started on aspirin 81 mg, ticagrelor 90 mg BID, intravenous heparin drip, and atorvastatin 80 mg QHS. Later on, metoprolol was also added after her blood pressure had improved.

An echocardiogram that was performed on the day of admission demonstrated severely reduced left ventricular systolic function with an estimated ejection fraction of 25%. There was inferior, inferolateral, and anterolateral left ventricular akinesis with near global hypokinesis. Right ventricular systolic function was normal. The patient's LV dysfunction was believed to be from cardiac ischemia/stunning related to a transient occlusion of the right coronary artery and the cardiac arrest. The patient had a complicated course over the next two weeks primarily related to anoxic brain injury from the cardiac arrest. She demonstrated myoclonic seizures and cortical blindness and was diagnosed with "Lance-Adams syndrome" and "Posterior Reversible Leukoencephalopathy syndrome," respectively. She was started on a combination of antiepileptic medications resulting in improvement of her myoclonic seizures. A repeat echocardiogram was performed two weeks after the initial presentation, which demonstrated that regional and global left ventricular function had returned to normal. Her discharge medications included aspirin 81 mg, ticagrelor 90 mg BID, and metoprolol ER 25 mg. Atorvastatin was discontinued given that she had nonatherosclerotic disease and her LDL was 44 with a total cholesterol of 102. At time of discharge, she had some residual cortical blindness but improved markedly over the course of the next few months and ultimately made a complete neurological recovery including cessation of seizure activity.

3. Discussion

Fibromuscular dysplasia is an idiopathic nonatherosclerotic, noninflammatory vascular disease that primarily involves renal and carotid arteries, although coronary and other arterial vasculature systems can also be affected [1]. The etiology of FMD is uncertain, but it has been postulated that hormonal, genetic, metabolic, and traumatic factors might have a role [2]. About 90 percent of cases are diagnosed in women which could suggest some hormonal etiology. Estrogen thus may play a role, but there is no concrete evidence regarding this possibility. A genetic association has also been suggested and, according to some reports, about 7% to 11% of first-degree relatives have FMD. It has been hypothesized that genetically abnormal encasement of the vasa vasorum by connective tissue leads to medial ischemia, proliferation of myofibroblasts, and weakening of vessel wall thus rendering them vulnerable to dissection [3]. Fibromuscular dysplasia has been found to have a close association with dissection of arteries and may be the main predisposing factor for spontaneous coronary artery dissection (SCAD) [4]. Saw et al. studied 50 patients with nonatherosclerotic SCAD over a period of six years and concluded that as many as 86% of patients diagnosed with SCAD have FMD [4]. Another relatively small study by Toggweiler and colleagues published in 2012 also supported this association and suggested that patients diagnosed with SCAD should undergo screening for FMD [5].

Spontaneous coronary artery dissection (SCAD) is a rare pathologic condition that usually presents as acute coronary syndrome (ACS) or sudden cardiac death. The first case was reported in 1931, when a coronary artery dissection was found in a 42-year-old woman during an autopsy [6]. The incidence is much more common during pregnancy and the postpartum period, with SCAD reportedly responsible for 27% of cases of myocardial infarction (MI) in pregnant or postpartum women. This rate is significantly higher than in the general population where it accounts for only 0.28–1.1% of MI cases [7]. The pathophysiology of SCAD is not fully understood, though it is postulated that an intimal tear disrupts the vessel wall leading to true and false lumens [4]. An alternative postulated mechanism is that rupture of the vasa vasorum results in the formation of intramural hematoma [4]. Eventually, the expansion of the false lumen or hematoma can cause occlusion of the true vessel lumen leading to myocardial ischemia [4]. The mortality for SCAD in earlier studies was described to be as high as 50%, but, over the years, survival has improved to 85% owing to better availability of coronary diagnostic and treatment modalities [8].

Coronary angiography is the most widely used test and should not be delayed if a diagnosis of SCAD is suspected. The angiographic findings in SCAD can be quite variable, from multiple and extensive dissections seen in an otherwise normal appearing coronary artery to a single short dissection in a vessel with severe atherosclerosis [9]. Invasive angiography has its limitations though and sometimes may not distinguish between atherosclerotic and nonatherosclerotic lesions [10]. Intravascular ultrasound (IVUS) can directly visualize the vessel wall and may be used during angiography to help differentiate between true and false lumens [10]. Optical Coherence Tomography (OCT) has higher resolution and is superior to IVUS in determining double lumen morphology, intimal tear location, and extent of dissection [9]. There is no consensus on the specific guidelines for management of SCAD. Management decisions should be based on the hemodynamic status of the patient, the extent of dissection, the degree of vascular stenosis, and the adequacy of coronary flow [9]. If a patient is asymptomatic with limited vascular stenosis and adequate coronary flow, a conservative approach is appropriate and the patient can be medically treated with aspirin, beta blockers, and IV heparin [9]. Medical management in such cases usually leads to natural healing of the dissection over the course of next few months [9]. Thrombolytic drugs are usually avoided since they can potentially lead to worsening of dissection as well as intramural hematoma [10]. However, atherosclerosis is a much more common cause of acute coronary syndrome than SCAD, and therefore thrombolytic therapy should not be withheld for patients with ST elevation myocardial infarction (STEMI) in remote centers where primary percutaneous coronary intervention (PCI) is not available [10]. A more aggressive approach is reasonable if the patient is hemodynamically unstable or if the dissection leads to severe vascular stenosis (70–99% occlusion), resulting in inadequate coronary blood flow [9]. Such cases may require coronary revascularization through PCI, though it comes with risk of progression of the dissection and thus total arterial occlusion [9, 10]. Bioresorbable vascular scaffolds are being touted as an important new advance in interventional cardiology. They seem to work by transient scaffolding of the vessel wall while eluting an antiproliferative drug to counteract constrictive remodeling and intimal hyperplasia. Over the long term, the scaffolds get resorbed into the vessel wall resulting in enlarged vessel lumen and diminished atherosclerotic plaque [11]. Recently, the use of vascular scaffolds has been expanded for the treatment of nonatherosclerotic lesions including SCAD. Cockburn and colleagues recently reported a case of successful treatment of SCAD involving the left circumflex artery with excellent long term results [12]. There seems to be promise regarding their use in the management of SCAD, but more studies will be needed to strengthen this argument. Moreover, lack of availability and high cost may be limiting factors, at least for the time being. Coronary artery bypass grafting is usually reserved for cases involving left main coronary artery, multivessel dissection, and patients with failed PCI [9].

The patient in our case report presented after suffering a cardiac arrest as a result of RCA dissection. She underwent PCI and ultimately did well. Timely intervention can prove to be crucial for the survival of such critically ill patients. Patients diagnosed with SCAD should be assessed individually for decisions regarding medical management versus need for coronary revascularization.

Conflict of Interests

All the authors report that there are no financial disclosures and no competing interests regarding the publication of this paper.

References

[1] C. J. Sperati, N. Aggarwal, A. Arepally, and M. G. Atta, "Fibromuscular dysplasia," *Kidney International*, vol. 75, no. 3, pp. 333–336, 2009.

[2] A. Camacho, A. Villarejo, T. Moreno, R. Simón, A. Muñoz, and F. Mateos, "Vertebral artery fibromuscular dysplasia: an unusual cause of stroke in a 3-year-old child," *Developmental Medicine & Child Neurology*, vol. 45, no. 10, pp. 709–711, 2003.

[3] K. C. Michelis, J. W. Olin, D. Kadian-Dodov, V. d'Escamard, and J. C. Kovacic, "Coronary artery manifestations of fibromuscular dysplasia," *Journal of the American College of Cardiology*, vol. 64, no. 10, pp. 1033–1046, 2014.

[4] J. Saw, D. Ricci, A. Starovoytov, R. Fox, and C. E. Buller, "Spontaneous coronary artery dissection: prevalence of predisposing conditions including fibromuscular dysplasia in a tertiary center cohort," *JACC: Cardiovascular Interventions*, vol. 6, no. 1, pp. 44–52, 2013.

[5] S. Toggweiler, M. Puck, C. Thalhammer et al., "Associated vascular lesions in patients with spontaneous coronary artery dissection," *Swiss Medical Weekly*, vol. 142, Article ID w13538, 2012.

[6] H. C. Pretty, "Dissecting aneurysm of coronary artery in a woman aged 42: rupture," *British Medical Journal*, vol. 1, no. 3667, p. 667, 1931.

[7] C. E. Appleby, A. Barolet, D. Ing et al., "Contemporary management of pregnancy-related coronary artery dissection: a single-centre experience and literature review," *Experimental and Clinical Cardiology*, vol. 14, no. 1, pp. e8–e18, 2009.

[8] H. P. Brantley, B. R. Cabarrus, and A. Movahed, "Spontaneous multiarterial dissection immediately after childbirth," *Texas Heart Institute Journal*, vol. 39, no. 5, pp. 683–686, 2012.

[9] D. Giacoppo, D. Capodanno, G. Dangas, and C. Tamburino, "Spontaneous coronary artery dissection," *International Journal of Cardiology*, vol. 175, no. 1, pp. 8–20, 2014.

[10] J. Saw, "Spontaneous coronary artery dissection," *Canadian Journal of Cardiology*, vol. 29, no. 9, pp. 1027–1033, 2013.

[11] Y. Onuma and P. W. Serruys, "Bioresorbable scaffold: the advent of a new era in percutaneous coronary and peripheral revascularization?" *Circulation*, vol. 123, no. 7, pp. 779–797, 2011.

[12] J. Cockburn, W. Yan, R. Bhindi, and P. Hansen, "Spontaneous coronary artery dissection treated with bioresorbable vascular scaffolds guided by optical coherence tomography," *Canadian Journal of Cardiology*, vol. 30, no. 11, pp. 1461.e1–1461.e3, 2014.

41

Acute Coronary Syndrome: An Unusual Consequence of GERD

Chui Man Carmen Hui,[1] Santosh K. Padala,[2] Michael Lavelle,[3] Mikhail T. Torosoff,[2] Xinjun Cindy Zhu,[4] and Mandeep S. Sidhu[2]

[1]Department of Medicine, Albany Medical Center, Albany, NY 12208, USA
[2]Department of Medicine, Division of Cardiology, Albany Medical Center, Albany, NY 12208, USA
[3]Albany Medical College, Albany, NY 12208, USA
[4]Department of Medicine, Division of Gastroenterology, Albany Medical Center, Albany, NY 12208, USA

Correspondence should be addressed to Santosh K. Padala; santoshpadala@gmail.com

Academic Editor: Kjell Nikus

We report a case of an 83-year-old man with history of coronary artery disease and gastroesophageal reflux disease (GERD) who presented with sudden onset nocturnal dyspnea. He was diagnosed with non-ST elevation myocardial infarction based on the electrocardiographic changes and cardiac biomarker elevation. Cardiac catheterization revealed chronic three-vessel coronary artery disease, with 2 patent grafts and 2 chronically occluded grafts. While at the hospital, the patient experienced a similar episode of nocturnal dyspnea, prompting a barium esophagram, which was suggestive of a stricture in the distal esophagus from long-standing GERD. We hypothesized that he had myocardial ischemia due to increased oxygen demand from uncontrolled GERD symptoms. He had no further ischemic episodes after increasing the dose of antireflux medication over a 6-month follow-up. After presenting our case, we review the literature on this atypical presentation of GERD causing acute coronary syndrome and discuss potential mechanisms.

1. Introduction

Gastroesophageal reflux disease (GERD) is a common gastrointestinal disorder in the western industrial world. Although GERD classically presents with symptoms of heartburn and regurgitation of food contents, some patients may present with less typical extraesophageal cardiac or respiratory symptoms. We report an unusual case of an acute coronary syndrome in an elderly male as a consequence of GERD.

2. Case Report

An 83-year-old Italian male presented with sudden onset of dyspnea associated with cough and diaphoresis that woke him up from sleep at midnight. The symptoms lasted for an hour and he was taken to the hospital due to persistent discomfort. Upon presentation to the Emergency Department, he denied any chest discomfort, palpitations, dizziness, orthopnea, or lower extremity swelling. He also denied any nausea, vomiting, or epigastric discomfort. Over the previous five

to six years, the patient experienced recurring episodes of nocturnal coughing and difficulty breathing during his sleep which was typically precipitated after intake of a heavy meal. Additional past medical history included extensive 3-vessel coronary artery disease (CAD) with two prior coronary artery bypass surgeries, hypertension, dyslipidemia, chronic obstructive pulmonary disease, and long-standing severe GERD. His home medications included esomeprazole, lisinopril, metoprolol succinate, aspirin, clopidogrel, and ezetimibe. Vital signs on admission revealed blood pressure of 146/95 mmHg, pulse of 90 bpm, respiratory rate of 18 per minute with 100% O_2 saturation on 2 L of oxygen via nasal cannula. Physical exam did not reveal evidence of heart failure, wheezing, or crackles. Admission 12-lead surface electrocardiogram (ECG) revealed normal sinus rhythm with 1-2 mm horizontal ST depressions in V3 to V5, which resolved within one hour. The troponin I levels peaked at 2.6 (normal <0.04 ng/mL) and creatinine kinase levels were within normal limits.

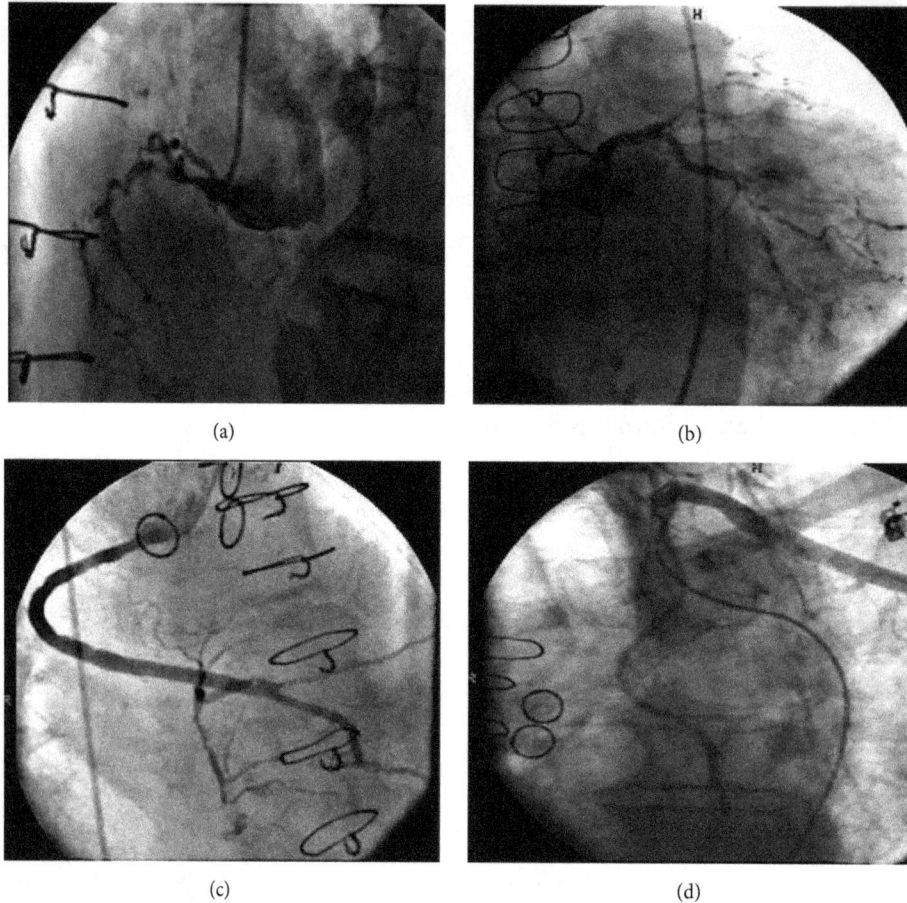

(a)

(b)

(c)

(d)

FIGURE 1: (a) Right coronary artery 100% occluded in the proximal segment. (b) Left anterior descending with 99% ostial and 100% mid occlusion and circumflex 99% distal occlusion. (c) Sequential vein graft to right posterolateral and posterior descending artery with 40% proximal disease. (d) Left internal mammary artery graft to distal left anterior descending widely patent.

Given extensive prior cardiac history, "anginal equivalent" symptoms, ischemic ECG changes, and elevated troponin I levels, non-ST elevation myocardial infarction (NSTEMI) was diagnosed and patient was started on appropriate optimal medical therapy for acute coronary syndrome. Subsequently, patient underwent an early invasive strategy of cardiac catheterization and angiography that revealed chronic, severe, native 3-vessel CAD (Figures 1(a) and 1(b)). He had patent sequential saphenous venous graft to right posterolateral and posterior descending artery and a patent left internal mammary artery to left anterior descending artery (Figures 1(c) and 1(d)). The saphenous venous grafts to the diagonal and circumflex artery were chronically occluded with evidence of collaterals. Based on the coronary anatomy the patient was managed conservatively with optimal medical therapy with no plan for percutaneous intervention or revascularization.

During the hospitalization, the patient had another episode of nocturnal dyspnea with chest tightness. He reported regurgitation and globus sensation described as "a lump in his throat with difficulty expanding his lungs." His vital signs recorded during this episode showed an abrupt rise in blood pressure to 159/85 mmHg, heart rate to 96 bpm,

and respiratory rate to 22–24 per minute, with an oxygen saturation of 98% on 2 L oxygen via nasal cannula. He denied any associated palpitations, dizziness, nausea, vomiting, or epigastric abdominal pain. ECG performed during this time showed ischemic changes, similar to his initial presentation.

The following day, the patient underwent a barium esophagram for evaluation of his symptoms, as an esophagogastroduodenoscopy (EGD) was deferred given recent NSTEMI. Barium esophagram demonstrated a smooth short narrowing in the distal esophagus proximal to the gastroesophageal junction, suggesting a stricture or spasm from yet controlled reflux disease (Figures 2(a) and 2(b)). In addition, he also had a flexible laryngoscopy showing normal nasopharynx, tongue, vallecula, epiglottis, and vocal cord motion. Given these findings suggesting poorly controlled reflux and the possibility of esophageal dysmotility, and temporal association of his symptoms with cardiac events, the esomeprazole dose was titrated up from 20 mg to 40 mg for symptomatic relief. The patient was stabilized with resolution of nocturnal symptoms and he was discharged home with plan to perform an outpatient upper EGD to evaluate for reflux and esophagitis. However, patient declined the elective EGD on his follow-up visit as he had no further episodes of

(a)

(b)

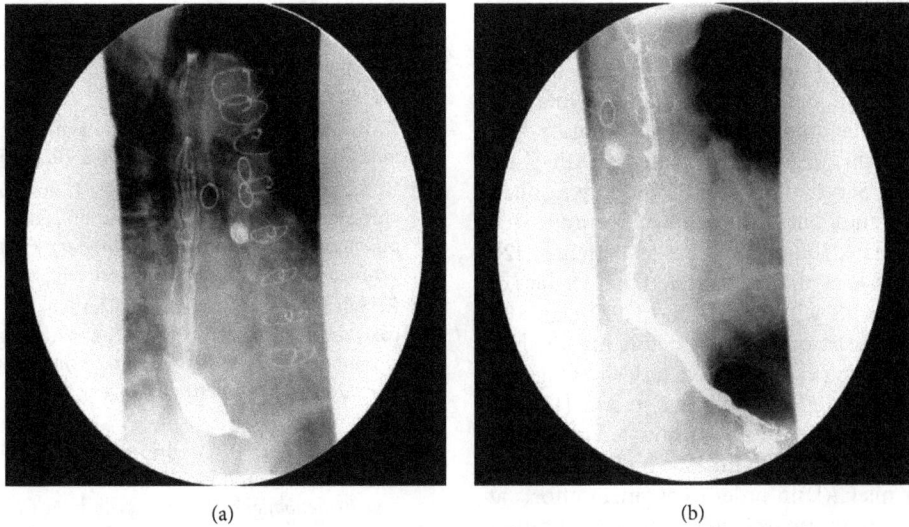

FIGURE 2: (a) Smooth short stricture in the distal esophagus slightly proximal to the gastroesophageal junction. This may represent a stricture or spasm related to reflux. (b) Multiple tertiary contractions of the distal esophagus suggestive of dysmotility.

nocturnal dyspnea on higher doses of antireflux medication. He remained symptom-free until 6-month follow-up visit.

3. Discussion

Gastroesophageal reflux disease (GERD) is a common gastrointestinal disorder with increasing prevalence worldwide. The prevalence of GERD ranged from 11% to 38.8% worldwide per Map of Digestive Disorders & Disease (MDD) with Mexico, Spain, Malaysia, and Yemen at the top quartile of prevalence, and Asian countries in the lowest quartile [1]. In USA, approximately 7 million people are affected [2]. According to National Digestive Disease Information Clearinghouse (NDDIC), 20% of the population had reflux symptoms at least once a week in 2004; 8.9 million ambulatory visits in 2009 and 4.7 million hospitalizations in 2010 were attributed to GERD [3]. Furthermore, the prevalence of GERD in patients with CAD is higher, with some studies reporting prevalence ranging from 40% to 78% [4].

GERD is caused by an impaired antireflux barrier and defective lower esophageal sphincter, leading to reflux of gastric acid into the esophagus. Typical GERD symptoms are heartburn and regurgitation of food contents. However, many patients with GERD may present with extraesophageal symptoms such as chest pain or discomfort mimicking angina, chronic cough, wheezing, dyspnea, globus sensation, hoarseness, or recurrent pneumonia as their primary presentation [5–7]. Identifying the cause and effect relationship between respiratory symptoms and GERD has been a clinical challenge. Two mechanisms have been proposed to be responsible for respiratory symptoms induced by gastric reflux: (1) vagal reflex response from stimulation of the vagus nerve by gastric acidic content, resulting in bronchoconstriction and (2) microaspiration of gastric contents causing direct irritation or trauma to the upper airway [5–7]. In a single-center study by Salvador et al., 30 patients with GERD underwent simultaneous 24-hour multichannel intraluminal impedance

pH monitoring and continuous O_2 saturation monitoring via pulse oximetry [8]. Approximately 60% of the reflux episodes were associated with oxygen desaturation. Furthermore, the high prevalence of O_2 desaturation was found mostly in GERD patients with primary respiratory complaints [8].

We present a case of an atypical presentation of GERD leading to NSTEMI, likely from demand ischemia in the setting of known severe 3-vessel native CAD as well as chronic total occlusions of venous grafts. Given the patient's extensive cardiac history and limited cardiac reserve, the physiologic response of elevated blood pressure, heart rate, respiratory rate, and transient hypoxia was likely significant enough to cause myocardial ischemia and injury. GERD may also lead to demand ischemia and cause NSTEMI through other mechanisms. It is well known that pain can cause an increase in myocardial oxygen demand through enhanced adrenergic activity with increased heart rate and blood pressure [9]. Pain from esophageal spasm is one distinct possibility for precipitating ischemia in this patient.

It is also possible that myocardial ischemia in our patient was due to "esophagocardiac reflex," which describes myocardial ischemia associated with chemical esophageal stimulation. Chauhan et al. demonstrated that esophageal acid stimulation in patients with documented CAD on angiogram resulted in typical chest discomfort and a significant reduction in coronary blood flow as measured by intracoronary Doppler in 9 of 14 (64%) patients [10]. In a study by Dobrzycki et al., 50 patients with angiographically proven CAD underwent simultaneous continuous ECG and esophageal pH monitoring for 24 hours to assess for ST-segment depression episodes and total duration of ischemic episodes [11]. Of 218 episodes of ST-segment depression, 45 (20.6%) correlated with pathologic reflux. Compared to patients without GERD, patients with GERD were found to have significantly higher number of ST-segment depression episodes and total ischemic burden. The authors also demonstrated significant improvement in ST-segment depression episodes and total ischemic burden following a 7-day course of proton pump therapy (PPI) in patients with GERD suggesting that restoring normal esophageal pH might eliminate acid-derived esophagocardiac reflex and hence myocardial ischemia [11]. Liu et al. reported similar findings of longer duration and higher incidence of ischemic events in patients with CAD and gastric reflux [12]. Short course of PPI not only resulted in fewer ischemic events, but also significantly improved the general health-related quality of life of patients [12]. Furthermore, Swiatowski et al. demonstrated that 14 days of PPI therapy in 34 patients with GERD and CAD caused a significant increase in the amount of time before maximal ST depression occurred during exercise stress test, showing that PPI therapy has a favorable effect on cardiac reserve [13].

For our patient, high dose of PPI was initiated to control his reflux symptoms along with further optimization of medical therapy for his CAD in order to augment efforts at secondary prevention of future ischemic events. Medication adjustment resulted in resolution of nocturnal symptoms, which were likely a manifestation of GERD and angina.

In conclusion, there is a high prevalence of GERD in patients with CAD. It is underappreciated that GERD can potentially cause myocardial ischemia by increasing myocardial oxygen demand or by decreasing myocardial oxygen supply (esophagocardiac reflex). Thus, it is critically important to recognize this association and initiate treatment with PPIs in appropriate patients with CAD and concomitant GERD as it might improve GERD and prevent future adverse cardiac events.

Conflict of Interests

The authors declare that there is no conflict of interests regarding the publication of this paper.

Authors' Contribution

Chui Man Carmen Hui and Santosh K. Padala contributed equally to the paper and share first authorship.

References

[1] F. Guarner, Lazaro, Gascon, Royo, Eximan, and Herrero, *Map of Digestive Disorders and Diseases*, World Gastroenterology Organization, 2008, http://www.worldgastroenterology.org/assets/downloads/pdf/wdhd/2008/events/map_of_digestive_disorders_2008.pdf.

[2] University of Florida, *Gastroesophageal Reflux Disease*, Office of Medical Informatics. University of Florida College of Medicine, 2012.

[3] Digestive Diseases Statistics for the United States—National Digestive Diseases Information Clearinghouse, March 2012, http://www.niddk.nih.gov/health-information/health-statistics/Pages/digestive-diseases-statistics-for-the-united-states.aspx.

[4] J. P. Liuzzo and J. A. Ambrose, "Chest pain from gastroesophageal reflux disease in patients with coronary artery disease," *Cardiology in Review*, vol. 13, no. 4, pp. 167–173, 2005.

[5] R. R. Gurski, A. R. Pereira Da Rosa, E. Do Valle, M. A. De Borba, and A. A. Valiati, "Extraesophageal manifestations of gastroesophageal reflux disease," *Jornal Brasileiro de Pneumologia*, vol. 32, no. 2, pp. 150–160, 2006.

[6] K. R. DeVault, "Extraesophageal symptoms of GERD," *Cleveland Clinic Journal of Medicine*, vol. 70, no. 5, pp. S20–S32, 2003.

[7] R. S. Irwin and J. M. Madison, "Diagnosis and treatment of chronic cough due to gastro-esophageal reflux disease and postnasal drip syndrome," *Pulmonary Pharmacology & Therapeutics*, vol. 15, no. 3, pp. 261–266, 2002.

[8] R. Salvador, T. J. Watson, F. Herbella et al., "Association of gastroesophageal reflux and O_2 desaturation: a novel study of simultaneous 24-h MII-pH and continuous pulse oximetry," *Journal of Gastrointestinal Surgery*, vol. 13, no. 5, pp. 854–861, 2009.

[9] M. J. Cousins, P. O. Bridenbaugh, D. B. Carr, and T. T. Horlocker, "Neural blockade: impact on outcome," in *Cousins and Bridenbaugh's Neural Blockade in Clinical Anesthesia and Pain Medicine*, C. L. Wu and S. S. Liu, Eds., pp. 144–46, Lippincott-Raven, Philadelphia, Pa, USA, 4th edition, 2009.

[10] A. Chauhan, P. A. Mullins, G. Taylor, M. C. Petch, and P. M. Schofield, "Cardioesophageal reflex: a mechanism for 'linked angina' in patients with angiographically proven coronary artery disease," *Journal of the American College of Cardiology*, vol. 27, no. 7, pp. 1621–1628, 1996.

[11] S. Dobrzycki, A. Baniukiewicz, J. Korecki et al., "Does gastroesophageal reflux provoke the myocardial ischemia in patients with CAD?" *International Journal of Cardiology*, vol. 104, no. 1, pp. 67–72, 2005.

[12] Y. Liu, S. He, Y. Chen et al., "Acid reflux in patients with coronary artery disease and refractory chest pain," *Internal Medicine*, vol. 52, no. 11, pp. 1165–1171, 2013.

[13] M. Swiatowski, B. Jacek, M. Klopocka et al., "Suppression of gastric acid production may improve the course of angina pectoris and the results of treadmill stress test in patients with coronary artery disease," *Medical Science Monitor*, vol. 10, no. 9, pp. CR524–CR529, 2004.

42

Instant Stent-Accentuated Three-Dimensional Optical Coherence Tomography Guided Selection of Proper Distal Cell for Side Branch Dilatation in Bifurcation Stenting

Fumiaki Nakao

Department of Cardiology, Yamaguchi Grand Medical Center, 77 Ohsaki, Hofu, Yamaguchi 747-8511, Japan

Correspondence should be addressed to Fumiaki Nakao; nakao-ymghp@umin.ac.jp

Academic Editor: Mohammad R. Movahed

In the bifurcation stenting, the distal rewiring for the side branch postdilatation confirmed by two-dimensional modalities may not lead to favorable results in some cases. If there are two distal cells divided by the link bridging from the carina, the rewiring through the larger distal cell may be recommended for the side branch postdilatation. Detailed confirmation of the rewired cell by the intraprocedural instant stent-accentuated three-dimensional optical coherence tomography is important.

1. Introduction

In the bifurcation stenting, the incomplete stent apposition (ISA) is a factor of poor prognosis and the proximal rewiring for the side branch (SB) postdilatation is a cause of the ISA [1]. Okamura et al. reported using the stent-enhanced three-dimensional optical coherence tomography (3D-OCT) in which jailed patterns of the SB ostium were divided into two types according to the presence of the link bridging from the carina (the free carina type, the connection to carina type), the distal rewiring was defined as the rewiring through the area which was enclosed by the carina and the stent strut having at least one distal top of the stent hoop located in front of the SB ostium, and both the free carina type and the distal rewiring lead to reducing the ISA after the SB postdilatation [2]. Detailed confirmation may be required to obtain a good result in the connection to carina type, because of the presence of two distal cells.

The instant stent-accentuated 3D-OCT (iSA3D-OCT) was developed to confirm the relation between stent struts and the jailed SB and the rewired cell in the bifurcation stenting [3]. It takes about 30 sec to automatically reconstruct the longitudinal cutaway view of the iSA3D-OCT from the original two-dimensional (2D) OCT by the offline computer with freeware ImageJ 1.47v (National Institutes of Health) and self-made macroprograms. The processing time and the

quality of images of the iSA3D-OCT are acceptable for the clinical use [3, 4].

2. Case Report

A 69-year-old man underwent percutaneous coronary intervention (PCI) for stenoses of the left anterior descending artery (LAD) (Figure 1). The ostial-mid LAD was stented with two platinum-chromium everolimus-eluting stents (Promus Premier, Boston Scientific Co.). Additional bail-out stenting was required for the proximal stent-edge dissection. The left main coronary artery-proximal LAD was stented with a 3.5 × 14 mm two-link ten-crown biolimus-eluting stent (Japanese design of Nobori, Terumo). After the guide wire was rewired to the left circumflex artery (LCx) (Figure 2(a)), intravascular ultrasonography (IVUS, OptiCross, Boston Scientific Co.) showed the distal rewiring (Figure 2(b) arrowheads). Intraprocedural iSA3D-OCT made from 2D-OCT (Dragonfly JP and ILUMIEN Optis, St. Jude Medical) showed two distal cells (the connection to carina type) and the rewiring through the smaller distal cell (Figure 2(c)). The larger distal cell located on counterclockwise direction for the smaller distal cell. The second rewiring was the same as the first rewiring. At the third rewiring (Figure 3(a)), the guide wire successfully passed through the larger distal cell

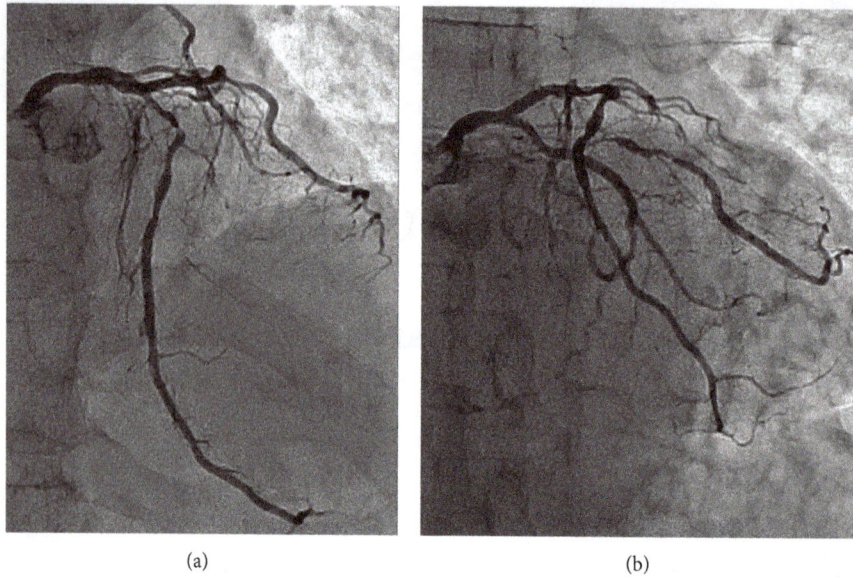

FIGURE 1: Baseline coronary angiography. (a) Cranial view and (b) caudal view.

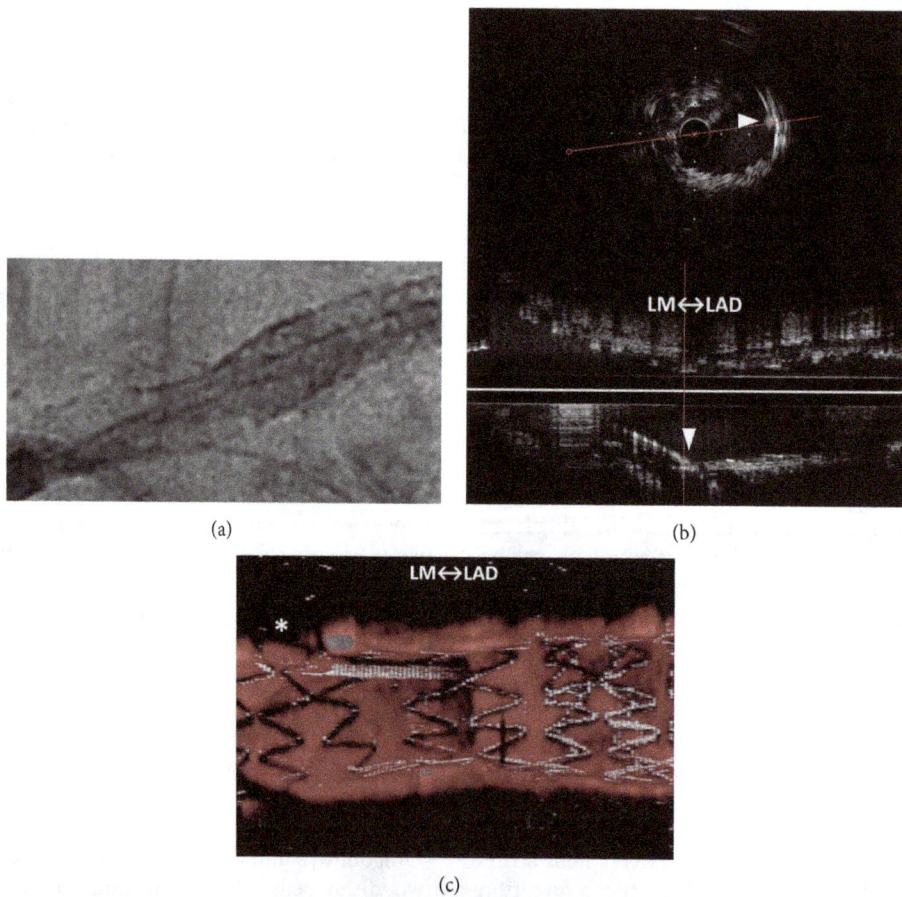

FIGURE 2: First rewiring. (a) X-ray fluorography, (b) intravascular ultrasonography showing the distal rewiring (arrowheads), and (c) intraprocedural instant stent-accentuated three-dimensional optical coherence tomography showing the rewiring through the smaller distal cell. LM: left main coronary artery, LAD: left anterior descending artery, and ∗: guide wire shadow artifact.

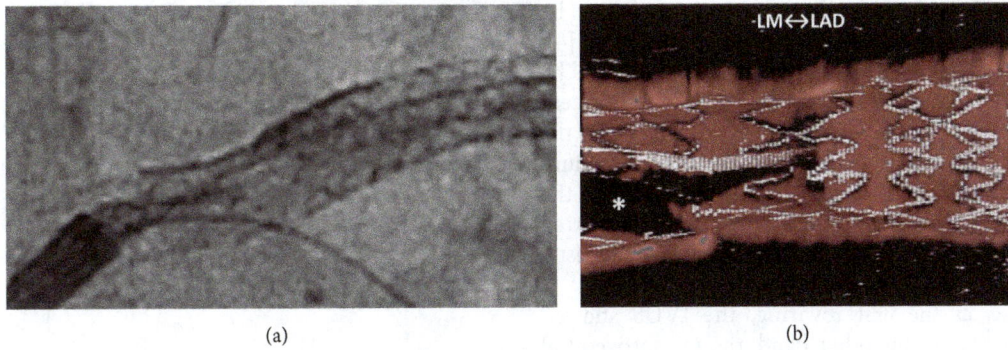

(a)   (b)

FIGURE 3: Third rewiring. (a) X-ray fluorography, (b) intraprocedural instant stent-accentuated three-dimensional optical coherence tomography showing the rewiring through the larger distal cell. LM: left main coronary artery, LAD: left anterior descending artery, and *: guide wire shadow artifact.

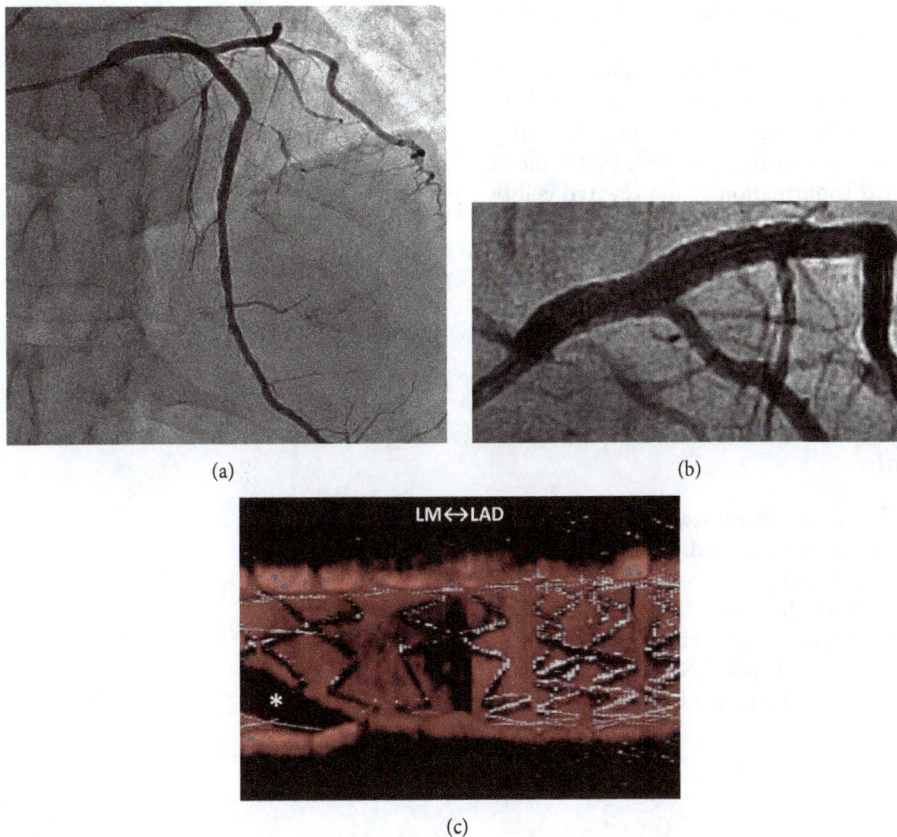

(a)   (b)

(c)

FIGURE 4: Final results. Cranial view (a) and caudal view (b) of final coronary angiography. (c) Final instant stent-accentuated three-dimensional optical coherence tomography showing minimized floating struts. LM: left main coronary artery, LAD: left anterior descending artery, and *: guide wire shadow artifact.

(Figure 3(b)). After the kissing balloon postdilatation was performed by simultaneously inflating 3.5 mm and 2.0 mm balloons, the final coronary angiography showed a good result (Figures 4(a) and 4(b)), and the final iSA3D-OCT showed minimized floating struts (Figure 4(c)).

3. Discussion

Although generally the distal rewiring on the SB ostium for the SB postdilatation has been recommended [5], the distal rewiring confirmed by 2D modalities may be insufficient to reduce the ISA. It is difficult to control the position of the link. In the connection to carina type that is present in 46% of the bifurcation stenting [2], there are two distal cells divided by the link bridging from the carina, and therefore further care may be required in addition to the distal rewiring. The rewiring through the larger distal cell is further advantageous than the smaller distal cell, in the point of the reduction of the ISA and the crossability to the SB lesion.

Another problem about the distal rewiring confirmed by 2D modalities is the rewiring through the far distal cell [4]. The far distal cell is defined as the area which is enclosed by the carina and the stent strut having no distal tops of the stent hoop located in front of the SB ostium. The dilatation of the far distal cell may lead to floating struts on the SB ostium and struts covering sparsely the distal main vessel. When the postdilatation of the SB ostium was required, the rewiring through the large center cell may be better than the far distal cell, even if the metallic carina is made.

In this case, at the first rewiring, the IVUS showed the distal rewiring. On the other hand, the intraprocedural iSA3D-OCT showed two distal cells and the rewiring through the smaller distal cell. The rewiring through the larger distal cell seemed to be advantageous for the postdilatation of the SB ostium. At the third rewiring, the guide wire was passed through the larger distal cell. In another day, there were no troubles in PCI for the LCx.

The distal rewiring confirmed by 2D modalities may not lead to favorable results in some cases. If there are two distal cells divided by the link bridging from the carina, the rewiring through the larger distal cell may be recommended for the SB postdilatation. Detailed confirmation of the rewired cell by intraprocedural iSA3D-OCT is important to find such cases.

Conflict of Interests

The author declares that there is no conflict of interests regarding the publication of this paper.

Acknowledgments

The author would like to thank Tooru Ueda, Takamasa Oda, Masashi Kanemoto, Yasuhiro Ikeda, and Takashi Fujii, from the Department of Cardiology, Ymaguchi Grand Medical Center, for their supports, and Jutaro Yamada, Takayuki Okamura, and Masafumi Yano, from the Division of Cardiology, Department of Medicine and Clinical Science, Yamaguchi University Graduate School of Medicine, for their helpful advice.

References

[1] G. F. Attizzani, D. Capodanno, Y. Ohno, and C. Tamburino, "Mechanisms, pathophysiology, and clinical aspects of incomplete stent apposition," *Journal of the American College of Cardiology*, vol. 63, no. 14, pp. 1355–1367, 2014.

[2] T. Okamura, Y. Onuma, J. Yamada et al., "3D optical coherence tomography: new insights into the process of optimal rewiring of side branches during bifurcational stenting," *EuroIntervention*, vol. 10, no. 8, pp. 907–915, 2014.

[3] F. Nakao, T. Ueda, S. Nishimura et al., "Novel and quick coronary image analysis by instant stent-accentuated three-dimensional optical coherence tomography system in catheterization laboratory," *Cardiovascular Intervention and Therapeutics*, vol. 28, no. 3, pp. 235–241, 2013.

[4] F. Nakao, "Importance of confirmation by instant stent-accentuated three-dimensional optical coherence tomography during bifurcation stenting: far distal rewiring of iSA3D-OCT," *AsiaIntervention*, vol. 1, no. 1, p. 71, 2015.

[5] E. Alegría-Barrero, N. Foin, P. H. Chan et al., "Optical coherence tomography for guidance of distal cell recrossing in bifurcation stenting: choosing the right cell matters," *EuroIntervention*, vol. 8, no. 2, pp. 205–213, 2012.

43

Noncompaction Cardiomyopathy with Charcot-Marie-Tooth Disease

Sherif Ali Eltawansy,[1] Andrea Bakos,[2] and John Checton[1,3]

[1]Internal Medicine Department, Monmouth Medical Center, Long Branch, NJ 07740, USA
[2]Drexel University College of Medicine, Philadelphia, PA 19129, USA
[3]Cardiology Department, Monmouth Medical Center, Long Branch, NJ 07740, USA

Correspondence should be addressed to Sherif Ali Eltawansy; seltawansy@barnabashealth.org

Academic Editor: Jesus Peteiro

We report a case of a 53-year-old female presenting with a new-onset heart failure that was contributed secondary to noncompaction cardiomyopathy. The diagnosis was made by echocardiogram and confirmed by cardiac MRI. Noncompaction cardiomyopathy (also known as ventricular hypertrabeculation) is a newly discovered disease. It is considered to be congenital (genetic) cardiomyopathy. It is usually associated with genetic disorders and that could explain the genetic pathogenesis of the non-compaction cardiomyopathy. Our case had a history of Charcot-Marie-Tooth disease. There is a high incidence of arrhythmia and embolic complications. The treatment usually consists of the medical management, defibrillator placement, and lifelong anticoagulation. Heart transplantation will be the last resort.

1. Case Presentation

We report a case of a 53-year-old Caucasian female who started to experience shortness of breath on exertion few months before presentation to us. She was admitted to a hospital in another state as she was on a trip due to worsening shortness of breathing. She was initially diagnosed as a case of congestive heart failure and was given furosemide and she improved. According to her medical records, she had a CT scan of the chest with angiography to exclude pulmonary embolism and it was negative. She was not known for any congenital heart disease, diabetes mellitus, or hypertension. She had a history of Charcot-Marie-Tooth disease with neuropathy. Her surgical history included uterine fibroid embolization 10 years ago and history of cat scratch disease 20 years ago. She went back home and was still taking oral furosemide. She was single and was working in a software company. She denied history of smoking, alcohol, or drug dependence. Review of system was negative apart from exertional dyspnea, orthopnea, and nocturnal dyspnea. Chronic foot pain with weakness and high arched foot was secondary to the history of Charcot-Marie-Tooth disease. By examination, body mass index was

$29.84\,kg/m^2$. By auscultation, there was a holosystolic murmur grade 2/6 in the lower left sternal border. There were no rales, rhonchi, or wheezes on auscultation at the time of presentation to us. The patient was then referred by her primary physician to the cardiologist office. EKG was done and showed sinus bradycardia with heart rate of 54/minute. There were nonspecific ST-T wave changes. Patient had an echocardiogram (Figure 1) showing left ventricle moderately dilated with severely reduced systolic function.

Ejection fraction was 25%. There was severe hypokinesis of the anteroseptal region with mild hypokinesia of the inferolateral wall. Right ventricle systolic function was moderately to severely reduced. There were severe mitral regurgitation, tricuspid regurgitation, dilated inferior vena cava, and increased right atrial pressure. Patient did a nuclear stress test showing abnormal myocardial perfusion of the left ventricle, left ventricular dilation, and area of thickening of the anterolateral portion of the left ventricle. It also showed severe global hypokinesia of the anterior wall and interventricular septum. The clinical, EKG, and hemodynamic response was normal. Patient was started by the cardiologist on carvedilol, lisinopril, vitamin D2, and warfarin for anticoagulation in addition to the furosemide.

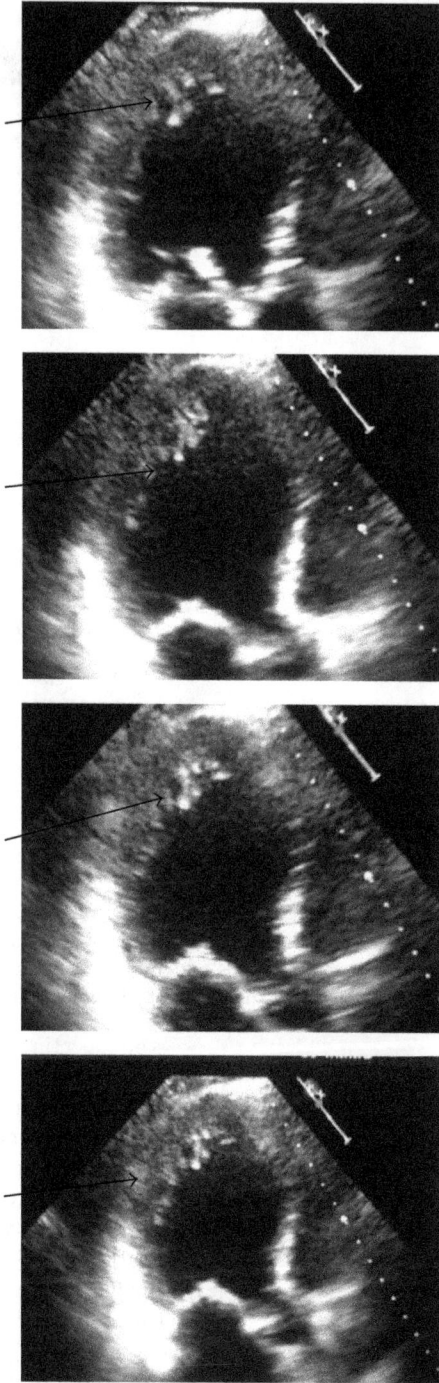

FIGURE 1: Echocardiogram.

assessment demonstrated mild systemic hypertension, moderately to severely elevated left ventricular end-diastolic pressure, severely depressed cardiac output, markedly elevated pulmonary capillary wedge pressure, mildly to moderately elevated systemic vascular resistance, and moderately elevated pulmonary vascular resistance. There were severe left sided failure and moderate to severe right sided failure. There was moderate pulmonary hypertension. There was no angiographic evidence for occlusive coronary artery disease. Global left ventricular function was severely depressed. EF calculated by contrast ventriculography was 22%, EF by echo was 25%, and EF by radionuclide angiography was 29%. The left ventricle was moderately dilated. There was no mural thrombus. The mitral valve exhibited severe regurgitation. Impression: the coronary anatomy is normal. Left ventricular function is markedly abnormal (noncompaction cardiomyopathy (NCC)). The patient had a Holter monitor showing infrequent premature ventricular contractions.

Cine MRI, morphology, phase-contrast, and contrast cardiac MRI were performed (Figure 2).

Left ventricle: LVED volume is 262 mL, LVES volume is 208 mL, and LVEF is 20%. There were severe LV dilatation with normal LV wall thickness, severe diffuse LV hypokinesis, no regional akinesis or dyskinesis, severe LV dilatation with normal LV wall thickness, and severe diffuse left ventricular hypokinesis. No regional akinesis or dyskinesis was found. Contrast late enhancement study showed no evidence of segmental or significant patchy late contrast enhancement of myocardial wall, no evidence of infarction or infiltration, and no evidence of large area of myocardial edema or myocarditis. Cardiac MRI findings showed Severe MR (mitral regurgitation) secondary to left ventricular dilatation, mitral annular dilatation, and left ventricular dysfunction. These findings were most consistent with dilated cardiomyopathy. After the revision with the cardiologist and given the previous echocardiographic results, it was found that the apex of LV is almost circumferentially heavily trabeculated with a ratio of trabeculated endocardial layer (noncompacted layer, 21 mm) to myocardial layer (compacted myocardium, 7 mm) of >3 though there is no involvement of apical septum; in the midlevel of LV the lateral wall and some part of inferior wall and anterolateral wall are heavily trabeculated with a ratio of noncompact (14 mm) to compact layer (6.5 mm) of >2; the basal segment of LV is mostly spared from trabeculation except lateral wall which is minimally/mildly trabeculated. The papillary muscles appear sponge-like with smaller muscle bundles. Left ventricle noncompaction is suspected with prominent lateral wall and most apical noncompact layer as well as sponge-like papillary muscle appearance. Left ventricle end-diastolic volume is 262 mL and left ventricle end-systolic volume is 208 mL.

The patient had a Medtronic single chamber AICD (automated implanted cardioverter defibrillator).

2. Discussion

Noncompaction cardiomyopathy (NCC), also called *spongiform cardiomyopathy*, is a rare congenital cardiomyopathy

Laboratory work included the following. Hemoglobin was 109 g/L, WBC was 8.8×10^9/L, platelets were 239×10^9/L, prothrombin time was 12.9 seconds, INR was 1.2, partial thromboplastin time (PTT) was 30.5 sec, serum creatinine was 61.83 μmol/L, blood urea nitrogen was 7.84 mmol urea /L, serum sodium [Na^+] was 143 mmol/L, and serum potassium [K^+] was 4.3 mmol/L. Cardiac enzymes: troponin I baseline was 0.02 μg/L. B-natriuretic peptide was 194 pg/mL.

Patient was scheduled for elective cardiac catheterization. The catheterization showed the following. Hemodynamic

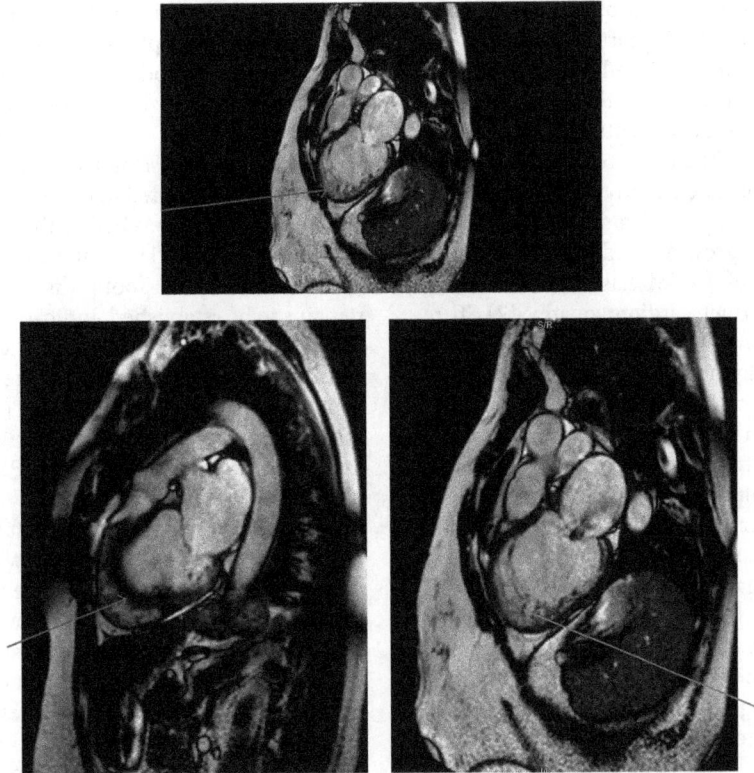

FIGURE 2: Cine MRI, morphology, phase-contrast, and contrast cardiac MRI.

that affects both children and adults [1]. It results from the failure of myocardial development during embryogenesis [2]. During early embryonic development, the myocardium is a loose network of interwoven fibers separated by deep recesses that link the myocardium with the left ventricular cavity. Gradual "compaction" of this spongy meshwork of fibers and intertrabecular recesses, or "sinusoids," occurs between weeks 5 and 8 of embryonic life, proceeding from the epicardium to endocardium and from the base of the heart to the apex. The coronary circulation develops concurrently during this process, and the intertrabecular recesses are reduced to capillaries [3]. The normal process of trabeculation appears to involve secretion of neuregulin growth factors from the endocardium and may also involve angiogenesis factors, such as vascular endothelial growth factor and angiopoietin-1 [4]. NVM (noncompaction of ventricular myocardium) was first described in association with other congenital anomalies, such as obstruction of the right or left ventricular outflow tracts, complex cyanotic congenital heart disease, and coronary artery anomalies [4]. The left ventricle is uniformly affected, but biventricular noncompaction has been reported, with right ventricular noncompaction described in less than one-half of patients [4]. Noncompaction cardiomyopathy was first identified as an isolated condition in 1984 by Engberding and Benber. They reported a 33-year-old female presenting with exertional dyspnea and palpitations. Investigations concluded persistence of myocardial sinusoids (now termed noncompaction) [5]. Trabeculation of the ventricles is normal, as are prominent, discrete muscular bundles greater than 2 mm.

In noncompaction, there are excessively prominent trabeculations. Chin et al. described echocardiographic method to distinguish noncompaction from normal trabeculation. They described a ratio of the distance from the trough and peak, of the trabeculations, to the epicardial surface. Noncompaction is diagnosed when the trabeculations are more than twice the thickness of the underlying ventricular wall [6]. Histologically, isolated noncompaction differs from noncompaction associated with other congenital heart diseases in that the deep intertrabecular recesses communicate with the left ventricular cavity in the former and with both the coronary circulation and the left ventricle in the latter [7]. Both familial and sporadic forms of noncompaction have been described. In the original report of INVM, which predominantly involved children, familial recurrence was seen in half of patients. Familial recurrence was seen in 18% in the largest reported adult population with INVM (isolated noncompaction of ventricular myocardium) [6, 7].

Bleyl et al. reported a family of 6 affected children with INVM and X-linked inheritance. In this family, genetic linkage localized INVM to a mutation in the G4.5 gene of the Xq28 chromosome region, where other myopathies with cardiac involvement have been localized, including Barth syndrome, Emery-Dreifuss muscular dystrophy, and myotubular myopathy [8]. The cardiac-specific gene CSX has been implicated in the development of some cases of INVM. Distal chromosome 5q deletion has been reported to cause loss of the gene [9].

In the initial case series of isolated noncompaction [6], the median age at diagnosis was 7 years. Subsequent case reports have described this finding in adults, including the elderly [7]. In the largest series of patients with INVM, the prevalence was 0.014% of patients referred to the echocardiography laboratory. The true prevalence is unclear [7]. Isolated noncompaction is currently categorized as an unclassified cardiomyopathy by the World Health Organization classification, but a growing body of literature on the characteristic features of INVM has led some to call for its designation as a distinct cardiomyopathy [7]. Three major clinical manifestations of noncompaction have been described: heart failure, arrhythmias, and embolic events [3]. Findings vary among patients, ranging from asymptomatic left ventricular dysfunction to severe, disabling congestive heart failure. Over two-thirds of the patients in the largest series with INVM had symptomatic heart failure [7]. Both systolic and diastolic ventricular dysfunctions have been described. Restrictive hemodynamics by cardiac catheterization as well as an initial presentation of INVM as a restrictive cardiomyopathy has been described in children with INVM [10]. Systolic dysfunction could be coming from subendocardial perfusion defect which has been described in INVM using cardiac magnetic resonance imaging (MRI) [11]. Positron emission tomography (PET) [12] and scintigraphy with thallium-201 [10] have demonstrated transmural perfusion defects correlating with areas of noncompacted myocardium in INVM. Junga et al. suggested that altered perfusion and coronary flow reserve in INVM may be related to failure of the coronary microcirculation to grow with the increasing ventricular mass, compression of the intramural coronary bed by the hypertrophied myocardium, or both processes [12]. Arrhythmias are common including atrial fibrillation, ventricular tachycardia, and sudden death [7, 13]. Embolic complications may be related to development of thrombi in the extensively trabeculated ventricle, depressed systolic function, or the development of atrial fibrillation [7]. An association between noncompaction and neuromuscular disorders has also been described, with as many as 82% of patients having some form of neuromuscular disorder [14]. Although echocardiography has been the diagnostic test of choice for noncompaction, other modalities have been used for the diagnosis, including contrast ventriculography, computed tomography [15], and MRI [12]. Standard medical therapy for systolic and diastolic ventricular dysfunction is warranted.

Cardiac transplantation has been used for those with refractory congestive heart failure. Only 6 cases of INVM leading to cardiac transplantation have been published to date [16]. Because of the frequency of ventricular tachycardia and significant risk of sudden cardiac death and systemic embolism, assessment for atrial and ventricular arrhythmias by ambulatory ECG monitoring should be performed annually. As more information is gathered about NVM and risk of sudden cardiac death, implantable defibrillator technology may have an expanded role [17]. Long-term prophylactic anticoagulation has been recommended [7]. Although the prognosis for patients with NVM varies, nearly 60% of patients described in one large series had either died or undergone

cardiac transplantation within 6 years of diagnosis. Two of 8 in the initially asymptomatic group of this series died during the follow-up period, both having documented sustained ventricular tachycardia and one with sudden cardiac death [3].

Our reported case had a history of Charcot-Marie-Tooth disease which is related to the noncompaction cardiomyopathy discovered later. Whether there is a causal or pathogenic relation between LVHT (left ventricular hypertrabeculation) and Charcot-Marie-Tooth disease in the present patient remains to be established. Indications for a causal relation are as follows [17]. Having reviewed the literature, it appears that cardiac abnormalities are more frequent in Charcot-Marie-Tooth patients than in controls [18]. Myocardial involvement in a case like Charcot-Marie-Tooth disease could be due to partial homology of the PMP22 protein with other proteins expressed in the heart, such as EMP or MP20. LVHT, dilated cardiomyopathy, left bundle branch block, and heart failure may be associated with Charcot-Marie-Tooth hereditary neuropathy type 1A due to the PMP22 duplication on chromosome 17p11.2-12. A causal relation between the cardiac abnormalities and the mutation remains elusive. If a patient with a neuromuscular disorder is investigated echocardiographically, special attention should be directed towards the detection of LVHT [19]. In the majority of the cases, LVHT occurs in association with various genetic disorders [20]. Whether the relation between these conditions and LVHT is causal or coincidental is unknown. The frequent occurrence together with genetic disease, however, suggests that, though unproven, there is a pathogenetic link between the various mutations and the occurrence of LVHT. Genetic disorders associated with LVHT include cardiac disease other than LVHT, NMDs (neuromuscular disorders) with cardiac involvement, noncardiac, non-NMD hereditary disorders, and chromosomal aberrations [21].

3. Conclusion

Noncompaction cardiomyopathy (also known as ventricular hypertrabeculation) is a rare form of cardiomyopathy that is usually diagnosed by echocardiogram or cardiac MRI. Misdiagnosis and underreporting of the disease make it difficult to fully understand and study that disease, especially that it is a newly discovered and described entity of the cardiomyopathy. Correlation has been reported with other genetic diseases like Charcot-Marie-Tooth disease in our case.

Conflict of Interests

The authors declare that there is no conflict of interests regarding the publication of this paper.

References

[1] R. H. Pignatelli, C. J. McMahon, W. J. Dreyer et al., "Clinical characterization of left ventricular noncompaction in children: a relatively common form of cardiomyopathy," *Circulation*, vol. 108, no. 21, pp. 2672–2678, 2003.

[2] N. Espinola-Zavaleta, M. E. Soto, L. M. Castellanos, S. Játiva-Chávez, and C. Keirns, "Non-compacted cardiomyopathy: clinical-echocardiographic study," *Cardiovascular Ultrasound*, vol. 4, no. 1, article 35, 2006.

[3] M. Ritter, E. Oechslin, G. Sütsch, C. Attenhofer, J. Schneider, and R. Jenni, "Isolated noncompaction of the myocardium in adults," *Mayo Clinic Proceedings*, vol. 72, no. 1, pp. 26–31, 1997.

[4] E. Zambrano, S. J. Marshalko, C. C. Jaffe, and P. Hui, "Isolated noncompaction of the ventricular myocardium: clinical and molecular aspects of a rare cardiomyopathy," *Laboratory Investigation*, vol. 82, no. 2, pp. 117–122, 2002.

[5] R. Engberding and F. Bender, "Identification of a rare congenital anomaly of the myocardium by two-dimensional echocardiography: persistence of isolated myocardial sinusoids," *The American Journal of Cardiology*, vol. 53, no. 11, pp. 1733–1734, 1984.

[6] T. K. Chin, J. K. Perloff, R. G. Williams, K. Jue, and R. Mohrmann, "Isolated noncompaction of left ventricular myocardium: a study of eight cases," *Circulation*, vol. 82, no. 2, pp. 507–513, 1990.

[7] E. N. Oechslin, C. H. A. Jost, J. R. Rojas, P. A. Kaufmann, and R. Jenni, "Long-term follow-up of 34 adults with isolated left ventricular noncompaction: a distinct cardiomyopathy with poor prognosis," *Journal of the American College of Cardiology*, vol. 36, no. 2, pp. 493–500, 2000.

[8] S. B. Bleyl, B. R. Mumford, M.-C. Brown-Harrison et al., "Xq28-linked noncompaction of the left ventricular myocardium: prenatal diagnosis and pathologic analysis of affected individuals," *The American Journal of Medical Genetics*, vol. 72, no. 3, pp. 257–265, 1997.

[9] R. M. Pauli, S. Scheib-Wixted, L. Cripe, S. Izumo, and G. S. Sekhon, "Ventricular noncompaction and distal chromosome 5q deletion," *American Journal of Medical Genetics*, vol. 85, no. 4, pp. 419–423, 1999.

[10] F. Ichida, Y. Hamamichi, T. Miyawaki et al., "Clinical features of isolated noncompaction of the ventricular myocardium: long-term clinical course, hemodynamic properties, and genetic background," *Journal of the American College of Cardiology*, vol. 34, no. 1, pp. 233–240, 1999.

[11] R. Soler, E. Rodríguez, L. Monserrat, and N. Alvarez, "MRI of subendocardial perfusion deficits in isolated left ventricular noncompaction," *Journal of Computer Assisted Tomography*, vol. 26, no. 3, pp. 373–375, 2002.

[12] G. Junga, S. Kneifel, A. Von Smekal, H. Steinert, and U. Bauersfeld, "Myocardial ischaemia in children with isolated ventricular non-compaction," *European Heart Journal*, vol. 20, no. 12, pp. 910–916, 1999.

[13] A. Rigopoulos, I. K. Rizos, C. Aggeli et al., "Isolated left ventricular noncompaction: an unclassified cardiomyopathy with severe prognosis in adults," *Cardiology*, vol. 98, no. 1-2, pp. 25–32, 2002.

[14] C. Stöllberger, J. Finsterer, and G. Blazek, "Left ventricular hypertrabeculation/noncompaction and association with additional cardiac abnormalities and neuromuscular disorders," *American Journal of Cardiology*, vol. 90, no. 8, pp. 899–902, 2002.

[15] D. J. Conces Jr., T. Ryan, and R. D. Tarver, "Noncompaction of ventricular myocardium: CT appearance," *American Journal of Roentgenology*, vol. 156, no. 4, pp. 717–718, 1991.

[16] V. Conraads, B. Paelinck, A. Vorlat, M. Goethals, W. Jacobs, and C. Vrints, "Isolated non-compaction of the left ventricle: a rare indication for transplantation," *Journal of Heart and Lung Transplantation*, vol. 20, no. 8, pp. 904–907, 2001.

[17] C. Stöllberger and J. Finsterer, "Left ventricular hypertrabeculation/noncompaction," *Journal of the American Society of Echocardiography*, vol. 17, no. 1, pp. 91–100, 2004.

[18] T. Stojkovic, J. de Seze, O. Dubourg et al., "Autonomic and respiratory dysfunction in Charcot-Marie-Tooth disease due to Thr124Met mutation in the myelin protein zero gene," *Clinical Neurophysiology*, vol. 114, no. 9, pp. 1609–1614, 2003.

[19] G. Corrado, N. Checcarelli, M. Santarone, C. Stöllberger, and J. Finsterer, "Left ventricular hypertrabeculation/noncompaction with PMP22 duplication-based charcot-marie-tooth disease type 1A," *Cardiology*, vol. 105, no. 3, pp. 142–145, 2006.

[20] J. R. Gimeno, J. Lacunza, A. García-Alberola et al., "Penetrance and risk profile in inherited cardiac diseases studied in a dedicated screening clinic," *The American Journal of Cardiology*, vol. 104, no. 3, pp. 406–410, 2009.

[21] J. Finsterer, "Left ventricular non-compaction and its cardiac and neurologic implications," *Heart Failure Reviews*, vol. 15, no. 6, pp. 589–603, 2010.

44

Tender Endothelium Syndrome: Combination of Hypotension, Bradycardia, Contrast Induced Chest Pain, and Microvascular Angina

Shivesh Goberdhan,[1] Soon Kwang Chiew,[2] and Jaffer Syed[2]

[1]*Department of Internal Medicine, Queens University, Kingston General Hospital, 76 Stuart Street, Kingston, ON, Canada K7L 2V7*
[2]*Department of Cardiology, McMaster University, St. Catharines Hospital, 1200 4th Avenue, St. Catharines, ON, Canada L2S 0A9*

Correspondence should be addressed to Shivesh Goberdhan; shivesh.goberdhan@gmail.com

Academic Editor: Kjell Nikus

Hypotension, bradycardia, and contrast induced chest pain are potential complications of cardiac catheterization and coronary angiography. Catheter-induced coronary spasm has been occasionally demonstrated, but its relationship to spontaneous coronary spasm is unclear. We describe a 64-year-old female who underwent coronary artery bypass surgery in 1998 on the basis of an angiographic diagnosis of severe left main disease, who recently presented with increasingly frequent typical angina. Repeat coronary angiography was immediately complicated by severe chest pain, hypotension, and bradycardia but demonstrated only mild disease of the left main artery and entire coronary tree with complete occlusion of her prior grafts. This reaction was almost identical to that observed during her original coronary angiogram. We now believe her original angiogram was complicated by severe catheter-induced left main spasm, with the accompanying contrast reaction attributed to left main disease, and the occlusion of coronary grafts explained by the absence of significant left main disease. The combination of these symptoms has not been documented in the literature. In this instance, these manifestations erroneously led to coronary bypass surgery. It is unknown whether routine, systematic injection of intracoronary nitroglycerin prior to angiography might blunt the severity of such reactions.

1. Introduction

Typical angina is defined by three features: substernal location chest discomfort, provocation by exertion or emotional stress, and relief by rest or nitroglycerin. When only two of the above criteria are met, atypical angina is suggested, while the presence of only one feature suggests noncardiac chest pain [1]. Epicardial coronary artery spasm also manifests as substernal chest pain but usually lacks a clear association with exertion and can be difficult to diagnose due to the fleeting nature of symptoms and wide range of electrocardiogram (ECG) findings, although transient ST elevation is most commonly seen [2]. Coronary microvascular dysfunction (CMVD) involves the coronary microcirculation, sparing the epicardial arteries. Microvascular angina (MVA) is a clinical manifestation of CMVD and can be seen in patients who present with anginal pain, without epicardial coronary disease [3]. Stable primary MVA refers to angina episodes related to effort without cardiac or systemic disease; but inclusive to this diagnosis are those with diabetes mellitus and uncomplicated hypertension. Risk factors for CMVD are similar to those for epicardial CAD and include dyslipidemia, diabetes mellitus, and smoking, yet the precise pathophysiology is poorly understood [3]. Coronary artery spasm is also reported in 1%–5% of percutaneous coronary interventions and can be induced via guide wire insertion. The mechanism surrounding this is believed to be a result of increased vasomotor tone and mechanical stimulation from the catheter tip [2, 4].

There are many adverse reactions that can occur during coronary angiography, involving both the catheterization process and the use of radiocontrast dye [5]. Catheter-induced vasospasm is uncommon but important to recognize and distinguish from atherothrombotic disease [6].

Hypotension and bradycardia are well known complications of coronary angiography and are directly correlated with the hyperosmolality of the contrast. Ionic contrast is associated with a greater incidence of mild to moderate adverse reactions than nonionic low-osmolar agents. These reactions include bradycardia, chest pain, transient hypotension, and elevation of left ventricular end diastolic pressure [5]. We report a case in which a patient presented with potential MVA, and, during coronary engagement with iohexol (nonionic, low osmolality contrast), the patient experienced hypotension, bradycardia, and extreme chest pain.

2. Case Report

A 64-year-old woman, with a history of double vessel coronary bypass surgery (CABG) in 1998, presented with five months of increasingly frequent exertional chest tightness and dyspnea. In 1998, the patient presented similarly with a few months' history of exertional chest heaviness, dyspnea, and jaw numbness. After a positive treadmill stress test demonstrating ST depressions, diagnostic coronary angiography was complicated by severe hypotension immediately upon catheter engagement of the left main artery, with blood pressure falling to less than 50 systolic and accompanied by severe chest pain. Limited angiographic images obtained demonstrated an 80% left main stenosis, with angiographically normal vessels in the remainder of the coronary tree. The patient was kept in hospital and sent for double vessel CABG, receiving a left internal thoracic artery (LITA) graft to LAD and saphenous vein graft to obtuse marginal. Since 1998, the patient had been relatively asymptomatic up until five months prior to current presentation.

Her current symptoms were similar, though not identical to her initial presentation in 1998, but they were still provoked by activity and relieved with nitroglycerin spray and rest. She also reported a significant decrease in energy and her usual activities were limited due to exertional dyspnea. Review of systems was otherwise noncontributory. Notably, she was an active user of tobacco, smoking half a pack a day for the past ten years, was a social drinker, and had a mother who died from a heart attack in her early 60s. Her medical history was significant for gastroesophageal reflux, hypertension, dyslipidemia, and hypothyroidism. Her medications included atenolol, ezetimibe, rosuvastatin, paroxetine, and l-thyroxine. She had also recently been placed on topical nitrate patch. Her new-onset symptoms prompted a referral for repeat coronary and graft angiography, and possible percutaneous intervention if appropriate. Based on her cardiovascular history and current suggestive symptoms, stress testing was decided against, due to her high pretest probability of having ischemic disease.

Prior to the procedure the patient had a benign physical examination with a resting ECG demonstrating sinus rhythm, with nonspecific T-wave inversions in V1 and V2. Access during the procedure was gained via right femoral artery where a 6-French sheath was inserted. Her baseline blood pressure was 110/70 mmHg. 6-French JL 4.0 and JR 4.0 catheters were used for selective coronary engagement. Immediately upon first injection of left coronary system with

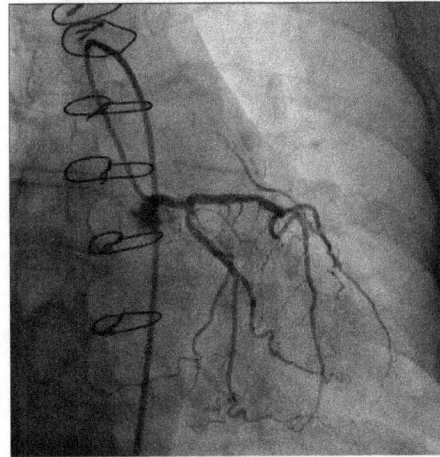

FIGURE 1: This is a selective injection of the left coronary system in the AP Caudal projection, demonstrating a large left main coronary artery free of obstructive narrowing, a mild proximal circumflex stenosis, and very minor disease of both ongoing circumflex and LAD. Retrograde filling of a small calibre LITA graft can be seen.

Omnipaque® (nonionic, low osmolality radiocontrast dye), she developed severe chest pain, hypotension (systolic blood pressure dropped to 80 mmHg), and bradycardia. Atropine 0.5 mg IV resulted in improvement of hemodynamics but had no impact on the severity of chest pain, which was reproduced with each contrast injection of the coronaries. Following atropine-related improvement in hemodynamics, intracoronary nitroglycerin was administered and she was able to tolerate completion of the procedure. Notably, chest pain severity was similar between injections of the right and left coronary systems. At case end, her hypotension and bradycardia had completely resolved; she was clinically pain-free and did not recall the pain during the procedure.

In contrast to her original catheterization procedure of 1998, selective coronary angiography failed to demonstrate evidence of hemodynamically significant stenosis within the left main coronary artery and remaining coronary tree (as shown in Figure 1). In addition, there was complete occlusion of the saphenous vein graft to the obtuse marginal (OM) and functional occlusion of the LITA graft to LAD, both of which appeared chronic (as shown in Figure 2). There was also normal left ventricular systolic function. Medical management was recommended, as well as risk factor modification, and she was strongly counseled on the importance of smoking cessation. The patient was discharged the same day and follow-up was arranged.

3. Discussion

This case report describes a patient presenting with typical angina without correlative angiographic findings, with unique features of procedural chest pain, bradycardia, and hypotension during selective coronary injection. These findings stand in contrast to those of her original procedure in one key respect: the absence of significant left main disease. We believe the original procedure to have been complicated

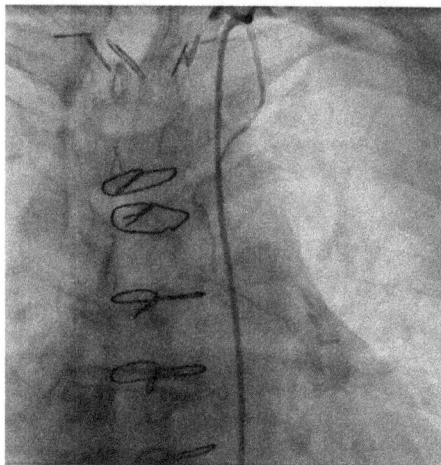

FIGURE 2: This is a selective injection of the LITA graft in the AP, demonstrating it to be of very small calibre and functionally occluded distally.

by severe catheter-induced spasm of the left main artery, but this was misinterpreted as a fixed stenosis resulting in the performance of coronary artery bypass surgery. Thus, the documented occlusion coronary grafts are easily explained by the patient's lack of obstructive, atherosclerotic CAD.

A wide range of adverse effects have been described with the use of contrast media during cardiac angiography, including allergic reactions, reduced myocardial contractility, hypotension, nausea, vomiting, bronchospasm, fatal arrhythmias, pulmonary edema, and embolic events [5, 7]. During our patient's recent coronary angiography, Omnipaque, a nonionic, low-osmolar contrast, was used. When compared to high osmolar ionic media, the use of Omnipaque has been associated with significantly reduced complications [8].

Cardiac catheterization has been commonly known to cause coronary ostial spasm, most typically the right coronary artery, in contrast to the left main coronary artery [9]. Catheter-induced spasm is often related to mechanical irritation and excessive catheter torque. Patient factors regarding catheter-induced spasm include excessive vasomotor tone, early endothelial dysfunction, and active smoking [9].

Interestingly, the chest pain experienced by the patient during the recent angiogram was unlike her presenting cardiac angina symptoms. In review of the literature, chest pain labeled as mild/moderate has been noted in patients receiving iopamidol and ioxaglate, although the frequency of this symptom was low (16/500 cases between the two contrast dyes) [5]. The mechanism of chest pain related to the injection of contrast is not established. Another study documents angina as an adverse effect of iohexol, observed in 27 patients out of 1077, although the anginal events were not specifically described or compared to their presenting symptoms [7].

Based on her typical clinical symptoms and lack of atherosclerotic disease at angiography, our patient is suspected of having microvascular angina (MVA). The diagnosis of MVA could be explored further in this patient and could involve vasodilator tests, response to vasoconstrictor stimuli,

and intracoronary Doppler studies but such tests have poor sensitivity and specificity and additional patient risk, and would likely not change clinical management [3]. Myocardial ischemia related to CMVD is not a well-understood phenomenon but as the abnormalities may not be uniformly distributed amongst a major coronary branch, objective evidence is difficult to obtain [3].

It was decided that our patient would be treated medically. Recommendations included discontinuing her beta-blocker, given the known propensity of such agents to worsen vasospastic phenomena, and she was aggressively counseled on the importance of smoking cessation and how this might improve her symptom control [3]. An increase in the dose of her topical nitrate and the addition of a calcium channel blocker were also discussed. While microvascular angina, catheter-induced spasm, and chest pain during coronary injection have individually been described, we believe the presence of all three features in a single patient represents a unique finding. Although routine administration of nitrates prior to angiography may not be feasible, possibly cases with left main ostial/shaft or right coronary ostial lesions could benefit from pretreatment. Systematic employment of intracoronary nitroglycerin, meticulous catheter technique, and an awareness of such issues are important for both clinicians and angiographers alike.

4. Conclusion

This is a unique case of a 64-year-old who erroneously underwent coronary bypass surgery after what now seems to be severe catheter-induced left main spasm. In combination with severe chest pain and hypotension with contrast injection, these symptoms together have not been seen in the literature. It is imperative to note that since the mechanisms of microvascular angina are not fully understood, it cannot be concluded as to whether all of these symptoms are connected. It is unknown whether routine, systematic injection of intracoronary nitroglycerin prior to angiography might blunt the severity of such reactions, and it is important for angiographers and clinicians to be aware of this potential combination.

Conflict of Interests

The authors declare that there is no conflict of interests regarding the publication of this paper.

References

[1] "2012 ACCF/AHA/ACP/AATS/PCNA/SCAI/STS Guidelines for the diagnosis and management of patients with stable ischemic heart disease," *Journal of the American College of Cardiology*, vol. 60, p. 24, 2012.

[2] S. Stern and A. B. De Luna, "Coronary artery spasm: a 2009 update," *Circulation*, vol. 119, no. 18, pp. 2531–2534, 2009.

[3] G. A. Lanza and F. Crea, "Primary coronary microvascular dysfunction: clinical presentation, pathophysiology, and management," *Circulation*, vol. 121, no. 21, pp. 2317–2325, 2010.

[4] D. Perera, S. J. Patel, and S. R. Redwood, "Catheter induced spasm: a trap for the unwary," *Heart*, vol. 89, no. 5, article 511, 2003.

[5] E. W. Gertz, J. A. Wisneski, R. Miller et al., "Adverse reactions of low osmolality contrast media during cardiac angiography: a prospective randomized multicenter study," *Journal of the American College of Cardiology*, vol. 19, no. 5, pp. 899–906, 1992.

[6] A. A. Mohammed, A. Yang, K. Shao et al., "Patients with left main coronary artery vasospasm inadvertently undergoing coronary artery bypass grafting surgery," *Journal of the American College of Cardiology*, vol. 61, no. 8, pp. 899–900, 2013.

[7] W. H. Matthai Jr., W. G. Kussmaul III, J. Krol, J. E. Goin, J. S. Schwartz, and J. W. Hirshfeld Jr., "A comparison of low- with high-osmolality contrast agents in cardiac angiography. Identification of criteria for selective use," *Circulation*, vol. 89, no. 1, pp. 291–301, 1994.

[8] K. Levorstad, K. Vatne, U. Brodahl, B. Laake, S. Simonsen, and T. Aakhus, "Safety of the nonionic contrast medium omnipaque in coronary angiography," *CardioVascular and Interventional Radiology*, vol. 12, no. 2, pp. 98–100, 1989.

[9] U. Lingegowda, J. Marmur, and E. Cavusoglu, "Catheter-induced spasm of the left main coronary artery anatomic "kinking" in its course," *Journal of Invasive Cardiology*, vol. 17, no. 3, pp. 192–194, 2005.

45

Anomalous Origination of Right Coronary Artery from Left Sinus in Asymptomatic Young Male Presenting with Positive Ischemic Response on Treadmill Test

Budi Yuli Setianto, Anggoro Budi Hartopo,
Putrika Prastuti Ratna Gharini, and Nahar Taufiq

Department of Cardiology and Vascular Medicine, Faculty of Medicine, Universitas Gadjah Mada and Dr. Sardjito Hospital,
Yogyakarta 55281, Indonesia

Correspondence should be addressed to Budi Yuli Setianto; budyuls@ugm.ac.id
and Anggoro Budi Hartopo; a_bhartopo@ugm.ac.id

Academic Editor: Aiden Abidov

Anomalous origination of coronary artery from the opposite sinus (ACAOS) is a rare coronary artery anomaly. Right ACAOS with interarterial course is a type of ACAOS, which conveys a high risk for myocardial ischemia or sudden death. We reported a case of right ACAOS with interarterial course in otherwise healthy young male. He was asymptomatic, until an obligatory medical check-up with treadmill test showed a sign of positive ischemic response. Further work-up revealed that he had right ACAOS with interarterial course. Watchful observation was applied to him, while strenuous physical activity and competitive sport were absolutely prohibited.

1. Introduction

Anomalous origination of coronary artery from the opposite sinus (ACAOS) is an uncommon coronary anomaly. Its incidence is reported to be around 1.07% [1]. It comprises anomaly of right coronary artery originated from left sinus (right ACAOS) and its opposite or left ACAOS. The incidence of right ACAOS is between 0.12% and 0.92% [1, 2]. Both right and left ACAOS have significant clinical consequence if the ectopic artery has an interarterial course or intramural intussusception [1]. Myocardial ischemia is clinical symptoms and signs frequently associated with ACAOS with interarterial course. A constant relationship is observed between left ACAOS and sudden death or ischemia during extreme exercise [1]. Right ACAOS with an interarterial course is a type of ACAOS which poses high risk for myocardial ischemia or sudden death as well [3]. However, most ACAOS does not reveal signs and symptoms; therefore the diagnosis is often found in postmortem autopsy. We described a case of asymptomatic young male who underwent treadmill test for

obligatory medical check-up and the result showed a positive ischemic response. Further investigation revealed that he suffered from right ACAOS with an interarterial course.

2. Case Report

A 28-year-old male was referred to cardiology unit of our hospital from a general practitioner due to positive ischemic response on treadmill test during his obligatory medical check-up. He underwent medical check-up as an obligation related to his career. The result of Bruce-method treadmill test was positive ischemic response, good physical fitness, and aerobic capacity of 14.37 Mets (Figure 1). During treadmill test, the patient did not complain of chest pain; however his electrocardiogram showed horizontal ST depression indicating myocardial ischemia. Anamnesis revealed no history of chest pain, dyspnea on effort, dyspnea at rest, syncope, palpitation at rest, and palpitation on activity. The patient had no family history of sudden death or similar abnormality. Physical examination was within normal limit. Laboratory

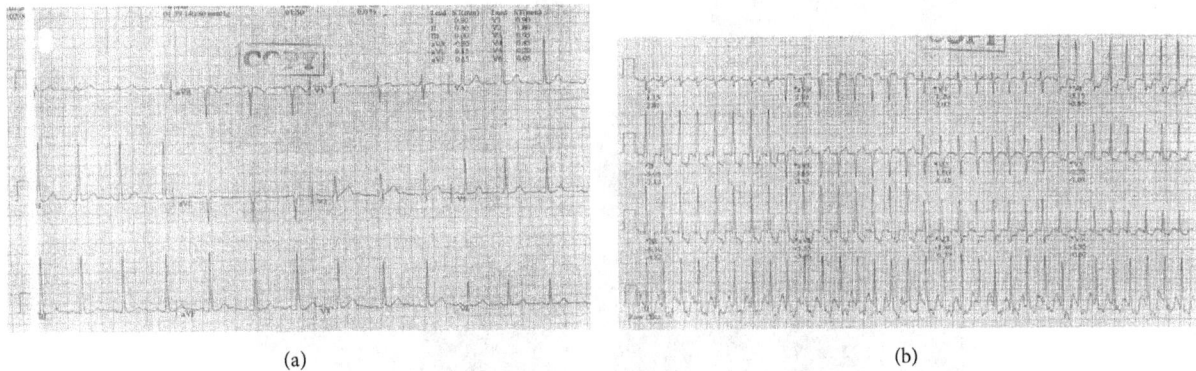

FIGURE 1: Electrocardiogram of the case before treadmill test (a) and during treadmill test showing ischemic sign (b).

examination showed normal value. Electrocardiogram at rest indicated sinus rhythm without sign of ischemia (Figure 1).

A noninvasive examination was performed with echocardiography. Transthorax echocardiogram showed normal cardiac chamber dimension, normal right ventricle and left ventricle wall thickness, normal left and right ventricle systolic and diastolic function, and normal left ventricular segmental and global wall motion. Mitral valve and tricuspid valve were anatomically and functionally normal. Aortic valve examination showed three cusps with normal anatomy and function. Ostium of left coronary artery (LCA) was apparent with diameter of 5 mm, whereas ostium of right coronary artery (RCA) was absent.

Coronary angiography was performed for the patient, started by cannulation into ostium of LCA with Tiger 6 F catheter via radial access. An LCAgraph by contrast agent showed normal left main (LM), normal left anterior descendent (LAD), and left circumflexus (LCx). On LCAgraph view of RAO 20 Caudal 20 and LAO 30 Cranial 15, an RCA was originated from left sinus near LM and coursed through the right aspect of heart (Figure 2). The caliber of RCA was small with normal bifurcation. Posterior descending artery was filled from LCx (left dominance).

The confirmation by cardiac multi slice CT (cMSCT) scan showed that RCA originated from left sinus of Valsalva with interarterial course between ascending aorta and pulmonary artery. The caliber of RCA was small with no sign of stenosis in the RCA (Figures 3 and 4). The small RCA runs through right atrioventricular sulcus and vascularized the right part of the heart. The proximal part of RCA passed through ascending aorta and pulmonary artery.

Based on the diagnostic work-up, the patient was diagnosed as right ACAOS with interarterial course. The evidence of myocardial ischemia, as depicted by positive ischemic response on treadmill test, was evident in the exercise electrocardiogram of this patient although asymptomatic. Right ACAOS with interarterial course was responsible for the ischemia sign. No other structural cardiac abnormalities were found in the patient; therefore the coronary anomaly was the most likely etiology of the ischemia sign. After in-depth consultation about the prognostic implication of this anomaly, the patient and family decided that surgical correction was not to be done then. Therefore, in this patient,

conservative management was employed. Watchful observation was applied to the patient, while strenuous physical activity and competitive sport were absolutely prohibited. Beta blocker as needed was given to the patient. During eight-month follow-up after the diagnosis, the patient reported no ischemic symptom during regular activity. He never took beta blocker medication then.

3. Discussion

We report a case of 28-year-old male who suffered from right ACAOS with interarterial course and the sign of myocardial ischemia. Close observation and limitation of strenuous activity were advised. Neither medication nor surgical revascularization was applied to the patient. Eight-month follow-up of this patient was uneventful.

Coronary artery anomaly is an uncommon condition with prevalence on coronary angiography between 0.61% and 5.64% [2]. The incidence of right ACAOS from coronary angiography is between 0.12% and 0.92% [1, 2]. Right ACAOS with interarterial course is a group of ACAOS with high risk for developing myocardial ischemia and sudden death [3]. Close and reliable relationship is observed between left ACAOS and the incidence of sudden death and ischemia during strenuous physical activity [1]. The clinical picture of ACAOS can be divided into two spectra: the first is sudden death in the young and after strenuous physical activity or sport and the second is atypical clinical picture [1]. Most of ACAOS patients are asymptomatic. Atypical chest discomfort is the most prevalent symptom urging patients to refer to the health facility and to perform the coronary angiography to detect ACAOS. Some patients come due to positive stress test or sign of ischemic heart disease on ECG [1]. In this case, patient was referred due to positive stress test without any ischemic symptoms previously.

Clinical implication of coronary artery anomaly can be divided into ischemic and nonischemic. Ischemic implication can be fixed or episodic ischemia [1]. Right ACAOS with interarterial course is associated with episodic myocardial ischemia. Interarterial course means that ectopic coronary artery runs through two big vessels arising from ventricle, that is, aorta and pulmonary artery. Three mechanisms are proposed regarding the proneness of right ACAOS with

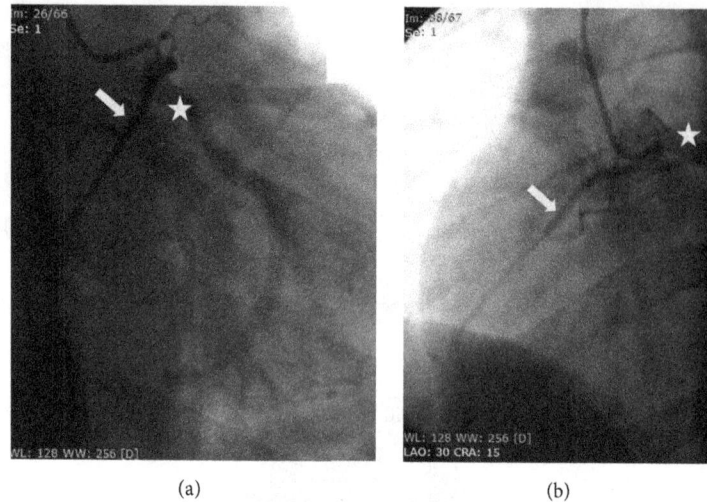

FIGURE 2: (a) and (b) Coronary angiography (RAO 20 Caudal 20 view and LAO 30 Cranial 15 view) shows RCA (arrow) originated from left sinus and its ostium was adjacent to LCA ostium (star). The caliber of RCA was small and coursed into right ventricles with normal bifurcation.

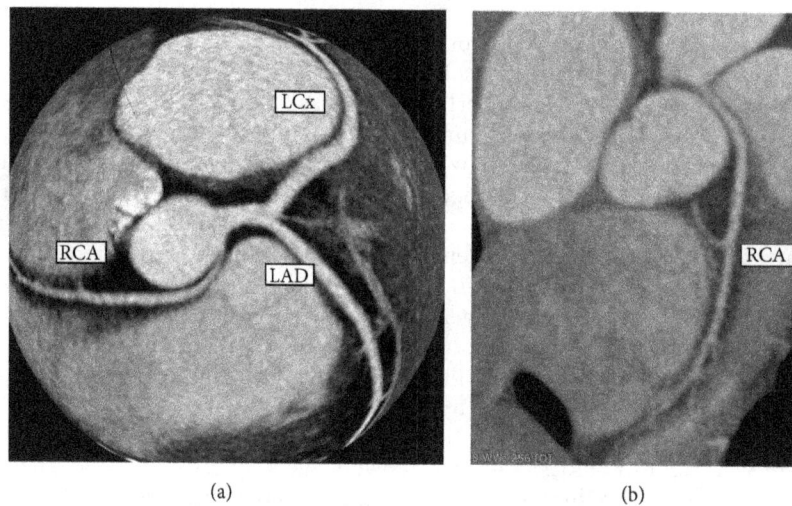

FIGURE 3: (a) and (b) Cardiac MSCT shows RCA originated from left sinus of Valsalva adjacent to LCA ostium with interarterial course between ascending aorta and pulmonary artery. The caliber of RCA was small and coursed into right atrioventricular sulcus.

interarterial course to develop ischemia or sudden death, that is, sharp angulation and kinking of coronary artery while running off from the opposite sinus, valve-like mechanism causing acute closure in the slit-like coronary artery ostium, and compression of narrowed segment of coronary artery by aorta or pulmonary artery particularly during strenuous activity [4]. Hard activity causes dilatation of aortic root and pulmonary trunk which compresses slit-like ostium or particular segment of ectopic coronary artery. This occurs especially in individuals with sufficient aortic distensibility, such as in young people or sportsmen [1]. In our case, the patient was still young and without any complaints during daily activity and regular excercise. Ischemic sign appeared in the treadmill test marked by down-slopping and horizontal ST-depression in stage 4 Bruce-method treadmill test. We speculated that compression of RCA by big vessels was responsible for the ischemic sign.

However, the unusual thing about this case is the fact that the RCA was not a dominant vessel because, based on angiogram and cMSCT, the PDA aroused from LCx. In most cases reported with ischemic symptoms associated with right ACAOS, the RCA is a dominant vessel; therefore obstruction of this vessel produces significant myocardial ischemia. Echocardiogram of the patient showed no other signs of structural cardiac abnormality; therefore the most likely source of ischemia was intramural course of the RCA anomaly. The left dominance nature of the patient prevented, so far, fatal ischemia. Furthermore, the caliber of anomalous RCA, which was small, may also account for the significant ischemic ECG changes developed during excercise test.

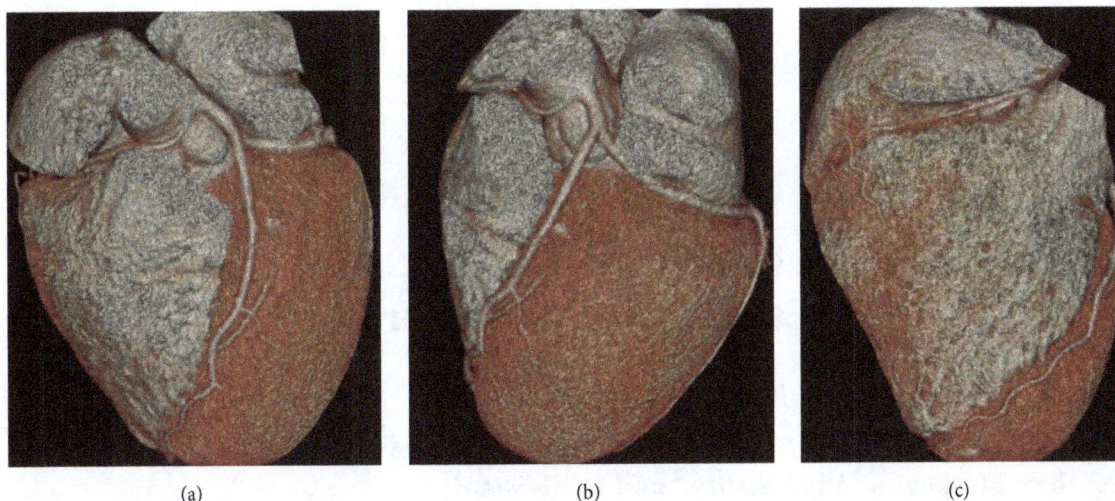

(a)   (b)   (c)

FIGURE 4: (a)–(c) Reconstruction 3D cardiac MSCT shows RCA originated from left sinus of Valsalva adjacent to LCA ostium with interarterial course between ascending aorta and pulmonary artery through right atrioventricular sulcus.

Treatment modalities for right ACAOS with signs and symptoms of ischemia are watchful observation and drugs and coronary angioplasty with stent and corrective surgery [5]. The goal of right ACAOS treatment is to prevent sudden death and improve quality of life [3]. In this patient, after being given several alternatives treatment modalities, watchful observation was selected by the patient and his family. Restriction of strenuous activity and competitive sport was encouraged since these may cause ischemic myocardial or sudden death. Maron and Zipes (2005) stated that right ACAOS patients without intervention should not involve in competitive sport and hard physical activity [6]. The report of close observation and medication with beta blocker within 2 and 5 years in ACAOS results in zero sudden death [7]. The ACC/AHA guideline in 2008 stated that conservative approach is reasonable in right ACAOS without evidence of ischemia [8]. However, since in this patient the evidence of ischemia was present, surgical coronary revascularization should be performed (level of evidence B) [8].

4. Conclusion

In conclusion, this is a case report of rare coronary artery anomaly, right ACAOS with interarterial course, with evidence of ischemic sign, that is, positive ischemic response in treadmill test, in otherwise asymptomatic young male. Wachthful observation and strenuous activity restriction were applied in this case.

Conflict of Interests

There is no conflict of interests.

References

[1] P. Angelini, "Coronary artery anomalies: an entity in search of an identity," *Circulation*, vol. 115, no. 10, pp. 1296–1305, 2007.

[2] M. Yurtdas and O. Gülen, "Anomalous origin of the right coronary artery from the left anterior descending artery: review of the literature," *Cardiology Journal*, vol. 19, no. 2, pp. 122–129, 2012.

[3] R. Barriales-Villa and C. M. Tassa, "Congenital coronary artery anomalies with origin in the contralateral sinus of valsalva: which approach should we take?" *Revista Espanola de Cardiologia*, vol. 59, no. 4, pp. 360–370, 2006.

[4] K. Tsujita, A. Maehara, G. S. Mintz et al., "In vivo intravascular ultrasonic assessment of anomalous right coronary artery arising from left coronary sinus," *The American Journal of Cardiology*, vol. 103, no. 5, pp. 747–751, 2009.

[5] P. Angelini, "Coronary artery anomalies—current clinical issues: definitions, classification, incidence, clinical relevance, and treatment guidelines," *Texas Heart Institute Journal*, vol. 29, no. 4, pp. 271–278, 2002.

[6] B. J. Maron and D. P. Zipes, "Introduction: eligibility recommendations for competitive athletes with cardiovascular abnormalities—general considerations," *Journal of the American College of Cardiology*, vol. 45, no. 8, pp. 1318–1321, 2005.

[7] M. B. Bixby, "Successful medical management of a patient with an anomalous right coronary artery who declined surgery," *American Journal of Critical Care*, vol. 7, no. 5, pp. 393–394, 1998.

[8] C. A. Warnes, R. G. Williams, T. M. Bashore et al., "ACC/AHA Guidelines for the management of adults with congenital heart disease: a report of the American College of Cardiology/American Heart Association Task Force on Practice Guidelines (Writing Committee to Develop Guidelines for the Management of Adults With Congenital Heart Disease)," *Circulation*, vol. 118, pp. e714–e833, 2008.

46

A Rare Case of Renal Infarct due to Noncompaction Cardiomyopathy: A Case Report and Literature Review

Karan Wats,[1] On Chen,[2] Nupur Nippun Uppal,[3] Syeda Atiqa Batul,[2] Norbert Moskovits,[2] Vijay Shetty,[2] and Jacob Shani[2]

[1]Internal Medicine, Maimonides Medical Center, Brooklyn, NY 11219, USA
[2]Department of Cardiology, Maimonides Medical Center, Brooklyn, NY 11219, USA
[3]Department of Nephrology, North Shore Long Island Jewish Hospital, New Hyde Park, NY 11040, USA

Correspondence should be addressed to Karan Wats; karanwats87@gmail.com

Academic Editor: Hiroaki Kitaoka

Left ventricular noncompaction cardiomyopathy is a rare myocardial disorder which results from failure of left ventricle to compact in embryogenesis. We present a case of a 53-year-old female who came because of abdominal pain and was found to have renal infarct secondary to noncompaction cardiomyopathy.

1. Introduction

Left ventricular noncompaction is a rare form of genetic cardiomyopathy that occurs due to arrest in the compaction of developing myocardium which leads to deep trabeculae and recesses giving the ventricle a spongiform appearance [1–4]. It has been grouped under "genetic cardiomyopathy" by the ACC/AHA [5]. While it most commonly presents as heart failure; ventricular arrhythmias, systemic embolism, or sudden death can occur [4, 6, 7]. While thromboembolic events are not uncommon, they usually present as cardioembolic stroke. We present a case of renal infarct in a middle aged female who presented with abdominal pain and was found to have noncompaction on echocardiography. In our search we found no cases of isolated renal emboli as a presentation of left ventricular noncompaction cardiomyopathy.

2. Case Presentation

A 53-year-old female with a history of hypertension presented with the complaints of left sided back pain and dysuria for 2 days. Patient denied any history of chest pain, shortness of breath, or any cardiac problems in the past. Physical examination was significant for bibasilar crackles and pedal edema but no costovertebral tenderness. There was no family history of cardiomyopathy or heart failure. Routine labs showed hemoglobin, 10.5; white cell count, 6.4; platelets, 391. Renal and liver functions tests were within normal limits. An EKG test was done on admission which showed normal sinus rhythm and left axis deviation but no significant ST-T wave changes. Urine analysis was done which was negative for urinary tract infection. CT scan of abdomen (Figures 1 and 2) showed multiple areas of wedge-shaped hypoenhancement in the left kidney with mild adjacent stranding consistent with renal infarcts.

Echocardiogram (Figures 3 and 4) showed a left ventricular ejection fraction, 25% with dilated left ventricle, prominent left ventricular trabeculations, and deep intertrabecular recesses communicating with the LV cavity, consistent with left ventricular noncompaction. Patient underwent an elective angiogram which revealed normal coronaries. Patient was started on heparin for renal emboli and bridged to Coumadin. She was discharged to home with a cardiologist follow-up and INR checks.

3. Discussion

Left ventricular noncompaction (LVNC) was first described in 1975 by Dusek et al. [1] in infant hearts as spongy myocardium. It was later described in adults by Engberding

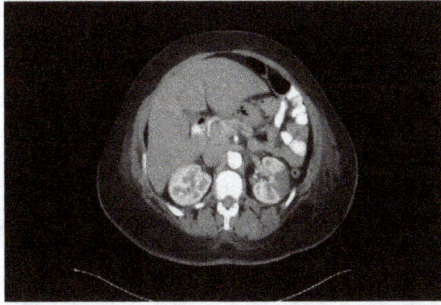

FIGURE 1: CT scan axial view showing wedge-shaped hypoenhancement in the left kidney marked with an arrow consistent with renal infarct.

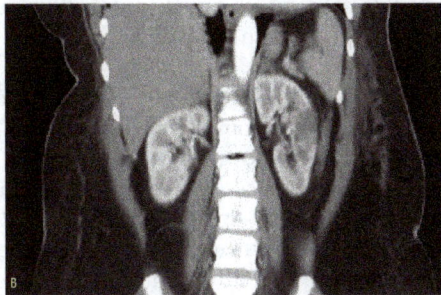

FIGURE 2: Coronal view of the abdomen showing an area of hypoenhancement marked by an arrow consistent with renal infarct.

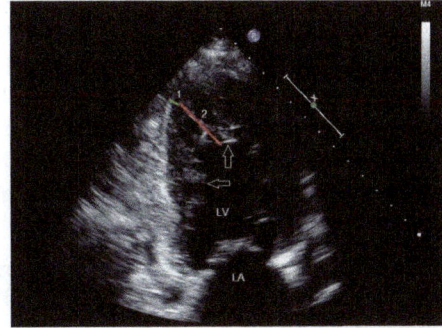

FIGURE 3: Echocardiographic 2 chamber view showing noncompacted myocardium in the left ventricle marked by yellow arrows. It also shows the ratio of noncompacted/compacted myocardium marked by red and green lines, respectively, with a ratio >2:1. LA: left atrium, LV: left ventricle, 1–0.59 cm and 2–2.14 cm as measured.

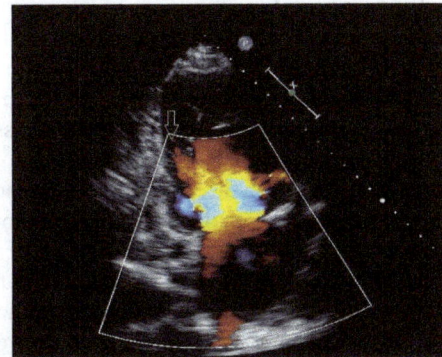

FIGURE 4: Color Doppler showing blood flow in sinusoids in the left ventricle.

and Bender [2] as lack of sinusoidal regression in embryogenesis. Isolated left ventricular noncompaction is a rare form of cardiomyopathy which has been grouped under the genetic cardiomyopathy by the American Heart Association which is caused by arrest of compaction of myocardial fibers during embryogenesis [2–5]. It is characterized by (1) an abnormal myocardial structure characterized by prominent trabeculae and deep intertrabecular recesses with two layers of myocardium, a compacted epicardial layer and a noncompacted endocardium. (2) There is continuity and blood flow from LV to these deep intertrabecular recesses which are filled with blood but there is no evidence of communication with the epicardial coronary artery system [8, 9].

LVNC is a genetically heterogeneous disorder and both familial and sporadic forms have been described. Mutations in various genes [10–12] have been described. Familial forms have been associated with mutations in mitochondrial, sarcomeric, and cytoskeletal genes. A study conducted by Murphy et al. [13] found 8 affected family members among 32 patients. Although genetic testing is not routinely recommended at this time, the Heart Failure Society of America practice guidelines [14] recommend clinical screening of all first-degree relatives of affected patients for LVNC.

The incidence of isolated noncompaction varies among different studies but has been noted to be anywhere between 0.014 and 1.3%. A lot of patients with LVNC are diagnosed during the neonatal period. A significant number of these patients have undulating phenotype in which they have transient recovery of function and present with symptoms later in adult life. Most of the times in children, LVNC usually coexists with other genetic conditions like Barth syndrome, Emery-Dreifuss muscular dystrophy, myotubular myopathy, and so forth, in contrast to adults where it has been known to occur in isolation. It is still unclear whether presentation of LVNC in adulthood represents a long standing condition or delayed manifestation of molecular pathology. With increasing awareness of this rare condition and better and more specific echocardiographic diagnostic parameters, the prevalence of this condition has increased.

The most common forms of presentation include heart failure, arrhythmias, and systemic embolism [4, 6, 7]. In a study of 34 adult patients conducted by Oechslin et al. [4], heart failure was the presenting symptom in 68% of patients and arrhythmias most commonly observed included nonsustained and sustained ventricular tachycardia in 41% of patients. Systemic embolism, most commonly cardioembolic stroke, was observed in 21% of patients. Other forms of embolic complication which have been observed include transient ischemic attack, pulmonary embolism, and mesenteric ischemia [8]. Our patient presented with complaints of abdominal and was eventually found to have a renal infarct which is not a common presentation for this rare disease entity.

Echocardiography with color follow Doppler has been considered as the diagnostic modality of choice for diagnosis of this rare cardiomyopathy and specific criteria for diagnosis have been put forward by various researchers [6, 15–18]. Jenni et al. proposed the following criteria for diagnosis of this condition which have been shown to be highly specific for this condition:

(1) A thickened ventricular wall consisting of two layers, a thin compacted epicardial layer and a markedly thickened endocardial layer with numerous trabeculations and deep recesses with a maximum ratio of noncompacted to compacted myocardium of >2 : 1 at the end systole in the parasternal short axis view.

(2) Color Doppler evidence of flow within the deep intertrabecular recesses.

(3) Prominent trabecular meshwork in the LV apex or midventricular segments of inferior and lateral wall

Our patient had an echocardiogram which showed a noncompacted to compacted myocardium ratio of >2 : 1 at the ventricular apex prominent trabecular meshwork in the LV apex and color Doppler evidence of flow in the recesses thus making a diagnosis of LVNC.

Cardiac magnetic resonance imaging (Cardiac MRI) has been increasingly used for diagnosis of noncompaction cardiomyopathy as it provides a detailed image of cardiac morphology. Cardiac MRI is particularly useful in patients in whom the apex is difficult to visualize with echocardiography or in whom the diagnosis is uncertain with conventional echocardiography. A noncompacted/compacted ratio >2.3 measured at end diastole is used as the diagnostic indicator for noncompaction cardiomyopathy [19]. A study comparing the use of echocardiography versus Cardiac MRI showed no significant difference at the end diastole but Cardiac MRI at end systole was able to better characterize the extent of compaction [20]. Despite this small difference, echocardiography continues to be the diagnostic modality of choice for noncompaction cardiomyopathy.

Symptoms of heart failure are the most commonly presenting symptoms in LVNC. Tian et al. [21] found in their retrospective review that 60% with LVNC were in New York Heart Association (NYHA) functional class III/IV and 79% had systolic dysfunction (left ventricular ejection fraction (LVEF) <50%). The treatment principles remain the same as any other patient presenting with heart failure. Conventional guidelines for management of heart failure by ACC/AHA should be used when managing patients with LVNC. Patients with symptoms despite optimal medical management should be considered for implantable cardioverter defibrillator (ICD) implantation.

Sudden cardiac death is another concern in these patients and should always be evaluated for presence of sustained/nonsustained ventricular tachycardia. The incidence of ventricular arrhythmias varies from 6% [22] to 62% [6] and can lead to sudden death. ICD therapy may be considered in such cases as measure of primary prevention and should also be used in patients who have sustained ventricular tachycardia or cardiac arrest for secondary prevention. According to the Device Based Therapy guidelines [23], implantation of ICD for the prevention of sudden death in patients with LVNC is a class IIb recommendation.

Systemic embolism is another complication associated with LVNC. Initially it was thought to result from stagnation of flow across the prominent trabeculations and deep recesses leading to clot formation in noncompacted layer. A retrospective review done by Stöllberger and Finsterer [24] found that the rate of clot formation and embolism in LVNC is related to the presence of concomitant conditions like low EF, presence of atrial fibrillation, or both rather than LVNC alone. Therefore, oral anticoagulation is recommended in patients with concomitant low EF, atrial fibrillation, history of systemic embolism, and so forth.

Studies on asymptomatic patients with normal EF failed to show any increased risk of systemic embolism and therefore use of anticoagulation in this patient population remains controversial [25].

Large case series done by Lofiego et al. [22] and Greutmann et al. [26] for outcomes in patients with isolated LV noncompaction has shown that the prognosis differed depending on the presence or absence of symptoms at presentation. During follow-up of 46 months and 32 months in these case series, respectively, cardiovascular death and heart transplantation needed to be done in 31% of the patients as compared to none in any of the asymptomatic patients.

A recent retrospective review done by Tian et al. [21] in 106 patients with LVNC showed that 28 (26%) patients died or underwent heart transplantation during a follow-up of 2.9 ± 2.1 years. The study also showed that advanced heart failure, a dilated left heart with systolic dysfunction, reduced systolic blood pressure, pulmonary hypertension, and right bundle branch block predict adverse outcomes of LVNC at the time of diagnosis.

Another recent study [27] done on pediatric population showed that children who had normal or mild left ventricular dysfunction had much better prognosis in terms of arrhythmia burden and sudden cardiac death incidence further strengthening the importance of left ventricular function at the time of diagnosis and its impact on future health and outcomes.

4. Conclusion

While LVNC is not common, its prevalence has increased due to better imaging modalities and more specific diagnostic criteria but still this disease may be underdiagnosed due to lack of awareness among clinicians. Our case illustrates an uncommon presentation of LVNC with renal infarction as the presenting manifestation which later leads to finding of severely decreased LV function and diagnosis of LVNC. It is important to recognize that this condition as the management of LVNC is slightly different from other causes of LV dysfunction such as the need to anticoagulate because of the high risk of thromboembolism and the familial inheritance requiring genetic counselling, screening among family members.

This makes the disease, its presentations, complications, and management important for the general internist and the cardiologist to know.

Abbreviations

ACC: American College of Cardiology
AHA: American Heart Association
LV: Left ventricle
EF: Ejection fraction
LVNC: Left ventricular noncompaction
ICD: Implantable cardioverter defibrillator
MRI: Magnetic resonance imaging
NYHA: New York Heart Association.

Conflict of Interests

The authors declare that there is no conflict of interests regarding the publication of this paper.

References

[1] J. Dusek, B. Ostadal, and M. Duskova, "Postnatal persistence of spongy myocardium with embryonic blood supply," *Archives of Pathology*, vol. 99, no. 6, pp. 312–317, 1975.

[2] R. Engberding and F. Bender, "Echocardiographical diagnosis of myocardial sinusoids," *Zeitschrift für Kardiologie*, vol. 73, no. 12, pp. 786–788, 1984.

[3] R. Jenni, N. Goebel, R. Tartini, J. Schneider, U. Arbenz, and O. Oelz, "Persisting myocardial sinusoids of both ventricles as an isolated anomaly: echocardiographic, angiographic, and pathologic anatomical findings," *Cardiovascular and Interventional Radiology*, vol. 9, no. 3, pp. 127–131, 1986.

[4] E. N. Oechslin, C. H. Attenhofer Jost, J. R. Rojas, P. A. Kaufmann, and R. Jenni, "Long-term follow-up of 34 adults with isolated left ventricular noncompaction: a distinct cardiomyopathy with poor prognosis," *Journal of the American College of Cardiology*, vol. 36, no. 2, pp. 493–500, 2000.

[5] B. J. Maron, J. A. Towbin, G. Thiene et al., "Contemporary definitions and classification of the cardiomyopathies: an American Heart Association Scientific Statement from the Council on Clinical Cardiology, Heart Failure and Transplantation Committee; Quality of Care and Outcomes Research and Functional Genomics and Translational Biology Interdisciplinary Working Groups; and Council on Epidemiology and Prevention," *Circulation*, vol. 113, no. 14, pp. 1807–1816, 2006.

[6] T. K. Chin, J. K. Perloff, R. G. Williams, K. Jue, and R. Mohrmann, "Isolated noncompaction of left ventricular myocardium. A study of eight cases," *Circulation*, vol. 82, no. 2, pp. 507–513, 1990.

[7] F. Ichida, Y. Hamamichi, T. Miyawaki et al., "Clinical features of isolated noncompaction of the ventricular myocardium: long-term clinical course, hemodynamic properties, and genetic background," *Journal of the American College of Cardiology*, vol. 34, no. 1, pp. 233–240, 1999.

[8] M. Ritter, E. Oechslin, G. Sütsch, C. Attenhofer, J. Schneider, and R. Jenni, "Isolated noncompaction of the myocardium in adults," *Mayo Clinic Proceedings*, vol. 72, no. 1, pp. 26–31, 1997.

[9] B. C. Weiford, V. D. Subbarao, and K. M. Mulhern, "Noncompaction of the ventricular myocardium," *Circulation*, vol. 109, no. 24, pp. 2965–2971, 2004.

[10] M. Vatta, B. Mohapatra, S. Jimenez et al., "Mutations in Cypher/ZASP in patients with dilated cardiomyopathy and left ventricular non-compaction," *Journal of the American College of Cardiology*, vol. 42, no. 11, pp. 2014–2027, 2003.

[11] Y. M. Hoedemaekers, K. Caliskan, D. Majoor-Krakauer et al., "Cardiac β-myosin heavy chain defects in two families with non-compaction cardiomyopathy: linking non-compaction to hypertrophic, restrictive, and dilated cardiomyopathies," *European Heart Journal*, vol. 28, no. 22, pp. 2732–2737, 2007.

[12] F. Ichida, S. Tsubata, K. R. Bowles et al., "Novel gene mutations in patients with left ventricular noncompaction or Barth syndrome," *Circulation*, vol. 103, no. 9, pp. 1256–1263, 2001.

[13] R. T. Murphy, R. Thaman, J. Gimeno Blanes et al., "Natural history and familial characteristics of isolated left ventricular non-compaction," *European Heart Journal*, vol. 24, pp. 187–192, 2005.

[14] R. E. Hershberger, J. Lindenfeld, L. Mestroni, C. E. Seidman, M. R. G. Taylor, and J. A. Towbin, "Genetic evaluation of cardiomyopathy—a Heart Failure Society of America Practice Guideline," *Journal of Cardiac Failure*, vol. 15, no. 2, pp. 83–97, 2009.

[15] R. Jenni, E. Oechslin, J. Schneider, C. Attenhofer Jost, and P. A. Kaufmann, "Echocardiographic and pathoanatomical characteristics of isolated left ventricular non-compaction: a step towards classification as a distinct cardiomyopathy," *Heart*, vol. 86, no. 6, pp. 666–671, 2001.

[16] B. S. Frischknecht, C. H. A. Jost, E. N. Oechslin et al., "Validation of noncompaction criteria in dilated cardiomyopathy, and valvular and hypertensive heart disease," *Journal of the American Society of Echocardiography*, vol. 18, no. 8, pp. 865–872, 2005.

[17] C. Gebhard, B. E. Stähli, M. Greutmann, P. Biaggi, R. Jenni, and F. C. Tanner, "Reduced left ventricular compacta thickness: a novel echocardiographic criterion for non-compaction cardiomyopathy," *Journal of the American Society of Echocardiography*, vol. 25, no. 10, pp. 1050–1057, 2012.

[18] C. Stöllberger, J. Finsterer, and G. Blazek, "Left ventricular hypertrabeculation/noncompaction and association with additional cardiac abnormalities and neuromuscular disorders," *American Journal of Cardiology*, vol. 90, no. 8, pp. 899–902, 2002.

[19] S. E. Petersen, J. B. Selvanayagam, F. Wiesmann et al., "Left ventricular non-compaction: insights from cardiovascular magnetic resonance imaging," *Journal of the American College of Cardiology*, vol. 46, no. 1, pp. 101–105, 2005.

[20] F. Thuny, A. Jacquier, B. Jop et al., "Assessment of left ventricular non-compaction in adults: side-by-side comparison of cardiac magnetic resonance imaging with echocardiography," *Archives of Cardiovascular Diseases*, vol. 103, no. 3, pp. 150–159, 2010.

[21] T. Tian, Y. Liu, L. Gao et al., "Isolated left ventricular noncompaction: clinical profile and prognosis in 106 adult patients," *Heart Vessels*, vol. 29, pp. 645–655, 2014.

[22] C. Lofiego, E. Biagini, F. Pasquale et al., "Wide spectrum of presentation and variable outcomes of isolated left ventricular non-compaction," *Heart*, vol. 93, no. 1, pp. 65–71, 2007.

[23] A. Epstein, J. DiMarco, K. Ellenbogen et al., "ACC/AHA/HRS 2008 guidelines for device-based therapy of cardiac rhythm abnormalities," *Journal of the American College of Cardiology*, vol. 51, no. 21, pp. 2085–2105, 2008.

[24] C. Stöllberger and J. Finsterer, "Thrombi in left ventricular hypertrabeculation/noncompaction—review of the literature," *Acta Cardiologica*, vol. 59, no. 3, pp. 341–344, 2004.

[25] D. Aras, O. Tufekcioglu, K. Ergun et al., "Clinical features of isolated ventricular noncompaction in adults long-term clinical course, echocardiographic properties, and predictors of left

ventricular failure," *Journal of Cardiac Failure*, vol. 12, no. 9, pp. 726–733, 2006.

[26] M. Greutmann, M. L. Mah, C. K. Silversides et al., "Predictors of adverse outcome in adolescents and adults with isolated left ventricular noncompaction," *American Journal of Cardiology*, vol. 109, no. 2, pp. 276–281, 2012.

[27] R. J. Czosek, D. S. Spar, P. R. Khoury et al., "Outcomes, arrhythmic burden and ambulatory monitoring of pediatric patients with left ventricular non-compaction and preserved left ventricular function," *The American Journal of Cardiology*, vol. 115, no. 7, pp. 962–966, 2015.

47

Amphetamine Abuse Related Acute Myocardial Infarction

Archana Sinha,[1] **O'Dene Lewis,**[2] **Rajan Kumar,**[1]
Sri Lakshmi Hyndavi Yeruva,[3] **and Bryan H. Curry**[4]

[1]*Division of Cardiology, Saint Luke's University Health Network, 801 Ostrum Street, Bethlehem, PA 18015, USA*
[2]*Division of Pulmonary Medicine, Howard University Hospital, 2041 Georgia Avenue, Washington, DC 20060, USA*
[3]*Division of Hematology-Oncology, Howard University Hospital, 2041 Georgia Avenue, Washington, DC 20060, USA*
[4]*Division of Cardiology, Howard University Hospital, 2041 Georgia Avenue, Washington, DC 20060, USA*

Correspondence should be addressed to Archana Sinha; sinha.archana7@gmail.com

Academic Editor: Filippo M. Sarullo

Amphetamine abuse is a global problem. The cardiotoxic manifestations like acute myocardial infarction (AMI), heart failure, or arrhythmia related to misuse of amphetamine and its synthetic derivatives have been documented but are rather rare. Amphetamine-related AMI is even rarer. We report two cases of men who came to emergency department (ED) with chest pain, palpitation, or seizure and were subsequently found to have myocardial infarction associated with the use of amphetamines. It is crucial that, with increase in amphetamine abuse, clinicians are aware of this potentially dire complication. Patients with low to intermediate risk for coronary artery disease with atypical presentation may benefit from obtaining detailed substance abuse history and urine drug screen if deemed necessary.

1. Introduction

Amphetamine is a potent central nervous system stimulant and a substance of widespread abuse. United Nations Office on Drugs and Crime ranks amphetamine-type stimulants such as MDMA (popularly known as Ecstasy or Molly) and methamphetamine as the world's second most widely used type of drug after cannabis [1]. According to the figures released by National Survey on Drug Use and Health, 1.4 million or 0.5 percent of individuals aged 12 years or older were nonmedical users of stimulants in 2013 [2]. The use of amphetamine appears to vary with gender and race. It is predominantly seen in unemployed single white men aged 20–35 years [3]. Data suggests that Caucasians use amphetamines more than African Americans [4]. The role of cocaine as a causative agent of AMI is well established [5, 6] but AMI due to amphetamine use or abuse has not been as widely recognized. Westover et al. showed modest, though statistically significant, association between amphetamine abuse and AMI in their population-based study [7]. The most popular amphetamines encountered in abuse include amphetamine, 3,4-methylenedioxymethamphetamine (MDMA), 4-methoxyamphetamine (PMA), 3,4-methylenedioxyamphetamine (MDA), 3,4-methylenedioxyethylamphetamine (MDEA), and 4-methylthioamphetamine (4-MTA) [8]. We report two cases of previously healthy men who presented with atypical chest pain and palpitations to the ED and later were diagnosed with AMI associated with use of amphetamines.

2. Case 1

A 41-year-old African American male was brought to our ED with worsening constant, central, pleuritic chest pain of one-day duration that woke him from sleep. He also complained of nausea, tingling, and numbness of both hands. He reported a history of few weeks of intermittent chest pain in the same location, with no aggravating or relieving factors. His past medical history was significant for dyslipidemia. He denied prescription or illicit drug use but gave a remote history of smoking, alcohol, and marijuana abuse. He had no known drug allergy. His father passed away from a myocardial infarction at 66 years of age. On presentation to the ED his blood pressure was 107/60 mm Hg,

TABLE 1: Laboratory data of cardiac enzyme trends.

Cardiac enzymes	Case 1			Case 2		
	1st set	2nd set	3rd set	1st set	2nd set	3rd set
CPK (35–230 IU/L)	2176	2174	4895	271	481	365
CK-MB (0.0–5.0 ng/mL)	55.5	40	9.7	29.4	56.5	23.8
Troponin (0.00–0.03 ng/mL)	2.22	1.3	0.31	1.73	9.57	6.74
Myoglobin (0–450 pg/mL)	467	139	287	79	55	19

CPK: creatine phosphokinase; CK-MB: creatine kinase (CK) MB isoenzyme.

TABLE 2: Laboratory data of the patients at admission in the hospital and during hospitalization.

Laboratory parameter (normal range)	Case 1	Case 2
Urea (7–25 mg/dL)	9	21
Creatinine (0.6–1.2 mg/dL)	0.9	1.5
Sodium (135–148 mEq/L)	137	137
Potassium (3.5–5.3 mEq/L)	4.0	3.5
Calcium (8.5–10.5 mg/dL)	9.1	9.0
Phosphorus (2.5–4.5 mg/dL)	2.9	4.7
Magnesium (1.7–2.5 mg/dL)	2.0	2.4
Prothrombin time (12.5–14.5 seconds)	13.0	14.8
Partial thromboplastin time (24–34 seconds)	31.5	31.6
International normalized ratio (1.12–1.46)	0.99	1.17
White blood cell (3.2–10.6) cells/liter	8	10.5
Hemoglobin (12.1–15.9 g/dL)	14.9	12.6
Mean corpuscular volume (77.8–94.0 fL)	87	91.9
Platelet (177000–406000/μL)	161	227
Erythrocyte sedimentation rate (0–10 mm/h)	20	—
Thyroid stimulation hormone (0.4–40 mU/mL)	—	3.14
Human immune deficiency virus	Nonreactive	Nonreactive
Total cholesterol levels (145–200 mg/dL)	199	150
Serum triglycerides (20–160 mg/dL)	151	102
LDL cholesterol (50–150 mg/dL)	135	99
HDL cholesterol (45–85 mg/dL)	30	46
Fasting blood sugar (60–110 mg/dL)	171	100

LDL: low-density lipoprotein; HDL; high-density lipoprotein.

heart rate was 78 beats per minute, respiratory rate was 16 per minute, and temperature was 97°F with an oxygen saturation of 99% on room air. Cardiovascular examination was unremarkable. His lungs were clear to auscultation and his abdominal examination was within normal limits. Electrocardiogram (EKG) showed sinus tachycardia with diffuse ST segment elevation suggestive of early repolarization (Figure 1). His initial set of cardiac enzymes showed markedly elevated CPK of 2176 U/L, CK-MB of 55.5 ng/mL, troponin I of 2.22 ng/mL, and myoglobin of 467 ng/mL (Table 1). He was admitted to the cardiac unit for hemodynamic monitoring, serial serum cardiac enzymes levels assays, serial EKGs, and assessment of left ventricular function. The rest of his laboratory values are listed in Table 2. The urine drug screen was positive for amphetamines and negative for cocaine, opiates, barbiturates, cannabinoids, benzodiazepines, and phencyclidine, methadone, and propoxyphene. Chest X-ray showed no acute pathology. A transthoracic echocardiogram showed normal left ventricular systolic function without any regional wall motion abnormalities. Cardiac catheterization revealed normal epicardial coronary arteries without any evidence of atherosclerotic disease. Serum troponin levels showed a downward trend on follow-up lab tests. The patient was started on amlodipine 10 mg for possible coronary vasospasm. He was discharged home after two days of hospitalization. The final diagnosis of AMI likely secondary to amphetamine-induced vasospasm was made.

3. Case 2

A 23-year-old African American male was brought to our ED with a seizure episode preceded by palpitations and diaphoresis. He was on a rigorous exercise regimen and had started taking an over-the-counter product called Shakeology one week before. At the time of admission, his blood

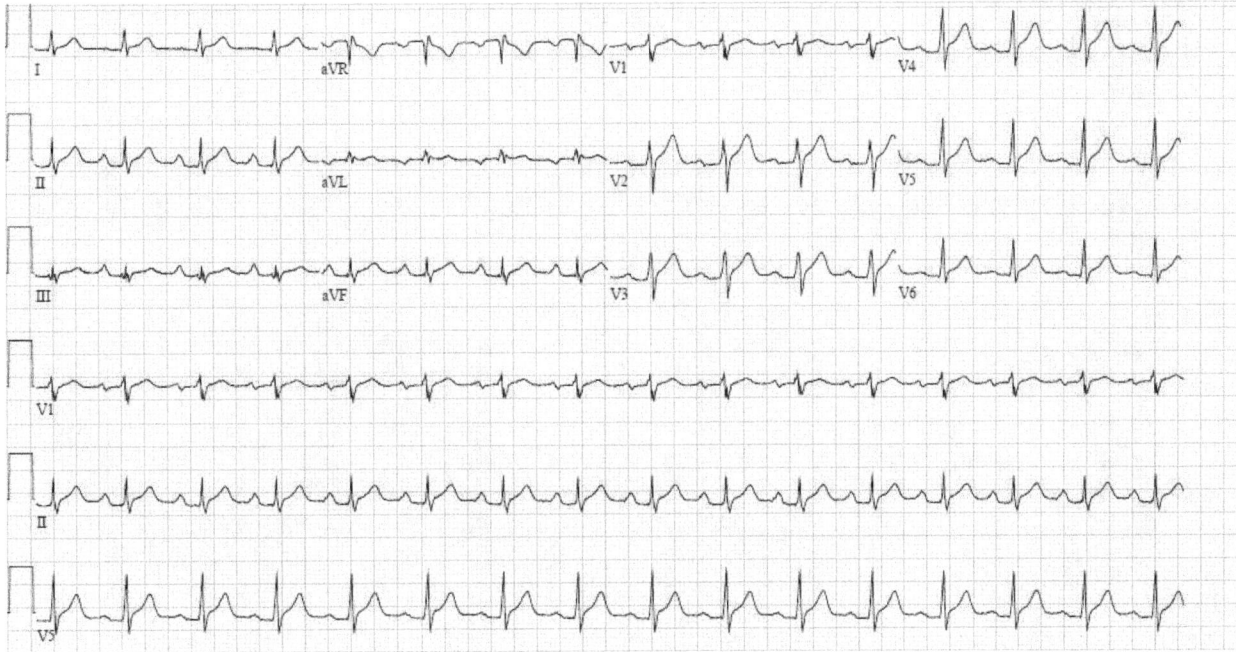

FIGURE 1: Sinus tachycardia and diffuse ST segment elevation suggestive of early repolarization.

pressure was 101/64 mm Hg, heart rate was 154 beats per minute, respiratory rate was 18 per minute, and temperature was 98°F with an oxygen saturation of 98% on room air. He denied prescription or illicit drug use but on the day of presentation he did drink some alcohol. He admitted to smoking two cigarettes per week and having a couple of beers on the weekend. His past medical history was unremarkable and he had no known drug allergies. There was no significant family history of any cardiac conditions. Cardiovascular examination revealed an irregularly irregular heart beat and the EKG showed atrial fibrillation without any significant ST changes (Figure 2(a)). His lungs were clear to auscultation and abdominal examination was within normal limits. His initial cardiac enzymes were elevated with CPK of 271 U/L, CK-MB of 29.4 ng/mL, troponin I of 1.73 ng/mL, and myoglobin of 79 ng/mL (Table 1). He was admitted to cardiac unit for further monitoring and management. Repeat EKG showed spontaneous conversion to normal sinus rhythm (Figure 2(b)). The rest of his laboratory values were normal (Table 2). Troponin I levels peaked at 9.57 ng/mL. No acute pathology was noted on chest X-ray. Cardiac CT angiogram with calcium scoring was done. It showed calcium score of 0 Agatston units and no evidence of coronary artery disease. The urine drug screen was positive for amphetamines and negative for cocaine, opiates, barbiturates, cannabinoids, benzodiazepines, and phencyclidine, methadone, and propoxyphene. Coronary vasospasm likely secondary to amphetamine was considered possible etiology and he was started on amlodipine 10 mg. He was discharged home on fourth day after resolution of his symptoms. The final diagnosis of atrial fibrillation and non-ST segment elevation myocardial infarction likely secondary to amphetamine-induced vasospasm was made.

4. Discussion

Amphetamine is a synthetic derivative of phenethylamine. Amphetamines are central nervous system stimulants that stimulate the release of catecholamines especially norepinephrine and dopamine from presynaptic nerve endings and prevent their reuptake, thus creating a hyperadrenergic state [9]. Its history of abuse dates back to its development more than 100 years ago. The last twenty-five years have seen a rapid surge in illicit use of amphetamine and related compounds in the United States. The routes of administration can be oral, intravenous (IV), and inhalation. With oral use there is approximately 1-hour delay in symptoms, whereas when inhaled or injected effects are seen within few minutes. The peak plasma concentration is achieved in 5 minutes with IV use and in 2 to 3 hours after ingestion. The rate of metabolism is highly variable and up to 30% of the parent compound can be excreted unchanged in the urine. Plasma half-life ranges from 5 to 30 hours depending on urine flow and pH [10].

The most common cardiovascular side effects of amphetamine abuse are hypertension and tachycardia [11]. Other common complaints can be chest pain, palpitations, and shortness of breath. There have been reports of serious cardiovascular complications like cardiomyopathy, cardiac dysrhythmia, myocardial infarction, cor pulmonale, myocarditis, necrotizing vasculitis, coronary rupture, and sudden cardiac arrest [11–14]. The exact pathophysiological mechanism of myocardial infarction following amphetamine use is unclear. Proposed mechanisms include coronary vasospasm, coronary spasm with intracoronary thrombus, prothrombotic activation [15, 16], increased myocardial oxygen demand induced by catecholamines [17], and catecholamine-mediated platelet aggregation with subsequent thrombus

(a)

(b)

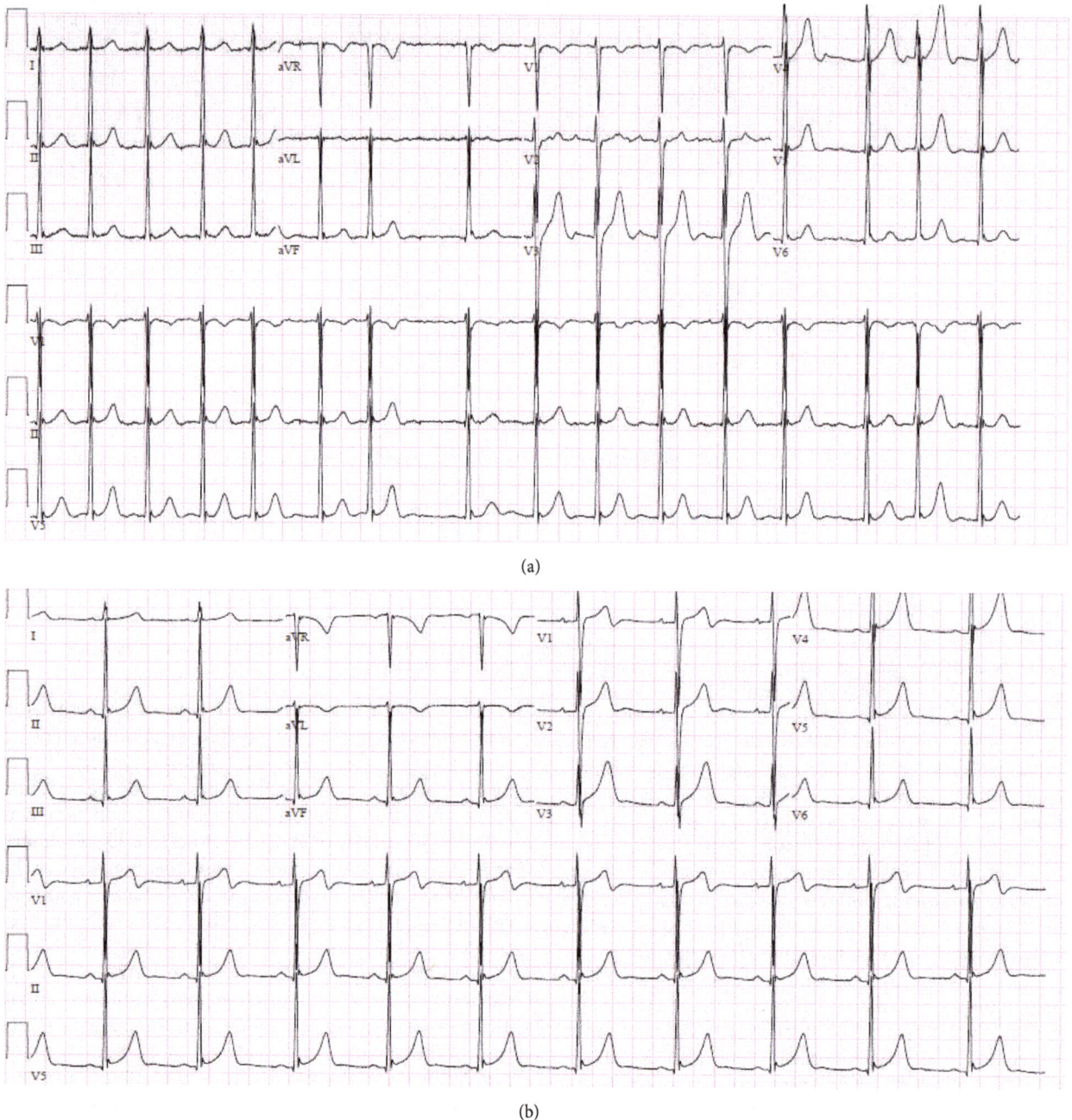

FIGURE 2: (a) Atrial fibrillation without any significant ST changes. (b) Normal sinus rhythm with early repolarization.

formation [18]. The role of amphetamine in inducing vaso-constriction and vasospasm is not completely explained by adrenergic stimulation [19].

Our patients had no therapeutic indication for amphet-amine-like substances and denied any recreational drug use. The exact route of intake could not be ascertained. 45% of the adults in a recent single centre study by Alghamdi et al. did not admit to substance abuse. Adults aged <40 years were more likely to admit to substance abuse [20]. Urine drug screens are generally performed using either immunoassays or gas chromatography-mass spectrometry (GC-MS) [21]. One major problem with immunoassays is false-positive

results. Therefore, a more specific confirmatory test such as GC-MS is needed to confirm a positive finding with an immunoassay. GC-MS is more accurate than an immunoas-say but it is more expensive and time-consuming [22]. Our patients were not on any drugs or dietary supplements that are known to cause false-positive immunoassay [23]. One of our limitations is absence of GC-MS urine drug screen or serum amphetamine levels for the patients.

Patient 2 had history of consumption of a meal replace-ment shake (Shakeology). Popular dietary supplements are known to cause false-positive urine drug screen for amphet-amine [23, 24] and also have been implicated in causing sudden cardiac death and AMI [25, 26]. Shakeology is not mentioned in the list of such dietary supplements released by the concerned agencies [27].

Patient 1 had normal sinus rhythm with early repolarization and patients 2 had atrial fibrillation with nonspecific ST changes. Serial cardiac biomarkers were elevated in both patients. Liebetrau et al. proposed diagnostic approach for AMI in patients with atrial fibrillation and symptoms suggestive of AMI. The specificity-optimized cut-off values higher than the 99th percentile concentration (0.032 ng/mL) and additional use of the 3-hour change in troponin concentration lead to a positive predictive value of more than 95%, facilitating identification of patients with AMI [28]. Patient 2 had atrial fibrillation that lasted for few minutes and resolved spontaneously. The maximal noted heart rate was 154 beats per minute. He did not have any evidence of hypotension. His troponin I on presentation was 1.73 ng/mL and subsequently increased to 9.57 ng/mL four hours later. It does not seem plausible that atrial fibrillation that was transient and without any hemodynamic compromise would lead to greater than fivefold increase in troponin on subsequent testing.

The treatment of AMI attributed to amphetamine abuse is not clearly defined [29, 30]. Calcium channel blockers may play an important role in the treatment of AMI due to amphetamines and as in our cases they may be effective in treatment of suspected coronary vasospasm. Beta-adrenergic receptor blocker administration should be avoided until the pathophysiology of this condition has been clarified as they may exacerbate coronary vasospasm. Thrombolytic therapy or intravenous anticoagulants may be used if coronary thrombus is present [19].

Patient 1 had cardiac catheterization while Patient 2 had CT coronary angiography given his low risk for coronary artery disease. No evidence of coronary artery disease was found in either subject. Both patients had good outcome and were discharged home to follow-up in cardiology clinic.

5. Conclusion

Amphetamine and related substances are now among the most commonly abused drugs worldwide. Amphetamine associated AMI may become more common in the acute care setting if the rate of amphetamine abuse continues to increase. Although the exact mechanism by which it does so is still unclear, there seems to be intricate interaction of host and drug factors that is responsible for the variability in clinical presentation and outcome. Clinically a number of areas need to be addressed, the most important being the appropriate therapeutic approach. Physicians working in the emergency departments as well as cardiologists should be sensitive to this complication, as early diagnosis can be the key to successful management of this potentially fatal complication.

Consent

Patients' consent was obtained for the publication.

Disclosure

Bryan H. Curry is a senior author.

Conflict of Interests

The authors report no financial relationships or conflict of interests regarding the content herein.

References

[1] UNODC, World Drug Report 2011, Sales no. E.11.XI.10, United Nations Publications, 2011.

[2] Substance Abuse & Mental Health Services Administration, Results from the 2013 National Survey on Drug Use and Health, http://www.samhsa.gov/data/NSDUH/2013SummNatFindDetTables/Index.aspx.

[3] B. Huang, D. A. Dawson, F. S. Stinson et al., "Prevalence, correlates, and comorbidity of nonmedical prescription drug use and drug use disorders in the United States: results of the National Epidemiologic Survey on Alcohol and Related Conditions," Journal of Clinical Psychiatry, vol. 67, no. 7, pp. 1062–1073, 2006.

[4] T. F. Borders, B. M. Booth, X. Han et al., "Longitudinal changes in methamphetamine and cocaine use in untreated rural stimulant users: racial differences and the impact of methamphetamine legislation," Addiction, vol. 103, no. 5, pp. 800–808, 2008.

[5] A. I. Qureshi, M. F. Suri, L. R. Guterman, and L. N. Hopkins, "Cocaine use and the likelihood of nonfatal myocardial infarction and stroke: data from the Third National Health and Nutrition Examination Survey," Circulation, vol. 103, no. 4, pp. 502–506, 2001.

[6] S.-S. Yao, H. Spindola-Franco, M. Menegus, M. Greenberg, M. Goldberger, and J. Shirani, "Successful intracoronary thrombolysis in cocaine-associated acute myocardial infarction," Catheterization and Cardiovascular Diagnosis, vol. 42, no. 3, pp. 294–297, 1997.

[7] A. N. Westover, P. A. Nakonezny, and R. W. Haley, "Acute myocardial infarction in young adults who abuse amphetamines," Drug and Alcohol Dependence, vol. 96, no. 1-2, pp. 49–56, 2008.

[8] W. Jacobs, "Fatal amphetamine-associated cardiotoxicity and its medicolegal implications," American Journal of Forensic Medicine and Pathology, vol. 27, no. 2, pp. 156–160, 2006.

[9] B. K. Yamamoto, A. Moszczynska, and G. A. Gudelsky, "Amphetamine toxicities: classical and emerging mechanisms," Annals of the New York Academy of Sciences, vol. 1187, pp. 101–121, 2010.

[10] D. J. Watts and L. McCollester, "Methamphetamine-induced myocardial infarction with elevated troponin I," The American Journal of Emergency Medicine, vol. 24, no. 1, pp. 132–134, 2006.

[11] J. Waksman, R. N. Taylor, G. S. Bodor, F. F. S. Daly, H. A. Jolliff, and R. C. Dart, "Acute myocardial infarction associated with amphetamine use," Mayo Clinic Proceedings, vol. 76, no. 3, pp. 323–326, 2001.

[12] J. Brinkman, N. Hunfeld, and P. Melief, "'Double arrest'—amphetamine fatality in a 31-year-old male: a case report," Netherlands Journal of Critical Care, vol. 18, no. 2, pp. 17–20, 2014.

[13] E. Khattab and A. Shujaa, "Amphetamine abuse and acute thrombosis of left circumflex coronary artery," International Journal of Case Reports and Images, vol. 4, no. 12, pp. 698–701, 2013.

[14] K. Brennan, S. Shurmur, and A. Elhendy, "Coronary artery rupture associated with amphetamine abuse," Cardiology in Review, vol. 12, no. 5, pp. 282–283, 2004.

[15] T. T. Bashour, "Acute myocardial infarction resulting from amphetamine abuse: a spasm-thrombus interplay?" *American Heart Journal*, vol. 128, no. 6, part 1, pp. 1237–1239, 1994.

[16] C. Gebhard, A. Breitenstein, A. Akhmedov et al., "Amphetamines induce tissue factor and impair tissue factor pathway inhibitor: role of dopamine receptor type 4," *European Heart Journal*, vol. 31, no. 14, pp. 1780–1791, 2010.

[17] E. O. Feigl, "Coronary physiology," *Physiological Reviews*, vol. 63, no. 1, pp. 1–205, 1983.

[18] J. I. Haft, P. D. Kranz, F. J. Albert, and K. Fani, "Intravascular platelet aggregation in the heart induced by norepinephrine: microscopic studies," *Circulation*, vol. 46, no. 4, pp. 698–708, 1972.

[19] G. M. Costa, C. Pizzi, B. Bresciani, C. Tumscitz, M. Gentile, and R. Bugiardini, "Acute myocardial infarction caused by amphetamines: a case report and review of the literature," *Italian Heart Journal*, vol. 2, no. 6, pp. 478–480, 2001.

[20] M. Alghamdi, B. Alqahtani, and S. Alhowti, "Cardiovascular complications among individuals with amphetamine-positive urine drug screening admitted to a tertiary care hospital in Riyadh," *Journal of the Saudi Heart Association*, 2016.

[21] K. E. Moeller, K. C. Lee, and J. C. Kissack, "Urine drug screening: practical guide for clinicians," *Mayo Clinic Proceedings*, vol. 83, no. 1, pp. 66–76, 2008.

[22] J. B. Standridge, S. M. Adams, and A. P. Zotos, "Urine drug screening: a valuable office procedure," *American Family Physician*, vol. 81, no. 5, pp. 635–640, 2010.

[23] A. Saitman, H.-D. Park, and R. L. Fitzgerald, "False-positive interferences of common urine drug screen immunoassays: a review," *Journal of Analytical Toxicology*, vol. 38, no. 7, Article ID bku075, pp. 387–396, 2014.

[24] A. J. Pavletic and M. Pao, "Popular dietary supplement causes false-positive drug screen for amphetamines," *Psychosomatics*, vol. 55, no. 2, pp. 206–207, 2014.

[25] M. J. Eliason, A. Eichner, A. Cancio, L. Bestervelt, B. D. Adams, and P. A. Deuster, "Case reports: death of active duty soldiers following ingestion of dietary supplements containing 1,3-dimethylamylamine (DMAA)," *Military Medicine*, vol. 177, no. 12, pp. 1455–1459, 2012.

[26] T. B. Smith, B. A. Staub, G. M. Natarajan, D. M. Lasorda, and I. G. Poornima, "Acute myocardial infarction associated with dietary supplements containing 1,3-dimethylamylamine and *Citrus aurantium*," *Texas Heart Institute Journal*, vol. 41, no. 1, pp. 70–72, 2014.

[27] Human Performance Resource Center, Dietary Supplements/Products Containing DMAA, http://HPRC-ONLINE.org.

[28] C. Liebetrau, M. Weber, S. Tzikas et al., "Identification of acute myocardial infarction in patients with atrial fibrillation and chest pain with a contemporary sensitive troponin I assay," *BMC Medicine*, vol. 13, article 169, 2015.

[29] A. S. Ragland, Y. Ismail, and E. L. Arsura, "Myocardial infarction after amphetamine use," *American Heart Journal*, vol. 125, no. 1, pp. 247–249, 1993.

[30] M. J. MacMahon and V. R. Tallentire, "Stimulating stuff: the pathological effects of cocaine and amphetamines on the cardiovascular system," *The British Journal of Diabetes and Vascular Disease*, vol. 10, no. 5, pp. 251–255, 2010.

48

Mobile Intracardiac Mass after Inguinal Hernia Repair: An Unresolved Treatment Dilemma

Fahad Almehmadi,[1,2] Mark Davis,[1] and Sheldon M. Singh[1]

[1]*Schulich Heart Center, Sunnybrook Health Sciences Center, University of Toronto, 2075 Bayview Avenue, Toronto, ON, Canada M4N 3M5*
[2]*King Saud Bin Abdulaziz University of Health Sciences, Jeddah, Saudi Arabia*

Correspondence should be addressed to Fahad Almehmadi; falmehma@gmail.com

Academic Editor: Mohammad R. Movahed

Right heart thrombi (RHT) are rare but well-described entity in literature. Their isolation has been considered as confirmatory for the diagnosis of venous thromboembolism (VTE). Even though their isolation aids the diagnosis, physicians are faced with a difficult management dilemma giving the paucity of data to support any treatment decision. We present a case of RHT in an 81-year-old man who presented to hospital with a large mobile right heart thrombus in transit seen on transthoracic echocardiogram (TTE). He was successfully treated with anticoagulation alone. This case highlights the importance of TTE in establishing the diagnosis and describes the interplay of factors influencing treatment decision.

1. Introduction

Right heart thrombi (RHT) are rare manifestation of venous thromboembolism (VTE); their presence is considered a marker for higher clot burden and worse outcome [1–3]. Guidelines for management of VTE are well established [4]. But little is known about the optimum treatment strategy for RHT.

We present a case of right heart thrombi discovered on TTE emphasizing the utility of TTE in the setting of VTE. We aim also to describe the interplay of multiple clinical factors that may aid in treatment decision-making.

2. Case Presentation

An 81-year-old man presented with syncope 3 days after inguinal hernia repair. His past medical history was significant for a deep venous thrombosis that was diagnosed 2 months earlier. Electrocardiogram on presentation demonstrated sinus tachycardia with a S1Q3T3 pattern (Figure 1). Pulmonary embolism was suspected. Given a low creatinine clearance and a documented contrast allergy contrast CT angiography was not possible. As such, a transthoracic echocardiogram was performed demonstrating a dilated, hypokinetic right ventricle with preservation of apical contractile function (Supplemental Video in the Supplementary Material available online at http://dx.doi.org/10.1155/2015/375089) which has been reported to be consistent with a pulmonary embolism (McConnell's sign). Additionally a mobile serpiginous intracardiac mass straddling the tricuspid valve was present representing a thrombus in transit (Figures 2(a) and 2(b), Supplemental Video). Multiple bilateral large perfusion defects were observed in a ventilation perfusion scan confirming pulmonary emboli. Bilateral lower extremity deep venous thromboses were also present with leg Doppler evaluation. Fibrinolysis was contemplated given the presence of a large clot burden, right ventricular compromise, and presentation with syncope. However, given the increased bleeding risk due to age and renal dysfunction, conservative therapy with intense anticoagulation was initiated. During the course of therapy the patient experienced a brief episode of dyspnea and hypoxia presumed to be related to additional pulmonary embolism from the right heart thrombus given the fact that the thrombus visualized within the right heart initially was no longer present subsequent to this event. The patient remained hemodynamically stable with preserved

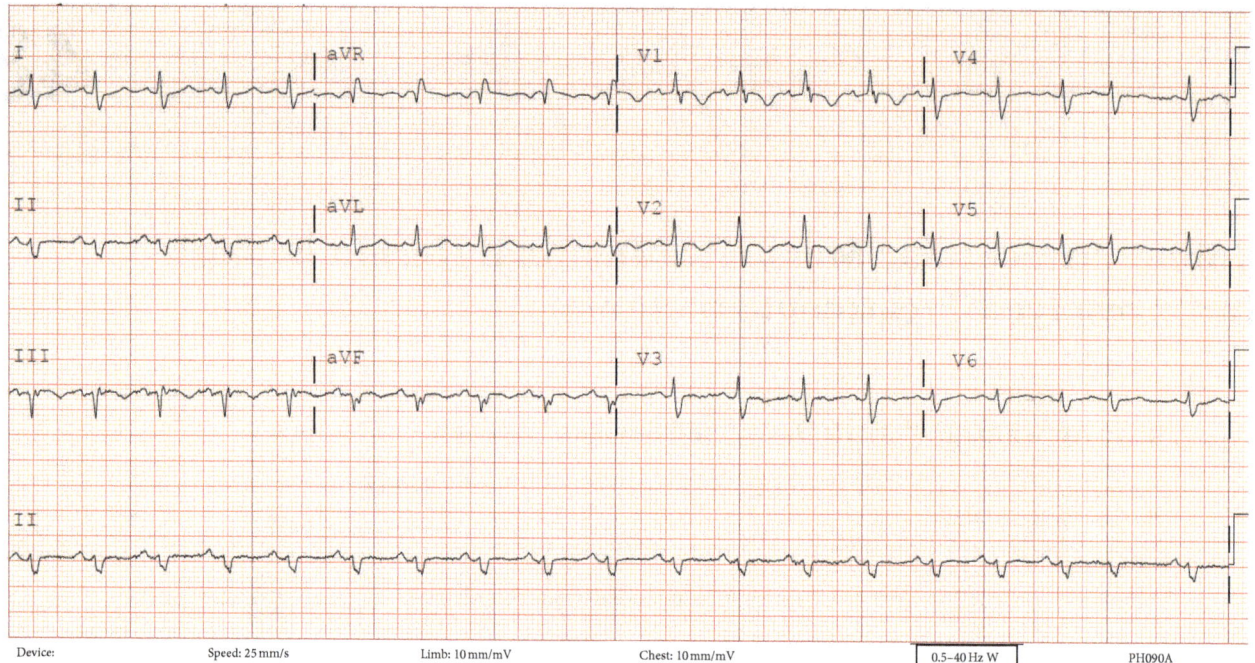

FIGURE 1: Electrocardiogram at presentation showing sinus tachycardia and S1Q3T3 pattern indicating right ventricular strain.

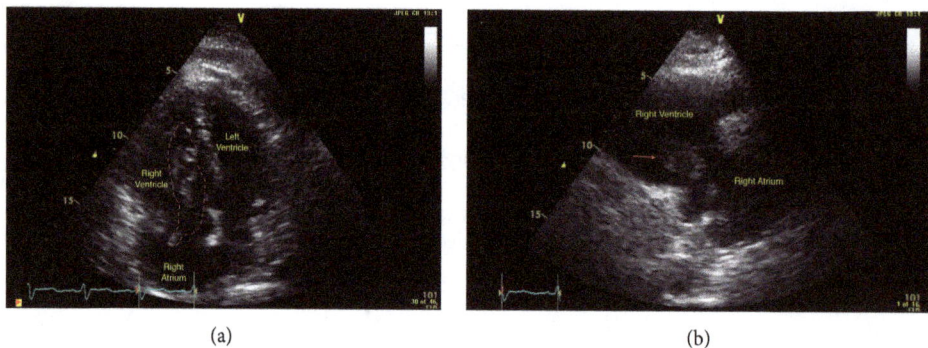

(a)

(b)

FIGURE 2: (a) An apical 4-chamber echocardiographic view of the heart showing the right heart thrombus protruding through the tricuspid valve. (b) A right ventricular inflow echocardiographic view of the heart showing the right heart thrombus protruding through the tricuspid valve.

oxygenation during his stay in the coronary care unit. He was subsequently discharged home.

3. Discussion

Right heart thrombi (RHT) can be one of many potential causes of a right heart mass including congenital structures (e.g., Chiari network, persistent Eustachian valve, and atrial septal aneurysm) and acquired causes (e.g., leads, vegetation, or tumors) [5, 6]. Clinical history and imaging will aid in diagnosis.

This case highlights the value of echocardiography with suspected pulmonary embolism. Although typical echocardiographic findings provide indirect evidence of pulmonary embolism, in the absence of prior cardiopulmonary disease these findings can be specific [7, 8]. Right heart thrombus (RHT) in transit has been reported in 4–10% of cases of

pulmonary embolism [9]. This finding confirms the diagnosis, indicates a higher clot burden, worse pulmonary hemodynamics, and functional class, and is associated with a 10-fold higher mortality than that of isolated pulmonary embolism [1–3].

Treatment of RHT represents a management dilemma, given the absence of clear consensus treatment guidelines. Indeed, the need for appropriate therapy is most evident by the high mortality observed in the first 24 hours and an overall mortality in untreated patients approaching 100% [3, 5].

Management strategies of varying risk have been proposed including pharmacological therapy with either intensive anticoagulation or thrombolysis and invasive therapy with either a catheter-based or surgical embolectomy. Comparative effectiveness studies evaluating these strategies have been limited by their small sample size and lack of randomization, both of which do not allow for a true understanding of the risks and benefits of each approach. For example, Finlayson described 38 cases of right heart thrombi where a similar and high (20–62%) in-hospital mortality was present regardless of the treatment modality used [5]. In contrast, Ryu et al. suggested that thrombolysis may have a mortality benefit over other therapeutic approaches with a mortality rate reported at 11% compared to 23% and 28% observed in patients treated with surgical embolectomy and anticoagulation, respectively [3].

Thrombolytic therapy has been advocated as the first treatment modality [1, 3, 5, 10–13] due to its widespread availability in clinical practice and its ability to hasten thrombus breakdown thereby lowering the overall thrombus burden and improve right and left ventricular hemodynamics [5, 10]. Successful thrombolysis has been reported with both slow and rapid infusion of Tissue Plasminogen Activator (tPA) [14]. Thrombolysis, however, does have the limitation of increased risk of bleeding, repeat embolization with subsequent sudden death, and chronic thromboembolic pulmonary hypertension [12, 15]. Surgical embolectomy has been advocated as a rescue therapy [12, 15, 16]. Surgery has its inherent risks including the need to transport to a more experienced facility, anesthesia risk, and the inability to clear distal pulmonary circulation emboli [15, 17]. Despite this, surgery may be the only option in a critically ill patient [18–20].

Catheter aspiration thrombectomy has also been used with success in few reported cases [17, 21]. This modality may only be feasible in few highly specialized centers. Even when it is available, gaining a safe access to the right atrium can be very challenging in the setting of VTE.

Anticoagulation is not advocated as a sole therapy [1, 3, 5, 22]. However, as demonstrated in the case, other clinical factors may prevent patients from receiving more aggressive therapy. As such, this approach may be the only one available to patients.

Given the limitations of each available therapy and lack of consensus on the management of patients with RHT, a personalized approach accounting for patient and institutional factors must be adopted for each patient.

Abbreviations

RHT: Right heart thrombi
VTE: Venous thromboembolism.

Conflict of Interests

The authors declare that there is no conflict of interests regarding the publication of this paper.

References

[1] V. Agarwal, N. Nalluri, M. A. Shariff et al., "Large embolus in transit—an unresolved therapeutic dilemma (case report and review of literature)," *Heart & Lung: The Journal of Critical Care*, vol. 43, no. 2, pp. 152–154, 2014.

[2] F. Casazza, C. Becattini, E. Guglielmelli et al., "Prognostic significance of free-floating right heart thromboemboli in acute pulmonary embolism: results from the Italian pulmonary embolism registry," *Thrombosis and Haemostasis*, vol. 111, no. 1, pp. 53–57, 2014.

[3] P. S. Rose, N. M. Punjabi, and D. B. Pearse, "Treatment of right heart thromboemboli," *Chest*, vol. 121, no. 3, pp. 806–814, 2002.

[4] C. Kearon, E. A. Akl, A. J. Comerota et al., "Antithrombotic therapy for VTE disease: Antithrombotic Therapy and Prevention of Thrombosis, 9th ed: American College of Chest Physicians Evidence-Based Clinical Practice Guidelines," *Chest*, vol. 141, pp. e419S–e494S, 2012.

[5] L. Chartier, J. Béra, M. Delomez et al., "Free-floating thrombi in the right heart: diagnosis, management, and prognostic indexes in 38 consecutive patients," *Circulation*, vol. 99, no. 21, pp. 2779–2783, 1999.

[6] S. Demirkol, F. G. Yesil, U. Bozlar, M. Unlu, S. Balta, and M. A. Sahin, "Multimodality imaging of a right atrial thrombus obliterating inferior vena cava," *Echocardiography*, vol. 30, no. 5, pp. E145–E147, 2013.

[7] J. H. Ryu, P. A. Pellikka, D. A. Froehling, S. G. Peters, and G. L. Aughenbaugh, "Saddle pulmonary embolism diagnosed by CT angiography: frequency, clinical features and outcome," *Respiratory Medicine*, vol. 101, no. 7, pp. 1537–1542, 2007.

[8] R. P. Sosland and K. Gupta, "Images in cardiovascular medicine: McConnell's sign," *Circulation*, vol. 118, no. 15, pp. e517–e518, 2008.

[9] G. N. Finlayson, "Right heart thrombi: consider the cause," *The Canadian Journal of Cardiology*, vol. 24, article 888, 2008.

[10] R. K. Shankarappa, R. S. Math, S. Papaiah, Y. M. Channabasappa, S. Karur, and M. C. Nanjappa, "Free floating right atrial thrombus with massive pulmonary embolism: near catastrophic course following thrombolytic therapy," *Indian Heart Journal*, vol. 65, no. 4, pp. 460–463, 2013.

[11] Y. Kato, Y. Fukuda, S.-I. Miura, and K. Saku, "Right heart thrombosis with pulmonary embolism," *Internal Medicine*, vol. 52, no. 15, pp. 1745–1746, 2013.

[12] Y. P. Yoo and K.-W. Kang, "Successful embolectomy of a migrated thrombolytic free-floating massive thrombus resulting in a pulmonary thromboembolism," *Journal of Cardiovascular Ultrasound*, vol. 21, no. 1, pp. 37–39, 2013.

[13] Ö. Şatiroğlu, M. Durakoğlugil, Y. Uğurlu et al., "Successful thrombolysis using recombinant tissue plasminogen activator in cases of severe pulmonary embolism with mobile thrombi in the right atrium," *Interventional Medicine & Applied Science*, vol. 6, no. 2, pp. 89–92, 2014.

[14] R. Arsanjani, S. Goldman, M. P. Habib, and M. R. Movahed, "Modified thrombolytic therapy for massive pulmonary emboli," *The American Journal of Medicine*, vol. 124, no. 8, pp. e7–e8, 2011.

[15] K. Hisatomi, T. Yamada, and D. Onohara, "Surgical embolectomy of a floating right heart thrombus and acute massive pulmonary embolism: report of a case," *Annals of Thoracic and Cardiovascular Surgery*, vol. 19, no. 4, pp. 316–319, 2013.

[16] G. M. Lohrmann, F. Peters, S. van Riet, and M. R. Essop, "Double trouble—a case report of mobile right atrial thrombus in the setting of acute pulmonary thromboembolism," *Heart, Lung & Circulation*, vol. 23, no. 10, pp. e214–e216, 2014.

[17] T. Momose, T. Morita, and T. Misawa, "Percutaneous treatment of a free-floating thrombus in the right atrium of a patient with pulmonary embolism and acute myocarditis," *Cardiovascular Intervention and Therapeutics*, vol. 28, no. 2, pp. 188–192, 2013.

[18] R. Yuan, "Neither here nor there: impending paradoxical embolism," *The American Journal of Medicine*, vol. 127, no. 12, pp. 1169–1171, 2014.

[19] A. Kessel-Schaefer, M. Lefkovits, M. J. Zellweger et al., "Migrating thrombus trapped in a patent foramen ovale," *Circulation*, vol. 103, no. 14, article 1928, 2001.

[20] T. Theologou, P. Tewari, K. Pointon, and I. M. Mitchell, "Pulmonary thromboembolism with floating thrombus trapped in patent foramen ovale," *Annals of Thoracic Surgery*, vol. 84, no. 6, pp. 2104–2106, 2007.

[21] J. Mukharji and J. E. Peterson, "Percutaneous removal of a large mobile right atrial thrombus using a basket retrieval device," *Catheterization and Cardiovascular Interventions*, vol. 51, no. 4, pp. 479–482, 2000.

[22] H. Akilli, E. E. Gül, A. Aribaş, K. Özdemir, M. Kayrak, and H. I. Erdogan, "Management of right heart thrombi associated with acute pulmonary embolism: a retrospective, single-center experience," *Anadolu Kardiyoloji Dergisi*, vol. 13, no. 6, pp. 528–533, 2013.

49

Constrictive Pericarditis: A Challenging Diagnosis in Paediatrics

Mariana Faustino,[1] Inês Carmo Mendes,[2] and Rui Anjos[2]

[1]*Cardiology Department, Hospital Fernando Fonseca, IC 19, Amadora, 2720-276 Lisbon, Portugal*
[2]*Pediatric Cardiology Department, Hospital de Santa Cruz, Avenida Professor Reinaldo dos Santos, Carnaxide, 2790-134 Lisbon, Portugal*

Correspondence should be addressed to Mariana Faustino; marianafaustino85@gmail.com

Academic Editor: Ramazan Akdemir

Constrictive pericarditis is an uncommon disease in children, usually difficult to diagnose. We present the case of a 14-year-old boy with a previous history of tuberculosis and right heart failure, in whom constrictive pericarditis was diagnosed. The case highlights the need to integrate all information, including clinical data, noninvasive cardiac imaging, and even invasive hemodynamic evaluation when required, in order to establish the correct diagnosis and proceed to surgical treatment.

1. Introduction

Constrictive pericarditis is characterized by the appearance of signs and symptoms of right heart failure due to loss of pericardial compliance and restricting diastolic filling [1]. It results from a chronic inflammatory process involving the parietal and visceral pericardial layers [2]. Idiopathic pericarditis, cardiac surgery, and radiotherapy are the most common causes in developed countries. Incomplete drainage of purulent pericarditis is a rare entity that should also be considered, but tuberculosis is still the most prevalent cause in developing countries, particularly in paediatric population [3, 4].

Constrictive pericarditis is not common in children and therefore not readily recalled, and the clinical picture often seems unrelated to the heart, so it sometimes may represent a diagnosis challenge [5].

2. Case Presentation

We present the case of a 14-year-old boy, born and resident in Angola. At 7 years of age he had fatigue, cough, fever, and no weight progression.

At 11 years of age pulmonary tuberculosis was diagnosed, confirmed in sputum cultures. He received quadruple antituberculosis therapy for 6 months. As heart failure symptoms and signs arose, with systemic and pulmonary congestion, the child was started on diuretics and evacuated to a Pediatric Cardiology Department in Portugal. The clinical examination revealed weight and height below the 3rd percentile, blood pressure and heart rate within normal limits, mild tachypnea, pulmonary auscultation with decreased sounds at the right inferior third and left basal crackles, and nonpulsatile hepatomegaly and ascites; jugular venous pulse was congestive until mandible angle; however the M-shaped pattern (prominent x and y descendants) was not evident. No kussmaul sign was present. No heart murmurs, pericardial rub, or pericardial knock was documented.

A chest radiography showed mild cardiac dilation and bilateral pulmonary effusion, predominantly in the right hemithorax (Figure 1). Electrocardiogram showed low voltage QRS in frontal leads compatible with effusion and/or constriction process (Figure 2). Laboratory tests revealed mild hypoalbuminemia (2.9 mg/dL), with normal liver enzymes; serum inflammatory markers were negative. Viral and autoimmune investigation was also negative.

Echocardiography showed significant enlargement of the right atria, inferior vena cava, and suprahepatic veins (Figures 3(a) and 3(b), clip 1 in Supplementary Material available online at http://dx.doi.org/10.1155/2015/402740); right ventricular systolic pressure and function were normal; Left ventricle function and volumes were normal. There was no

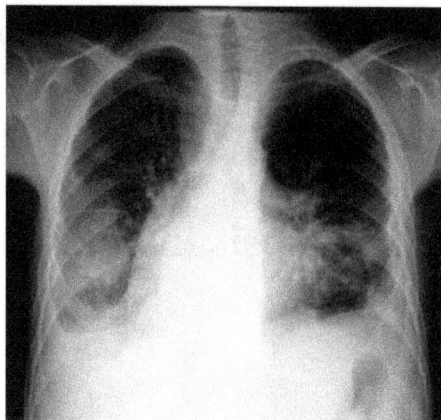

FIGURE 1: Posteroanterior chest radiography: mild cardiac dilation and bilateral pulmonary effusion, predominantly in the right hemithorax.

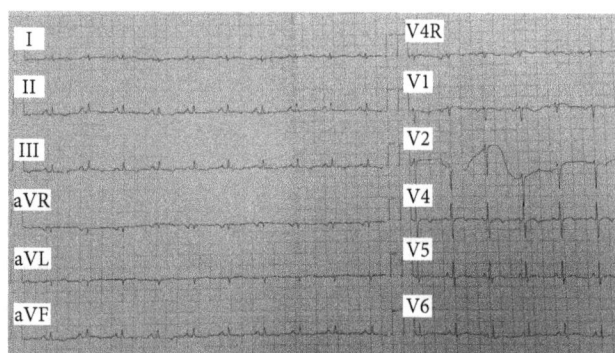

FIGURE 2: Twelve-lead electrocardiogram: heart rate of 90 beats/min; low voltage QRS in frontal leads; nonspecific alterations of ventricular repolarization.

pericardial effusion, but signs of ventricular interaction were found, septal bounce and significant respiratory variation in transvalvular flow (transmitral flow increasing by 50% during expiration) (Figure 3(c)). Unfortunately, hepatic vein respiratory variation was not possible to adequately assess. Dilatation of the right chambers and the flow pattern through the atrio-ventricular valves, in the absence of pulmonary hypertension, nor systolic left ventricle dysfunction, suggested pericardial constriction. Protodiastolic mitral annulus velocity was preserved (E' = 14 cm/s), and the ratio E/E' was low (annulus paradoxus). Septal E' velocity was higher than medial E' velocity (annulus reversus). This findings were also suggestive of pericardial disease, and not restrictive cardiomyopathy (Figure 3(d)).

In the presence of this clinical history and physical examination, authors suspected constrictive pericarditis. Echocardiography parameters were also suggestive of constrictive physiology but however considered not enough to establish the diagnosis. For confirmation, magnetic resonance was performed. As the patient was uncooperative only anatomic imaging was performed, and constrictive physiology was not demonstrated.

In spite of a high clinical and echocardiographic suspicion, in order to confirm the diagnosis, before proposing a surgery with no negligible risks, cardiac catheterization was performed (Figure 4). Several parameters were suggestive of constriction: elevated and equalized telediastolic pressures in both ventricles; telediastolic pressure in right ventricle (20 mmHg) higher than one-third of its systolic pressure (42 mmHg); increased mean right atrial pressure (17 mmHg); systolic area index of 1.29, suggesting ventricular interdependence. The ventricular filling pattern was suggestive of the classic square root sign (dip and plateau).

Patient was referred for pericardiectomy. Pericardium was thickened and adherent, not calcified, and it was excised from phrenic to phrenic nerve (Figure 5). There was an immediate decrease in right atria mean pressure (25 to 12 mmHg). Pathologic study of the surgical specimen revealed extensive fibrosis without active inflammation, compatible with chronic fibrous constrictive pericarditis. We assume that Tuberculosis was the cause of the constrictive pericarditis. The postoperative period was uneventful, with fast and complete regression of all signs of heart failure.

3. Discussion

The long lasting symptoms of this patient were very likely related to tuberculosis, which progressed with pericardial involvement and constriction, not reversible with antituberculosis therapy.

Although constrictive pericarditis is rare in children, it should be considered in the differential diagnosis of right heart failure. It is possible that this low incidence in children is due, in part, to subdiagnosis and also to the insidious character of this disease and its complications [5].

A high index of suspicion is necessary to establish the diagnosis of constrictive pericarditis [5]. It is necessary to integrate clinical evaluation with data from the several available methods and to have a critical approach position when eventual discrepancy arises.

Transthoracic echocardiography is usually the first diagnostic investigation performed for suspected constrictive pericarditis and can be very useful in the presence of the typical findings: septal bounce, dynamic respiratory variation in flow (transtricuspid, transmitral, and hepatic vein), and enhanced ventricular interaction [3]. In this way echocardiography has an important role in the differential diagnosis of constrictive pericarditis with other causes of heart failure, namely, restrictive cardiomyopathy, the most challenging entity to differentiate from constrictive pericarditis [1, 6]. However echocardiography might not be confirmatory in all cases, since some of these typical findings may not be present [5].

Cardiac magnetic resonance, despite being the imaging method of choice to evaluate the pericardium, was not useful and potentially confounding in this patient. Contrast enhanced CT angiography, being also a noninvasive investigation, is more tolerable and easier to perform in children than cardiac magnetic resonance and could have been a better

(a)

(b)

(c)

(d)

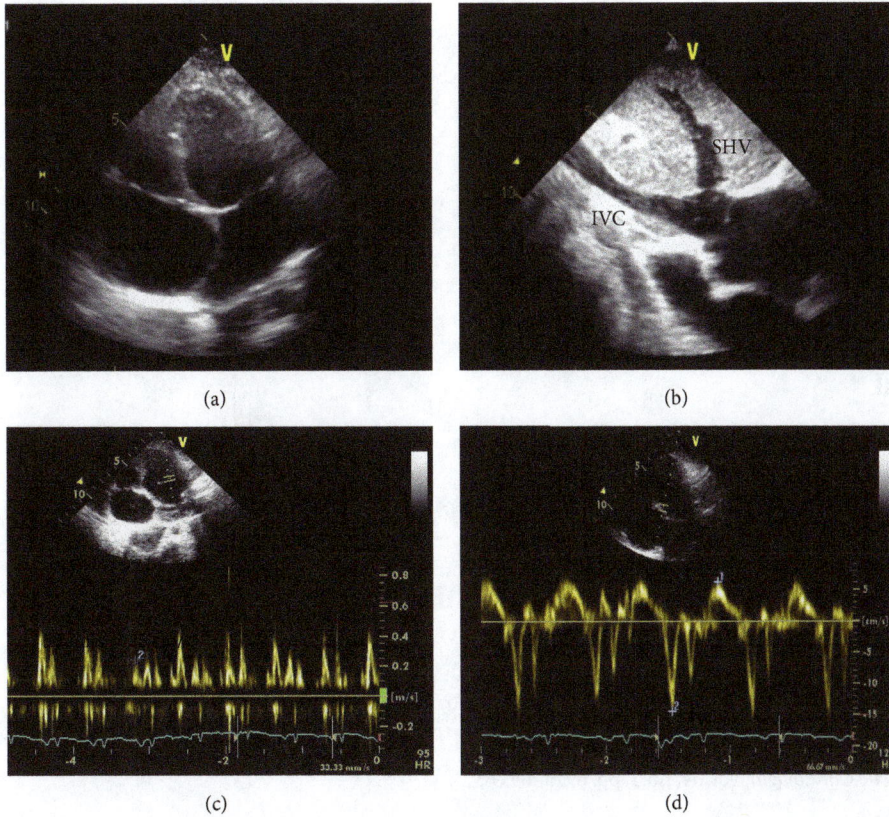

FIGURE 3: (a) Apical 4-chamber view with dilated right atria (RA), left deviated atrial septum; (b) subcostal view of dilated inferior vena cava (IVC) and suprahepatic veins (SHV); (c) significant (50%) transmitral flow variation with breathing, increasing during expiration (∗) and decreasing during inspiration (+); (d) high protodiastolic mitral annulus velocity (septal 14 cm/s, higher than lateral).

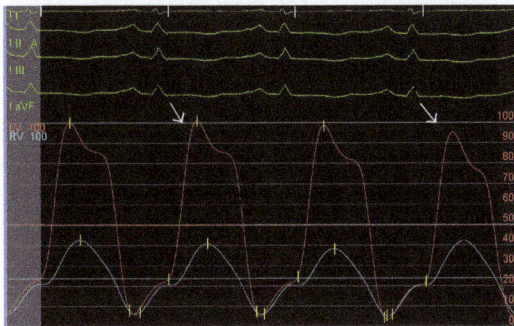

FIGURE 4: Elevated and equalized telediastolic pressure in ventricles (20 mmHg, arrow head); systolic area index calculated as the ratio between right ventricle/left ventricle systolic area in inspiration and right ventricle/left ventricle systolic area in expiration: $(114/473)/(107/572) = 1.29$.

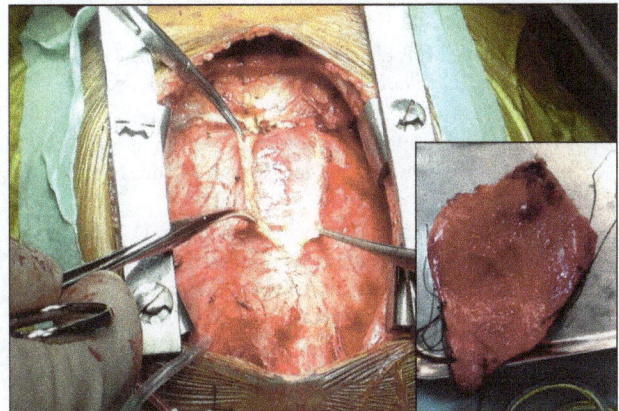

FIGURE 5: Thickened and adherent pericardium during and immediately after pericardiectomy.

option for this patient. It is useful to identify pericardial thickness and effusion, to detect enlargement of the mediastinal lymph nodes, and to evaluate lung parenchyma, which may be important in patients suspected to have tuberculosis [3].

Cardiovascular catheterization, although an invasive method and not always necessary, is the gold standard for the diagnosis of constriction and was crucial to confirm the diagnosis. A recent described criteria is the systolic area index, ratio of right ventricle to left ventricle systolic area during inspiration and expiration, that predicts ventricular interdependence with 97% sensitivity and 100% positive predictive power, when higher than 1.1 [7].

The case highlights the need to integrate all information, including clinical data, electrocardiography, chest radiography, cardiac imaging data, and even invasive hemodynamic evaluation. Cardiac catheterization is usually reserved for patients in whom there is significant diagnostic doubt after noninvasive evaluation, since the confirmation of the diagnosis is decisive for the therapeutic approach, in order to ensure that the expected benefit outweighs the potential risk.

A correct and early diagnosis of constrictive pericarditis is extremely important, since successful pericardiectomy can be curative [3]. In advanced disease, surgery results are suboptimal and mortality is higher, which is also related to poor preoperative general condition and advanced preoperative NYHA class [3].

Ethical Approval

The identity of the patient was absolutely preserved.

Conflict of Interests

The authors declare that there is no conflict of interests regarding the publication of this paper.

References

[1] L. Marta, M. Alves, M. Peres et al., "Effusive-constrictive pericarditis as the manifestation of an unexpected diagnosis," *Revista Portuguesa de Cardiologia*, vol. 34, no. 1, pp. 69.e1–69.e6, 2015.

[2] S. M. A. G. Ferreira, A. G. Ferreira Jr., A. do Nascimento Morais, W. S. Paz, and F. A. A. Silveira, "Constrictive chronic pericarditis in children," *Cardiology in the Young*, vol. 11, no. 2, pp. 210–213, 2001.

[3] S. Talwar, V. V. Nair, S. K. Choudhary et al., "Pericardiectomy in children <15 years of age," *Cardiology in the Young*, vol. 24, no. 4, pp. 616–622, 2014.

[4] P. P. Sengupta, M. F. Eleid, and B. K. Khandheria, "Constrictive pericarditis," *Circulation Journal*, vol. 72, no. 10, pp. 1555–1562, 2008.

[5] J. Guitti, "Constrictive pericarditis in a 19-month-old child," *Arquivos Brasileiros de Cardiologia*, vol. 74, no. 1, pp. 47–54, 2000.

[6] D. Silva, L. Sargento, M. Gato Varela, M. Lopes, D. Brito, and H. Madeira, "Pericardite constritiva—constrictive pericarditis—new methods in the diagnosis of an old disease: a case report," *Revista Portuguesa de Cardiologia*, vol. 31, pp. 677–682, 2012.

[7] D. R. Talreja, R. A. Nishimura, J. K. Oh, and D. R. Holmes, "Constrictive pericarditis in the modern era. Novel criteria for diagnosis in the cardiac catheterization laboratory," *Journal of the American College of Cardiology*, vol. 51, no. 3, pp. 315–319, 2008.

50

A Practical Method for No-Reflow Treatment

Mustafa Cetin,[1] Emrullah Kiziltunc,[1] Zehra Güven Cetin,[2] Harun Kundi,[1] Birsen Gulkan,[1] and Hülya Cicekcioglu[1]

[1]Cardiology Department, Numune Education and Research Hospital, Cardiology Department, 06100 Ankara, Turkey
[2]Cardiology Department, Dr. Nafiz Korez State Hospital, 06100 Ankara, Turkey

Correspondence should be addressed to Emrullah Kiziltunc; e.kiziltunc@gmail.com

Academic Editor: Manabu Shirotani

No-reflow is an undesirable result of percutaneous coronary interventions. Vasoactive drug administration at the distal part of the coronary artery is suggested as a therapeutic option for no-reflow treatment. Here, we represent two cases of successful no-reflow management with previously used monorail balloon at the same procedure as a hand-made distal infusion catheter.

1. Introduction

No-reflow is an undesirable result of percutaneous coronary interventions (PCI) [1]. Intracoronary (IC) vasodilators such as verapamil, nitroprusside, or adenosine are being administered for the treatment of no-reflow via the guiding catheter [2], but sometimes distal flow restoration is not satisfactory especially in patients with TIMI 0 flow. Vasoactive drug administration at the distal part of the coronary artery is suggested as a treatment option for no-reflow and some distal infusion catheters [3] and over-the-wire (OTW) balloon catheters [4] are being used for this purpose. However, OTW catheters need long guide wires and changing a short wire with a long wire has the risk of wire loss. Distal infusion catheters are special catheters for drug infusion at various vascular sites, but these catheters are not always available. Monorail balloon catheters are the most widely used catheters in routine clinical practice. Here, we describe two cases of successful no-reflow management by previously used monorail balloon at the same procedure as a hand-made distal infusion catheter.

2. Case 1

A 50-year-old male patient was taken to catheterization laboratory at the third hour of his pain with the diagnosis of acute posterolateral myocardial infarction (MI). The patient was pretreated with acetylsalicylic acid 300 mg, prasugrel 60 mg, and unfractionated heparin 100 mg/kg. Infarct related artery was first obtuse marginalis (OM) (Figure 1(a)). Total occlusion was crossed with a 0.014 inch floppy wire and the lesion was predilated with a 2.5/20 mm monorail balloon at 12 atm pressure. Control angiography revealed a thrombus shift to circumflex artery (Cx) which ceased the distal flow (Figure 1(b)). The occlusion was crossed with a second 0.014-inch floppy wire and the occlusion site was dilated with a 1.5/20 mm monorail balloon at 16 atm pressure (Figure 1(c)). After balloon angioplasty no-reflow developed. Intracoronary adenosine (250 mcg) was administered, but distal flow could not be restored (Figure 1(d)). Therefore we decided to give adenosine at the distal part of Cx and the previously used 1.5/20 mm monorail balloon was retrieved and perforated with a needle at four different sites. The perforated balloon was flushed from the hub with adenosine solution (1 cc/100 mcg) and bubbles were removed (Figures 2(a) and 2(b)). Then it was inserted to the distal part of the Cx and 250 mcg adenosine was injected via the balloon. Control angiography revealed TIMI 3 flow (Figure 1(e)). First OM was stented with a 3.5/12 mm bare metal stent and the procedure was terminated without any other complication.

3. Case 2

An 87-year-old female patient admitted with acute inferior MI and complete AV block at the thirteenth hour of her symptoms. The patient was taken to catheterization laboratory for primary PCI. She was pretreated with acetylsalicylic acid 300 mg, ticagrelor 180 mg, and 85 mg/kg unfractionated

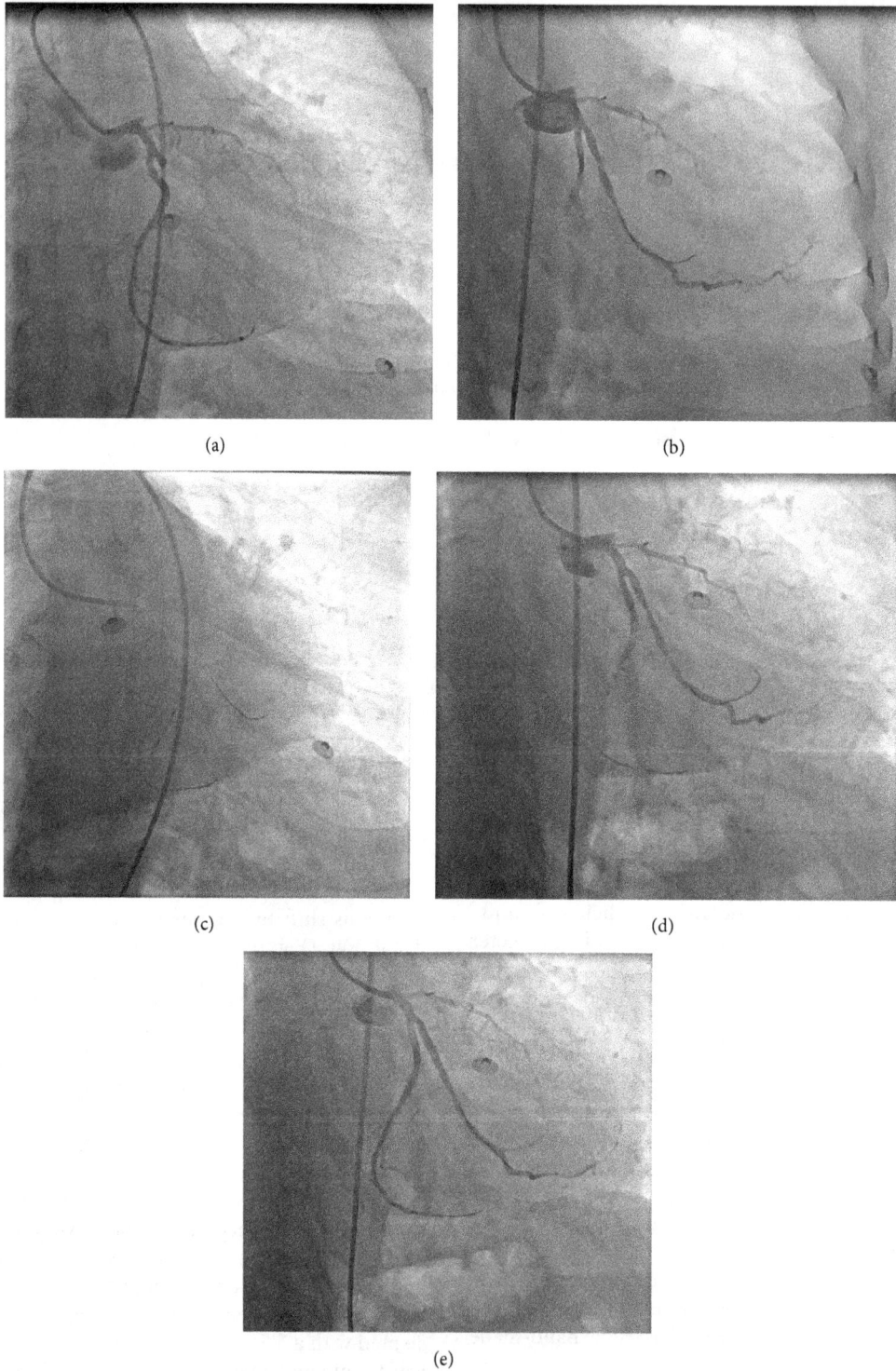

FIGURE 1: (a) The first angiogram of the patient. (b) After balloon dilatation to the first OM, Cx midportion was totally occluded due to thrombus shift. (c) A 1.5/20 mm monorail balloon was dilated at the Cx occlusion. (d) No-reflow developed. (e) 1.5/20 mm monorail balloon was perforated and was inserted to the distal part of the Cx; afterwards 250 mcg adenosine was injected via the balloon. Successful distal flow was restored. OM: obtuse marginalis, Cx: circumflex artery.

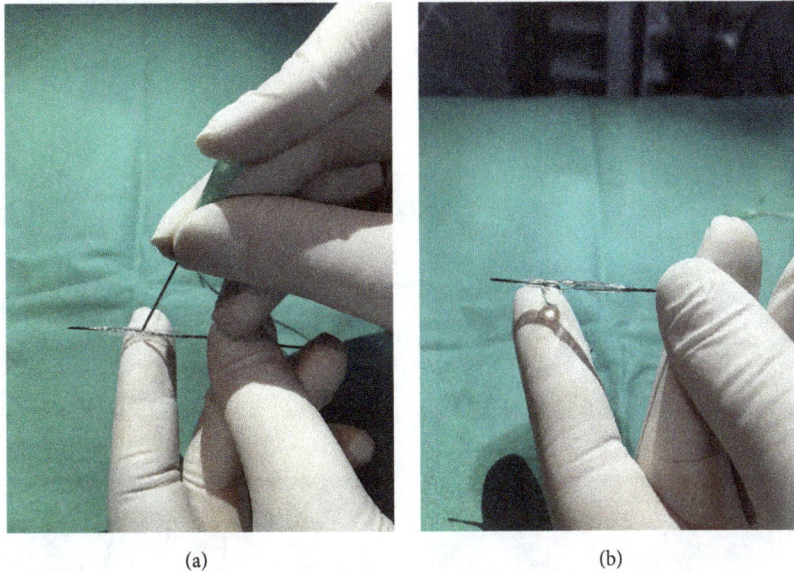

FIGURE 2: Preparation of balloon before distal infusion. (a) First the balloon is filled with saline and perforated with a needle from perpendicular four different sites. It is important to not cross the opposite layer of the balloon. (b) The perforated balloon is flushed from the hub with adenosine solution and the bubbles are removed.

heparin. Right coronary artery (RCA) was totally occluded at the midportion. A 0.014-inch floppy wire was inserted to the distal part of the RCA. The lesion was predilated with 1.20/12 mm and 3.0/15 mm monorail balloons, respectively, and a 3.0/18 mm drug eluting stent was implanted at 16 atm (Figure 3(a)). No-reflow developed after stent deployment. We administered 250 mcg adenosine via the guiding catheter but could not achieve any distal flow (Figure 3(b)). Afterwards, previously used 1.20/12 mm monorail balloon was perforated and flushed with adenosine solution (1 cc/100 mcg) and bubbles were removed. Then it was inserted to the distal part of the RCA and 250 mcg adenosine was injected via the balloon (Figure 3(c)). TIMI 3 flow was restored (Figure 3(d)).

4. Discussion

No-reflow increases mortality and hospital stay in acute MI patients [5]. Distal microembolisation, endothelial dysfunction, and reperfusion injury (by increasing the microvascular resistance) are the proposed mechanisms of no-reflow [6]. Antiplatelet agents, thrombus aspiration, distal embolic protection devices, and vasodilator drugs can be used for prevention and treatment of no-reflow [7]. IC vasodilator administration through the guiding catheter is frequently performed to resolve no-reflow. But it is obvious that administered vasodilator agents cannot penetrate to the coronary microcirculation especially in patients with TIMI 0 flow because there is no blood flow at the distal part of the vessel during no-reflow period. In addition, when vasodilator drug is administered by the guiding catheter, it penetrates to other coronary territories and the vasodilator drug concentration dilutes.

Administration of the vasodilator drugs at the distal part of the coronary can deal with these problems and vasoactive drug utility can be increased at the distal part of the coronary artery. OTW balloon catheters [8] and distal infusion

catheters [9, 10] have been using for this purpose and positive results were reported with distal vasodilator drug injection. However these two types of catheters have some disadvantages. Distal infusion catheters (like ClearWay, Atrium Medical Corporation, Hudson, NH, USA/multifunction probing catheter, Boston Scientific Corporation, Boston, MA) are suitable for drug administration at the distal part of coronary artery, but these catheters are not routinely found in most of the laboratories. OTW balloons are not the first choices in daily practice and need a long guidewire. Wire exchange for OTW balloon usage has the risk of wire loss and failure of rewiring, a very annoying situation for the operator. Monorail balloons are frequently used in daily practice. They are easily retrievable and they can be used with short guidewires. Here, we described successful usage of a monorail balloon for distal vasodilator drug infusion. There may be some safety concerns about inserting a perforated balloon to the distal part of the coronary and drug infusion through this balloon, but we did not encounter any complication with this method and reached successful results. Flushing the perforated balloon from the hub takes away the risk of air bubble embolism. Perforating the balloon form multiple sites reduces the risk of coronary dissection due to saline flow because injected saline's pressure is reduced by multiple holes. In addition, this method does not impose an additional cost to the procedure. Health expenditure is very important all around the world. We think that distal drug infusion with this method is safe and effective at least like other catheters; therefore using a new catheter and rising the cost of the procedure are unnecessary. In conclusion, perforation of a monorail balloon with a needle and using as a distal infusion catheter can be used for no-reflow treatment. We achieved favorable results with this off-label usage. This method is always available, easy, and safe and has no additional cost.

(a)

(b)

(c)

(d)

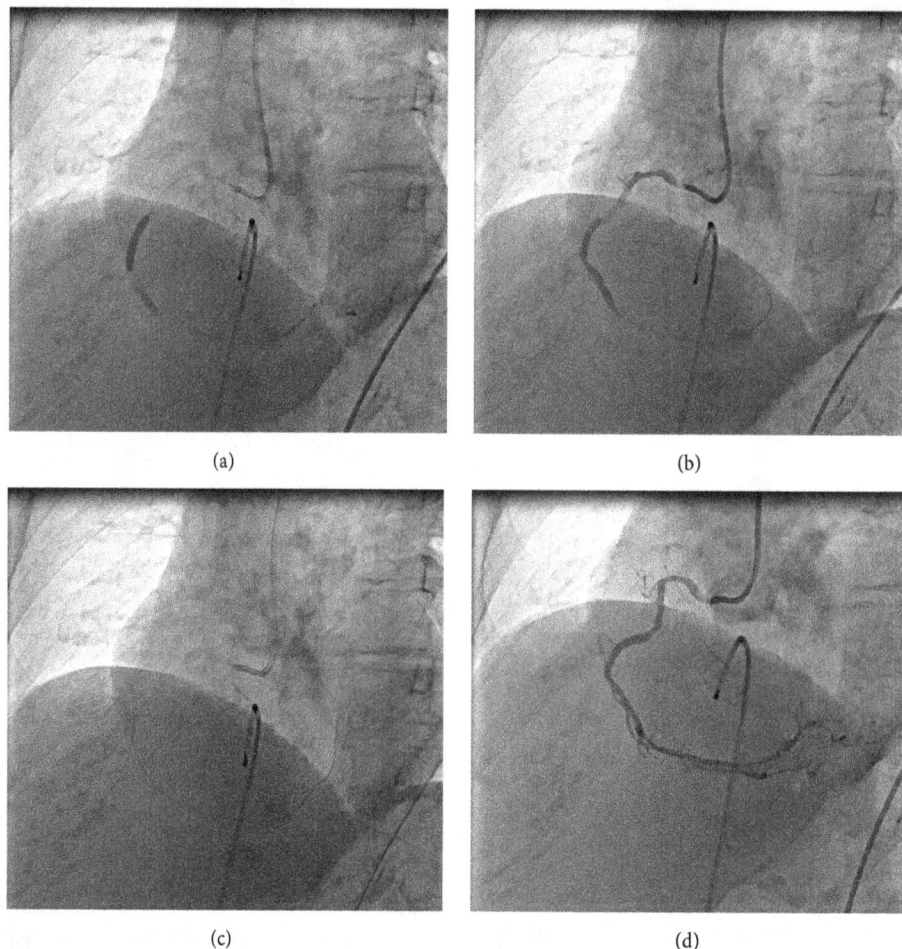

FIGURE 3: (a) 3.0/18 mm drug eluting stent deployment. (b) After stent deployment no-reflow developed. (c) 250 mcg adenosine was injected via the previously used perforated 1.20/12 mm monorail balloon to the distal part of the RCA. (d) TIMI 3 distal flow was restored. RCA: right coronary artery, TIMI: thrombolysis in myocardial infarction.

Conflict of Interests

The authors declare that there is no conflict of interests regarding the publication of this paper.

References

[1] G. Ndrepepa, K. Tiroch, M. Fusaro et al., "5-year prognostic value of no-reflow phenomenon after percutaneous coronary intervention in patients with acute myocardial infarction," *Journal of the American College of Cardiology*, vol. 55, no. 21, pp. 2383–2389, 2010.

[2] A. Q. Guo, L. Sheng, X. Lei, and W. Shu, "Pharmacological and physical prevention and treatment of no-reflow after primary percutaneous coronary intervention in ST-segment elevation myocardial infarction," *Journal of International Medical Research*, vol. 41, no. 3, pp. 537–547, 2013.

[3] W. Wilson and D. Eccleston, "How to manage no reflow phenomenon with local drug delivery via a rapid exchange catheter," *Catheterization and Cardiovascular Interventions*, vol. 77, no. 2, pp. 217–219, 2011.

[4] M.-R. Movahed and G. Baweja, "Distal administration of very high doses of intracoronary adenosine for the treatment of resistant no-reflow," *Experimental and Clinical Cardiology*, vol. 13, no. 3, pp. 141–143, 2008.

[5] F. S. Resnic, M. Wainstein, M. K. Y. Lee et al., "No-reflow is an independent predictor of death and myocardial infarction after percutaneous coronary intervention," *American Heart Journal*, vol. 145, no. 1, pp. 42–46, 2003.

[6] G. Galasso, S. Schiekofer, C. D'Anna et al., "No-reflow phenomenon: pathophysiology, diagnosis, prevention, and treatment. A review of the current literature and future perspectives," *Angiology*, vol. 65, no. 3, pp. 180–189, 2014.

[7] R. Jaffe, A. Dick, and B. H. Strauss, "Prevention and treatment of microvascular obstruction-related myocardial injury and coronary no-reflow following percutaneous coronary intervention: a systematic approach," *JACC: Cardiovascular Interventions*, vol. 3, no. 7, pp. 695–704, 2010.

[8] M. Marzilli, E. Orsini, P. Marraccini, and R. Testa, "Beneficial effects of intracoronary adenosine as an adjunct to primary angioplasty in acute myocardial infarction," *Circulation*, vol. 101, no. 18, pp. 2154–2159, 2000.

[9] G. Amit, C. Cafri, S. Yaroslavtsev et al., "Intracoronary nitro-prusside for the prevention of the no-reflow phenomenon after primary percutaneous coronary intervention in acute myocardial infarction. A randomized, double-blind, placebo-controlled clinical trial," *American Heart Journal*, vol. 152, no. 5, pp. 887.e9–887.e14, 2006.

[10] G. Maluenda, I. Ben-Dor, C. Delhaye et al., "Clinical experience with a novel intracoronary perfusion catheter to treat no-reflow phenomenon in acute coronary syndromes," *Journal of Interventional Cardiology*, vol. 23, no. 2, pp. 109–113, 2010.

51

Stenting of Variant Left Carotid Artery Using Brachial Artery Approach in a Patient with Unusual Type of Bovine Aortic Arch

Emre Gürel,[1] Zeki Yüksel Günaydın,[2] Ahmet Karagöz,[3] Osman Bektaş,[2] Adil Bayramoğlu,[2] Abdullah Çelik,[4] and Aslı Vural[3]

[1]*Department of Cardiology, Ordu State Hospital, 52200 Ordu, Turkey*
[2]*Department of Cardiology, Ordu University Hospital, 52200 Ordu, Turkey*
[3]*Department of Cardiology, Giresun University Hospital, 28200 Giresun, Turkey*
[4]*Department of Cardiovascular Surgery, Giresun University Hospital, 28200 Giresun, Turkey*

Correspondence should be addressed to Ahmet Karagöz; drahmetkgz@hotmail.com

Academic Editor: Kuan-Rau Chiou

Bovine aortic arch is the most frequently encountered variation in human aortic arch branching. A 63-year-old Asian male presented with symptomatic severe stenosis of left carotid artery originating from the brachiocephalic trunk. Selective engagement to the left carotid artery was unsuccessful using transfemoral approach. We reported on a successful left carotid artery stenting case using right brachial artery approach in a bovine aortic arch. This paper is worthy of reporting in terms of guiding physicians for interventional procedures in these types of challenging cases.

1. Introduction

"Bovine aortic arch" refers to the most common variant of aortic arch branching in humans. This configuration can be found in approximately 27% of the population and can be further divided into 2 subtypes. In the less usual subtype (7%), the left common carotid artery (CCA) originates directly from the innominate artery, while the more usual subtype can be described as the common origin of the innominate artery and the left CCA and can be found in approximately 20% of the population [1]. However, the actual bovine arch pattern, found in cattle, is different and has no resemblance to any of the above described human aortic arch patterns. A single great vessel originates from the aortic arch which gives two subclavians for either side and a bicarotid trunk. The bicarotid trunk then divides into the left and right CCA [2].

In these anatomic variants, selective cannulation of the left CCA is often technically difficult from the transfemoral approach. We report on a successful left carotid stenting case using right brachial artery approach in a patient with "bovine aortic arch."

2. Case Presentation

A 63-year-old Asian male with hypertension was admitted due to recent attacks of transient right upper extremity weakness and numbness, lasting 3 to 5 min. On admission, his blood pressure was high at 170/90 mmHg and heart rate was 80 beats/min. Neurologic examination was normal. Doppler ultrasound examination showed normal right internal carotid artery velocities (0.92 m/s of peak systolic velocity) and elevated velocities in the left internal carotid artery (2.79 m/s of peak systolic velocity) suggesting critical stenosis. Six months before this admission, he had undergone arch aortography at an outside institution using a femoral artery approach, which confirmed critical stenosis in the proximal right internal carotid artery (ICA), variant origin of the left CCA from the proximal brachiocephalic trunk, and also critical stenosis in the proximal left ICA (Figure 1). After selective cannulation of right CCA, successful carotid stent placement had been performed with distal protection at the bifurcation level (Figure 2). Left carotid stenosis had not been stented at that time. Because of the right sided transient

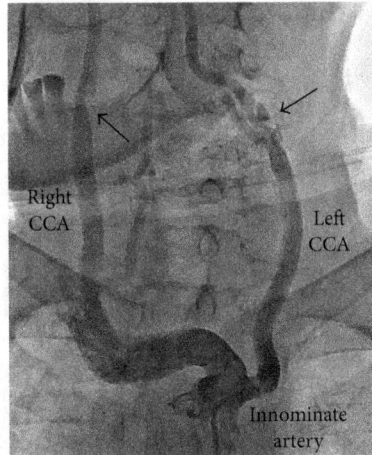

FIGURE 1: Aortic arch angiogram revealed critical stenosis in the proximal right internal carotid artery (black arrow), variant origin of the left common carotid artery from the innominate artery, and also critical stenosis in the proximal left internal carotid artery (black arrow) (CCA: common carotid artery).

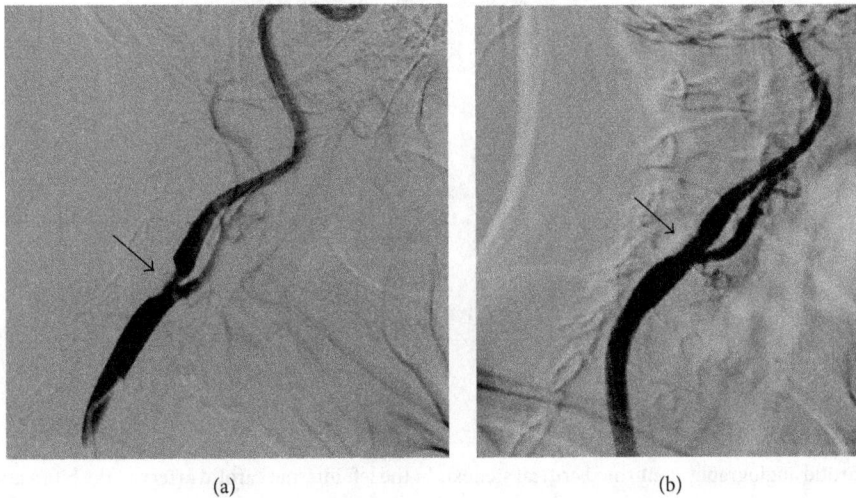

(a)   (b)

FIGURE 2: Selective right carotid angiography confirmed critical stenosis (black arrows) in the right internal carotid artery at the bifurcation level (a). Successful carotid stent placement was performed without residual stenosis (b).

ischemic attack episodes on admission to our institution, we decided to perform stenting to the stenosis in left ICA. Firstly, femoral approach was tried. However, selective engagement to the left CCA could not be possible in this way using standard catheters and Simmons catheter; therefore, right brachial approach was considered.

After pretreatment with aspirin (325 mg daily) and clopidogrel (75 mg daily) for five days, a 7 Fr sheath was inserted in the right brachial artery. A 5 Fr hydrophilic coated vertebral catheter (Merit Medical Systems, Inc., Utah, USA) was then advanced into the brachiocephalic trunk to engage selectively the left CCA (Figure 3). 0.035″ flexible guidewire (Merit Medical Systems, USA) was positioned at the left external carotid artery using this vertebral catheter and exchanged with a 0.035″ Amplatz extra-support guidewire. After that, a 7 Fr Asahi Zenyteex guiding catheter (Asahi-Intecc, USA) was positioned at the left common carotid artery and

extra-support guidewire was removed. Selective left carotid angiography confirmed critical stenosis at the bifurcation level of ICA (Figure 4). Distal embolic protection system (Emboshield, Abbot, IL, USA) was deployed in the distal ICA under fluoroscopic guidance. A 6 × 9 × 40 mm Sinus Carotid (Optimed, Ettlingen, Germany) self-expandable stent was successfully deployed in the left common and internal carotid artery, and postdilation was performed using a 5 × 20 mm Pyxis-c balloon (Stron Medical, Winsen, Germany) with the inflation at 10 atm for 10 sec (Figure 5). After postdilation, the follow-up angiogram showed complete coverage of the lesion without residual stenosis or dissection (Figure 6). The embolic protection system was removed and moderate debris was identified. The brachial artery sheath was removed and excellent hemostasis was achieved. The patient tolerated the procedure well and did not suffer any complications. He was discharged within 24 hours without any neurologic deficit

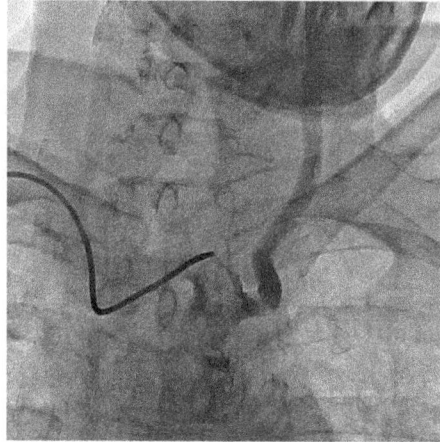

FIGURE 3: A 5 Fr hydrophilic coated vertebral catheter was advanced into the brachiocephalic trunk to engage selectively the left common carotid artery.

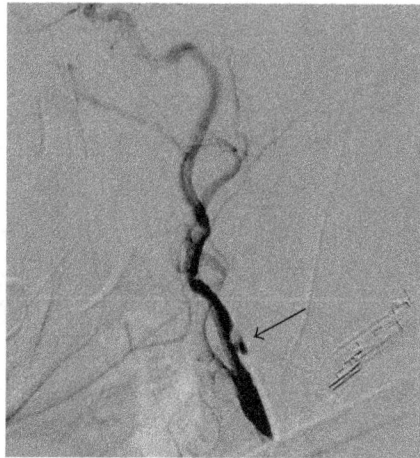

FIGURE 4: Selective left carotid angiography confirmed critical stenosis in the left internal carotid artery at the bifurcation level (black arrow).

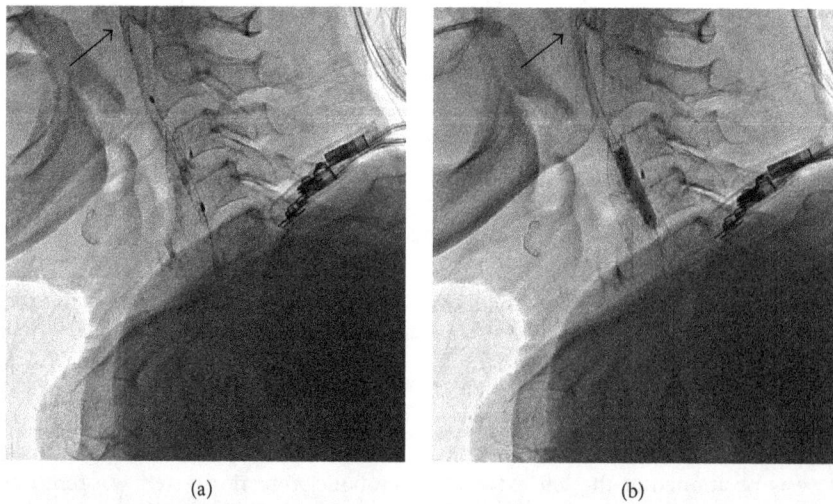

(a)

(b)

FIGURE 5: Self-expandable stent deployment (a) and postdilation (b) was performed after placement of the distal embolic protection system (black arrows) in the left internal carotid artery.

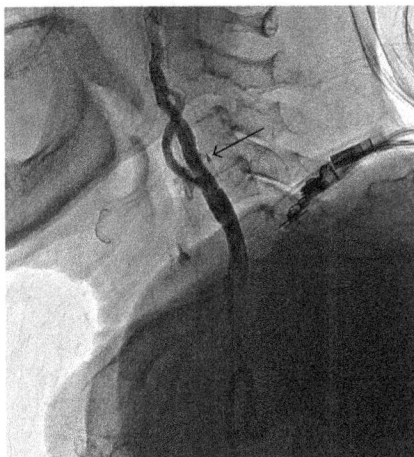

FIGURE 6: Left carotid angiography after stent deployment shows no residual stenosis in the internal carotid artery (black arrow).

and is now followed up at the outpatient clinic in a stable condition.

3. Discussion

Percutaneous carotid artery stenting represents a minimally invasive and less traumatic alternative to conventional surgical repair for managing carotid artery stenosis in selected patients, particularly those with younger (less than 70 years) and/or higher surgical risk [3, 4]. However, it is reported that transfemoral intervention is difficult in 1-2% of cases due to occlusive disease of the aorta and the iliofemoral arteries [5]. Alternative vascular access routes, such as the brachial artery, radial artery, or the direct route using the carotid artery, have been used in these cases [6–8]. Recent experiences with transbrachial carotid procedures have demonstrated that the brachial artery is a safe, feasible, and useful access route when the transfemoral procedure is difficult [9]. In our patient, the origin of the left CCA from the brachiocephalic trunk made the femoral approach less desirable. This bovine variant can be seen in 7% of the general population and is distinct from the more common bovine arch configuration that occurs in 27% involving a common origin of the brachiocephalic trunk and the left common carotid artery from the aortic arch. Although we used Simmons catheter containing complex curves in addition to standard catheters, selective cannulation of the left CCA could not be possible. For this reason, brachial access was considered. While performing the brachial approach, the guiding catheter position was stable and allowed the successful introduction of the balloon catheter and stent. This case showed that the right brachial access might be useful alternative for stenting of variant left carotid artery in patients with unusual type of bovine aortic arch. Carotid artery angioplasty and stenting procedures are technically difficult from the transfemoral approach in variant aortic arch branching such as "bovine aortic arch." We performed a right brachial artery approach for selective cannulation of a variant left CCA originating

from the brachiocephalic trunk and performed successful carotid stenting with distal protection.

Conflict of Interests

The authors declare that there is no conflict of interests regarding the publication of this paper.

References

[1] K. F. Layton, D. F. Kallmes, H. J. Cloft, E. P. Lindell, and V. S. Cox, "Bovine aortic arch variant in humans: clarification of a common misnomer," *American Journal of Neuroradiology*, vol. 27, no. 7, pp. 1541–1542, 2006.

[2] R. E. Habel and K. D. Budras, "Thoracic cavity," in *Bovine Anatomy: An Illustrated Text*, pp. 62–65, Schlütersche GmbH & Co, Hanover, Germany, 2003.

[3] V. A. Mantese, C. H. Timaran, D. Chiu, R. J. Begg, and T. G. Brott, "The carotid revascularization endarterectomy versus stenting trial (CREST): stenting versus carotid endarterectomy for carotid disease," *Stroke*, vol. 41, supplement 10, pp. S31–S34, 2010.

[4] T. G. Brott, R. W. Hobson II, G. Howard et al., "Stenting versus endarterectomy for treatment of carotid-artery stenosis," *The New England Journal of Medicine*, vol. 363, no. 1, pp. 11–23, 2010.

[5] M. H. Wholey, M. Wholey, P. Bergeron et al., "Current global status of carotid artery stent placement," *Catheterization and Cardiovascular Diagnosis*, vol. 44, no. 1, pp. 1–8, 1998.

[6] H. Sievert, R. Ensslen, A. Fach et al., "Brachial artery approach for transluminal angioplasty of the internal carotid artery," *Catheterization and Cardiovascular Diagnosis*, vol. 39, no. 4, pp. 421–423, 1996.

[7] F. J. Criado, E. P. Wilson, J. A. Martin, S. C. Patel, and H. Gnanasekeram, "Access strategies for carotid artery intervention," *Journal of Invasive Cardiology*, vol. 12, no. 1, pp. 61–68, 2000.

[8] F. Castriota, A. Cremonesi, R. Manetti, M. Lamarra, and G. Noera, "Carotid stenting using radial artery access," *Journal of Endovascular Surgery*, vol. 6, no. 4, pp. 385–386, 1999.

[9] C.-J. Wu, C.-I. Cheng, W.-C. Hung et al., "Feasibility and safety of transbrachial approach for patients with severe carotid artery stenosis undergoing stenting," *Catheterization and Cardiovascular Interventions*, vol. 67, no. 6, pp. 967–971, 2006.

52

Takotsubo Syndrome: A Pathway through the Pituitary Disease

Rui Plácido,[1] **Ana Filipa Martins,**[2] **Susana Robalo Martins,**[1] **Sónia do Vale,**[2]
Ana G. Almeida,[1] **Fausto Pinto,**[1] **and João Martin Martins**[2]

[1]*Hospital Santa Maria, Cardiology Department, Lisbon Academic Medical Centre, CCUL, Lisbon, Portugal*
[2]*Hospital de Santa Maria, Avenida Professor Egas Moniz, 1649-035 Lisboa, Portugal*

Correspondence should be addressed to Rui Plácido; placidorui@gmail.com

Academic Editor: Man-Hong Jim

Takotsubo cardiomyopathy (TTC) is characterized by reversible left ventricular apical and/or midventricular hypokinesia with unknown etiology. The clinical presentation is similar to acute myocardial infarction in the absence of significant obstructive coronary artery disease. Various predisposing factors have been related to TTC, such as acute neurological illnesses, endocrine diseases, pain, and emotional stress. We present the first description of an association between TTC cardiomyopathy and panhypopituitarism. This case reinforces the connection between the hormonal and cardiovascular systems. Furthermore, it supports the importance of a comprehensive and integrated medical history in the approach of a patient with cardiac disease, towards clinical decision-making.

1. Introduction

Takotsubo cardiomyopathy (TTC) is a novel cardiomyopathy that has been firstly described by Sato et al. [1] as an important consideration in the differential diagnosis of acute coronary syndrome. The presenting features of TTC are similar to those of myocardial ischemia after acute plaque rupture, but the characteristic distinctions are regional wall motion abnormalities that extend beyond a single coronary vascular bed and the absence of epicardial coronary occlusion. A preceding emotional or physical stressor is common [2]. The presentation can include life-threatening symptoms and hemodynamic compromise. Recently a substantial rate of death and complications after the acute phase of TTC was shown, with a long-term follow-up revealing a significant rate of death from any cause (5.6% per patient-year) and a rate of major adverse cardiac and cerebrovascular events (9.9% per patient-year) [2].

Marked increased levels of catecholamines and metanephrines are found in the acute phase and they probably account for a possible acute coronary spasm and/or focal myocardial dysfunction with contraction band necrosis/myocytolysis underlying the clinical condition [3]. Since the prognosis is much better and a different pharmacologic approach is required, angiotensin-converting–enzyme inhibitors or angiotensin receptor blockers are preferred [2], while inotropes should be avoided; the differential diagnosis is crucial [4]. Little is known about individual susceptibility to TTC. However increased sympathetic autonomic activity might be casually related. More rarely it may be related to a diseased hypothalamic-pituitary-adrenal axis (HPA), probably requiring chronic increased compensatory hyperactivity of the sympathetic autonomic system [5]. We report a clinical case supporting that association.

2. Case Presentation

A 74-year-old man presented at the emergency department with chest pain, palpitations, and progressive dyspnea within the last 24 hours. He had a past history of high blood pressure and dyslipidemia and was being treated with lisinopril/hydrochlorothiazide and simvastatin; an acquired atrioventricular block was managed with DDDR pacing. In the last year, fatigue, asthenia, adynamia, cold intolerance, loss of muscular strength, anorexia, decreased libido, and loss of male hair pattern distribution were also reported, with blood pressure decreasing whereat lisinopril/hydrochlorothiazide was interrupted. On physical examination, blood pressure was 102/84 mmHg, heart rate 65 beats per minute, respiratory rate 28 breaths per minute, and normal oxygen saturation

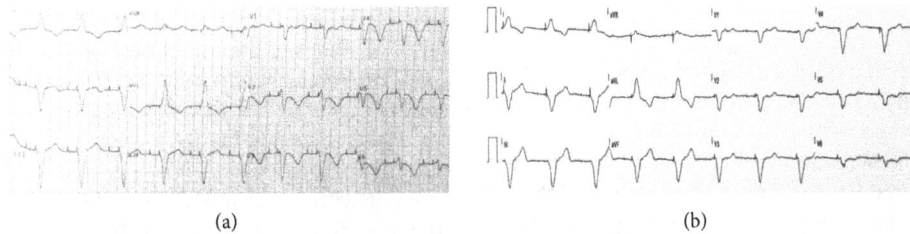

(a)

(b)

FIGURE 1: (a) Initial electrocardiogram showing an atrioventricular sequential paced rhythm with left bundle branch block morphology complexes, no ST-segment deviation, deeply inverted T waves on DI, aVL and precordial leads, and a prolonged QTc interval (560 ms). (b) Electrocardiogram 3 months after discharge.

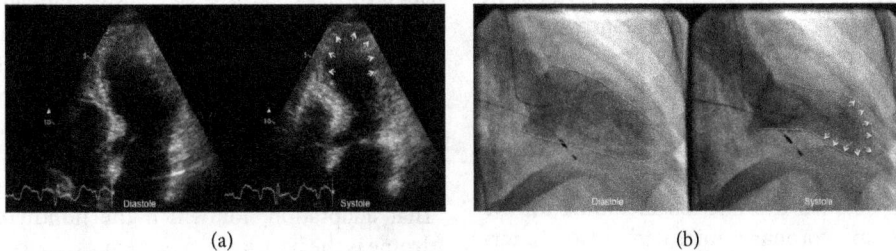

(a)

(b)

FIGURE 2: (a) Transthoracic echocardiography (apical four-chamber view) during the initial admission, demonstrating apical ballooning (white arrows). (b) Left ventriculography images in diastole and systole, showing typical type of takotsubo cardiomyopathy with apical ballooning, dyskinesia (white arrows), and left ventricle basal hypercontractility.

(ambient air) and temperature 36.6°C. He had signs of heart failure (jugular venous distention, peripheral edema, and pulmonary congestion) and cardiac auscultation was remarkable for a protodiastolic gallop.

Electrocardiogram showed an atrioventricular sequential paced rhythm with left bundle branch block morphology complexes, no ST-segment deviation, deeply inverted T waves on DI, aVL and precordial leads, and a prolonged QTc interval (560 ms) (Figure 1(a)). Complete blood count, serum electrolytes, renal function parameters, and glycaemia were normal. Troponin I (<0.07 ng/mL) was mildly elevated (0.79 ng/mL). Echocardiography showed a nondilated left ventricle with apical dyskinesia and hyperdynamic basal contraction assuming a systolic ballooning pattern, and a moderately depressed (37%) ejection fraction (Figure 2(a); Video 1 in Supplementary Material available online at http://dx.doi.org/10.1155/2016/9219018).

Acute coronary syndrome and TTC were considered in the differential diagnosis. Coronarography showing no significant coronary artery disease and a left ventriculogram revealing the typical apical ballooning (Figure 2(b); Video 2) favor the former hypothesis. Cardiac magnetic resonance was not performed given the presence of a noncompatible pacemaker.

During hospitalization the patient was managed with diuretics, beta-blocker, and angiotensin-converting enzyme inhibitor. Laboratory data showed a peak troponin I of 1,38 ng/mL. Pheochromocytoma/paraganglioma was excluded by urinary meta- and normetanephrines measurement (High Performance Liquid Chromatography) and the patient was referred for endocrine consultation.

A formal pituitary dynamic test was performed after an overnight fast: growth hormone-releasing hormone 100 μg, corticotropin-releasing hormone 100 μg, thyrotropin-releasing hormone 200 μg, and gonadotropin-releasing hormone 100 μg bolus (intravenous) at time 0; baseline/peak hormone levels were as follows: growth hormone (<2 ng/mL): 0.15/0.18; prolactin (2–18 ng/mL): 21/35; cortisol (4–23 μg/dL): 1.5/4.1; follicle-stimulating hormone (1–18 U/L): 2.2/2.8; luteinizing hormone (3–35 U/L): 0.3/1.1; other baseline values were insulin-like growth factor 1 (48–188 ng/mL): 33; adrenocorticotropin (0–46 pg/mL): 31; triiodothyronine (60–181 ng/dL): 81; thyroxine (4.5–10.9 μg/dL): 2.2; free thyroxine (0.89–1.80 ng/dL): 0.42; total testosterone (188–772 ng/dL): <10. All measurements were obtained with standardized chemiluminescence immunoassays; age and gender specific reference values at 8.00–10.00 h am after an overnight fast are presented within square brackets. Thyroid autoantibodies were negative.

Brain magnetic resonance imaging revealed a normal sized and positioned pituitary gland with no morphological abnormalities and a centered pituitary stalk.

A diagnosis of idiopathic panhypopituitarism was established and the patient was prescribed hydrocortisone 20 + 10 mg daily (oral), levothyroxine 100 μg daily (oral), and testosterone enanthate 250 mg every fortnight (intramuscular). The usual instructions were given orally and by writing regarding stressful conditions.

After 3 months of optimized heart failure treatment the patient showed clinical improvement, normalization of left ventricular function, and reversibility of T waves changes and QT prolongation (Figure 1(b)). Interestingly, in this case, the repolarization changes were clearly interpretable notwithstanding the presence of a right ventricular paced rhythm. In that time, lost weight was recovered and the patient regained normal physical vigour without other complaints.

3. Discussion

This case begins with an unusual presentation of TTC. There was no record for any particular acute emotional or physical stress; the patient is male while TTC is much more common in women and the presentation is that of an acute coronary syndrome with marked left ventricular dysfunction [3, 6].

TTC is an acute, reversible dysfunction of the left ventricle in the absence of significant obstructive coronary disease. Recently, Templin et al. [2] prospectively showed that the most common pattern was the apical type (81.7%) followed by the midventricular (14.6%), the basal (2.2%), and the focal (1.5%) types. The condition is especially prevalent in postmenopausal women but the true prevalence of TTC remains uncertain because of its underrecognition. The long-term prognosis is generally favorable. The pathophysiology of TTC is not established but is likely multifactorial, involving the vascular, endocrine, and central nervous systems. Several mechanisms have been postulated to link the sympathetic hyperactivity and myocardial dysfunction including diffuse coronary artery spasm, coronary microcirculation alterations, and direct catecholamine mediated myocyte injury [3, 7]. In 70% of the documented cases there is an apparent trigger leading to catecholamine-induced myocardial injury [6]. Further investigation is needed to define the connection between these triggers and their effect on the vulnerable myocardium.

In the acute phase, TTC is sometimes indistinguishable from acute myocardial infarction with respect to clinical symptoms, ECG changes, and cardiac biomarkers such as troponin and creatine kinase. Fast and accurate diagnosis on admission remains challenging, and exclusion of significant obstructive coronary artery disease is mandatory. Thus, there is a need for sensitive and specific biomarkers for the early diagnosis of TTC. MicroRNAs are a class of highly conserved and small noncoding posttranscriptional regulators of diverse cellular processes that have been recently considered as biomarkers in cardiovascular disease [8]. Jaguszewski et al. [9] recently described a signature of circulating microRNAs for sensitive and specific identification of TTC in the acute phase. The significant upregulation of stress- and depression-related microRNAs suggested a role of central and/or peripheral nervous system in TTC.

Retrospectively the patient of our case presented complains suggesting pituitary failure—low blood pressure, cold intolerance, loss of physical vigour and motivation, decreased libido, scanty body hair—although this is a rare condition, and these symptoms are by themselves rather common in older men [7]. Endocrine evaluation unequivocally revealed complete anterior pituitary failure, but the reason is not apparent. Combined pituitary failure by itself is a very rare condition—estimated prevalence 46/100.000 and estimated annual incidence 4/100.000—and at least in adult/old patients most commonly depends on pituitary tumors [10, 11]. Other less common causes include head trauma [12], for which the patient had no recollection and besides pituitary stalk section generally occurs; hemochromatosis and other metabolic conditions, for which no evidence was found in this case (iron, transferrin, and ferritin levels were normal

and the pituitary was not enlarged); vascular, that would be likely in this age group, namely, subarachnoid, hemorrhage [13]. However, there was no evidence for pituitary apoplexy at the CT scan. In fact most other conditions leading to combined pituitary failure, namely, infections, inflammatory, granulomatous, immune, or neoplastic disorders, generally present with structural abnormalities in the pituitary gland that can be shown by MRI [7, 10, 11]. Of course a congenital or genetic and functional defect is mostly unlikely, given patient age and clear evidence for previous normal growth and development, including two fathered children. In short, unequivocal combined pituitary failure is present but the reason is unclear. This occurs in around 10–20% of the cases, and an etiology sometimes is apparent only many years later [14]. An acute and transient defect is also unlikely since the patient had previous evidence of pituitary failure and maintained that condition for as long as two years of follow-up requiring substitutive therapy. Also, the possibility of a neuroendocrine adaptation to an acute/chronic condition may be discarded. That adaptation, for which the nonthyroidal patient syndrome is the best-known pattern, is associated with increased cortisol levels [15]. By the same token, a drug effect is unlikely.

Besides some perplexing features, a most interesting point can be made that progressive multiple pituitary failure may require an increased sustained sympathetic activity to cope with daily life physical and emotional challenges, since it is by itself certainly a stressful condition. Curiously enough, to our knowledge, other reports of TTC and endocrine disease always resolve around the theme of pheochromocytoma [16] or failure of the HPA axis [5, 17, 18]; to our knowledge, this is the first report of the association of TTC with adult onset multiple pituitary hormonal failure. Chronic activation of the sympathetic nervous system may on the other hand favor the development of TTC, as has been suggested by some reports regarding behavioral medicine [3]. Regarding combined pituitary failure, increased sympathetic drive may be particularly deleterious, since androgens may downregulate the stress response and may present direct vasodilator effects on coronary arteries [19], and low testosterone predicts the development of atherosclerosis and cardiovascular events [20] while glucocorticoids may play a supportive role on myocardial function [21] and hypothyroidism may impair coronary blood flow [22].

TTC represents an acute heart failure syndrome that is associated with a substantial risk for adverse events. The great variety of triggering factors in this disease needs to be illuminated and new investigations are required. Furthermore, a heightened vigilance in the treatment of these patients is crucial to improve prognosis.

In a way, the gap is narrowing between "Voodoo death" [23] as described by Sir Cannon in the 40s and TTC reported in the 90s. It remains to be seen if this association of combined pituitary failure and TTC is also reported by other authors. TTC by itself was also a long present but unknown condition until Sato first formally described it.

Conflict of Interests

The authors declare that there is no conflict of interests regarding the publication of this paper.

References

[1] H. Sato, H. Tateishi, T. Uchida et al., "Takotsubo type cardiomyopathy due to multivessel spasm," in *Clinical Aspect of Myocardial Injury: From Ischemia to Heart Failure*, K. Kodama, K. Haze, and M. Hon, Eds., pp. 56–64, Kagaku Hyoronsha, Tokyo, Japan, 1990.

[2] C. Templin, J. R. Ghadri, J. Diekmann et al., "Clinical features and outcomes of takotsubo (stress) cardiomyopathy," *The New England Journal of Medicine*, vol. 373, pp. 929–938, 2015.

[3] I. S. Wittstein, D. R. Thiemann, J. A. C. Lima et al., "Neurohumoral features of myocardial stunning due to sudden emotional stress," *The New England Journal of Medicine*, vol. 352, no. 6, pp. 539–548, 2005.

[4] J. R. Ghadri, F. Ruschitzka, T. F. Lüscher, and C. Templin, "Takotsubo cardiomyopathy: still much more to learn," *Heart*, vol. 100, no. 22, pp. 1804–1812, 2014.

[5] S. Sakihara, K. Kageyama, T. Nigawara, Y. Kidani, and T. Suda, "Ampulla (takotsubo) cardiomyopathy caused by secondary adrenal insufficiency in ACTH isolated deficiency," *Endocrine Journal*, vol. 54, no. 4, pp. 631–636, 2007.

[6] K. A. Bybee, T. Kara, A. Prasad et al., "Transient left ventricular apical ballooning: a syndrome that mimics ST-segment elevation myocardial infarction," *Annals of Internal Medicine*, vol. 141, no. 11, pp. 858–865, 2004.

[7] M. G. Burt and K. K. Y. Ho, "Hypopituitarism and growth hormone deficiency," in *Endocrinology. Adult and Pediatric*, J. L. Jameson, L. J. De Groot, D. M. Kretser et al., Eds., chapter 11, pp. 188–208, Elsevier Saunders, Philadelphia, Pa, USA, 7th edition, 2016.

[8] S. K. Gupta, C. Bang, and T. Thum, "Circulating MicroRNAs as biomarkers and potential paracrine mediators of cardiovascular disease," *Circulation: Cardiovascular Genetics*, vol. 3, no. 5, pp. 484–488, 2010.

[9] M. Jaguszewski, J. Osipova, J.-R. Ghadri et al., "A signature of circulating microRNAs differentiates takotsubo cardiomyopathy from acute myocardial infarction," *European Heart Journal*, vol. 35, no. 15, pp. 999–1006, 2014.

[10] M. Regal, C. Páramo, J. M. Sierra, and R. V. Garci-Mayor, "Prevalence and incidence of hypopituitarism in an adult Caucasian population in northwestern Spain," *Clinical Endocrinology*, vol. 55, no. 6, pp. 735–740, 2001.

[11] M. O. van Aken and S. W. J. Lamberts, "Diagnosis and treatment of hypopituitarism: an update," *Pituitary*, vol. 8, no. 3-4, pp. 183–191, 2005.

[12] E. Richmond and A. D. Rogol, "Traumatic brain injury: endocrine consequences in children and adults," *Endocrine*, vol. 45, no. 1, pp. 3–8, 2014.

[13] I. Kreitschmann-Andermahr, "Subarachnoid hemorrhage as a cause of hypopituitarism," *Pituitary*, vol. 8, no. 3-4, pp. 219–225, 2005.

[14] H. F. Nyström, A. Saveanu, E. J. L. Barbosa et al., "Detection of genetic hypopituitarism in an adult population of idiopathic pituitary insufficiency patients with growth hormone deficiency," *Pituitary*, vol. 14, no. 3, pp. 208–216, 2011.

[15] G. Van den Berghe, "Endocrine aspects of critical care medicine," in *Endocrinology. Adult and Pediatric*, J. L. Jameson, L. J. De Groot, D. M. Kretser et al., Eds., chapter 114, pp. 1987–1999, Saunders Elsevier, Philadelphia, Pa, USA, 7th edition, 2016.

[16] E. Lassnig, T. Weber, J. Auer, R. Nömeyer, and B. Eber, "Pheochromocytoma crisis presenting with shock and takotsubo-like cardiomyopathy," *International Journal of Cardiology*, vol. 134, no. 3, pp. e138–e140, 2009.

[17] C. Ukita, H. Miyazaki, N. Toyoda, A. Kosaki, M. Nishikawa, and T. Iwasaka, "Takotsubo cardiomyopathy during acute adrenal crisis due to isolated adrenocorticotropin deficiency," *Internal Medicine*, vol. 48, no. 5, pp. 347–352, 2009.

[18] M. Murakami, N. Matsushita, R. Arai et al., "Isolated adrenocorticotropin deficiency associated with delirium and takotsubo cardiomyopathy," *Case Reports in Endocrinology*, vol. 2012, Article ID 580481, 5 pages, 2012.

[19] R. D. Jones, K. M. English, T. Hugh Jones, and K. S. Channer, "Testosterone-induced coronary vasodilatation occurs via a non-genomic mechanism: evidence of a direct calcium antagonism action," *Clinical Science*, vol. 107, no. 2, pp. 149–158, 2004.

[20] Z. Hyde, P. E. Norman, L. Flicker et al., "Low free testosterone predicts mortality from cardiovascular disease but not other causes: the Health in Men study," *Journal of Clinical Endocrinology and Metabolism*, vol. 97, no. 1, pp. 179–189, 2012.

[21] R. Ren, R. H. Oakley, D. Cruz-Topete, and J. A. Cidlowski, "Dual role for glucocorticoids in cardiomyocyte hypertrophy and apoptosis," *Endocrinology*, vol. 153, no. 11, pp. 5346–5360, 2012.

[22] S. J. Lee, J. G. Kang, O. K. Ryu et al., "The relationship of thyroid hormone status with myocardial function in stress cardiomyopathy," *European Journal of Endocrinology*, vol. 160, no. 5, pp. 799–806, 2009.

[23] W. B. Cannon, "'Voodoo' death," *American Anthropologist*, vol. 44, pp. 169–181, 1942.

53

Coronary Thrombosis without Dissection following Blunt Trauma

Archana Sinha,[1] Michael Sibel,[2] Peter Thomas,[3] Francis Burt,[1]
James Cipolla,[3] Peter Puleo,[1] and Keith Baker[2]

[1]Division of Cardiovascular Disease, Saint Luke's University Health Network, Bethlehem, PA 18015, USA
[2]Department of Emergency Medicine, Saint Luke's University Health Network, Bethlehem, PA 18015, USA
[3]Department of Trauma Surgery, Saint Luke's University Health Network, Bethlehem, PA 18015, USA

Correspondence should be addressed to Archana Sinha; sinha.archana7@gmail.com

Academic Editor: Manabu Shirotani

Blunt trauma to the chest resulting in coronary thrombosis and ST elevation myocardial infarction (STEMI) is a rare but well-described occurrence in adults. Angiography in such cases has generally disclosed complete epicardial coronary occlusion with thrombus, indistinguishable from the findings commonly found in spontaneous plaque rupture due to atherosclerotic disease. In all previously reported cases in which coronary interrogation with intravascular ultrasound (IVUS) was performed in association with acute revascularization, coronary artery dissection was implicated as the etiology of coronary thrombosis. We present the first case report of blunt trauma-associated coronary thrombosis without underlying atherosclerosis or coronary dissection, as documented by IVUS imaging.

1. Introduction

Cardiac injury is an uncommon complication of blunt trauma; in most cases of cardiac dysfunction following blunt trauma injury, cardiac contusion is implicated. Arrhythmic death has been reported in children following blunt force injuries to the chest. In rare cases, coronary thrombosis and STEMI have been associated with blunt trauma to the chest in adults [1–3]. Angiography in such cases has generally disclosed complete epicardial coronary occlusion with thrombus, indistinguishable from the findings commonly found in spontaneous plaque rupture due to atherosclerotic disease [1–3]. In all previously reported cases in which coronary interrogation with IVUS was performed in association with acute revascularization, coronary artery dissection was implicated as the etiology of coronary thrombosis [4–8]. We present the first case report of blunt trauma-associated coronary thrombosis without underlying atherosclerosis or coronary dissection, as documented by IVUS imaging performed at the time of primary percutaneous revascularization.

2. Case Report

A 25-year-old previously healthy woman presented to the Emergency Department after sustaining a kick to her lower chest by a horse. She initially complained of epigastric pain and nausea; she also reported substernal chest discomfort that became progressively more prominent. She had no coronary atherosclerotic risk factors and did not use oral contraceptives. She had stable vital signs; physical examination was notable only for abrasions of the chest wall. An ECG revealed sinus bradycardia at 56 beats/min with ST segment elevation in leads V1, V2, and aVL and ST segment depressions in leads II, III, aVF, V5, and V6 (Figure 1). CT imaging of the chest, abdomen, and pelvis disclosed a small left pneumothorax, focal myocardial hypoattenuation suggesting the possibility of cardiac contusion, and soft tissue attenuation of the subhepatic porta hepatis indicating hemorrhage. An echocardiogram demonstrated severe hypokinesis of the mid and distal anteroseptal segments and the apex, with an estimated left ventricular ejection fraction of 45%. The aortic root was

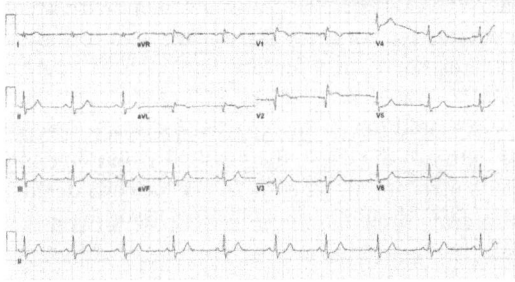

FIGURE 1: EKG showing ST segment elevation in leads V1, V2, and aVL and ST segment depressions in leads II, III, aVF, V5, and V6.

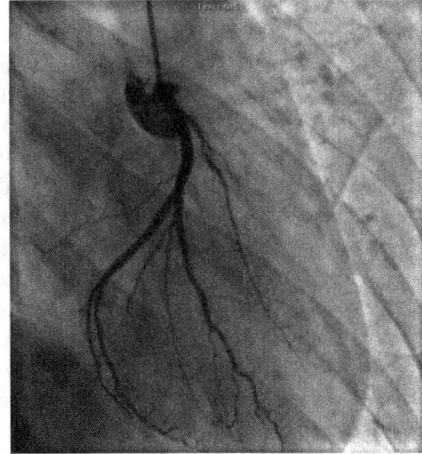

(a)

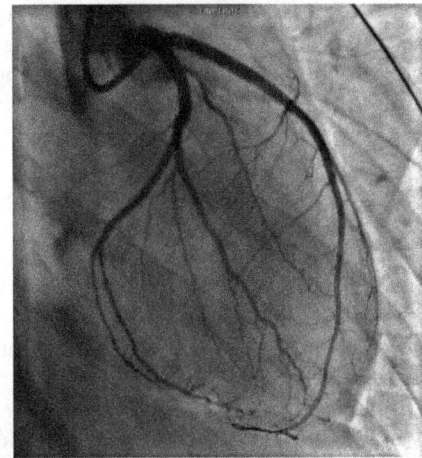

(b)

FIGURE 2: (a) Coronary angiogram showing total occlusion of LAD. (b) Restoration of normal flow following balloon dilation and stent deployment.

without evidence of dissection; there was no pericardial fluid or aortic valvular insufficiency. Because of the ECG and echo findings, emergent cardiac catheterization was performed. Coronary angiography via the right radial artery disclosed a total occlusion of the left anterior descending artery 2 mm from its origin (Figure 2(a)). All other epicardial vessels appeared to be normal. Antiplatelet and antithrombotic therapies with aspirin, clopidogrel, and bivalirudin were administered. A coronary wire was passed to the distal LAD, and balloon dilation with an undersized 2.5 mm balloon was performed, restoring normal antegrade flow. IVUS was then performed. Thrombus was evident adherent to the vessel wall in the proximal LAD. No dissection or atherosclerotic plaque was present (Figure 3/Video in Supplementary Material, available online at http://dx.doi.org/10.1155/2016/8671015). A 4.0 × 23 mm everolimus-eluting stent was deployed across the site of total occlusion (Figure 2(b)). Repeat IVUS imaging disclosed a lack of full stent apposition, and postdilation was performed with a 4.5 mm noncompliant balloon. Following PCI, antegrade flow was normal. CT angiography disclosed no evidence of aortic dissection. The patient exhibited mild pulmonary congestion on the following day that responded to diuretic therapy. Maximum serum troponin I level was 69.1 ng/mL. Hypercoagulability evaluation, including homocysteine, anti-nuclear antibody screen, antithrombin III, protein C, free and total protein S, protein S activity, Factor V Leiden mutation analysis, prothrombin 20210GA mutation, lupus anticoagulant profile, and anticardiolipin antibody, was negative. She was discharged on the 5th hospital day. Repeat echocardiography 2 weeks after her initial injury showed improvement in LV function, with residual mild to moderate hypokinesis of the mid to apical anterior wall and an ejection fraction of 50%.

3. Discussion

A wide variety of cardiovascular pathologies have been associated with blunt trauma injury, including myocardial contusion, aortic transection or less often aortic dissection, trauma-induced ventricular arrhythmia or commotio cordis in young children [9], hemopericardium with tamponade, and aortic valve leaflet avulsion [10–12]. Acute myocardial infarction (AMI) is a rare but well-described complication of blunt trauma to the chest. Since the advent of primary percutaneous

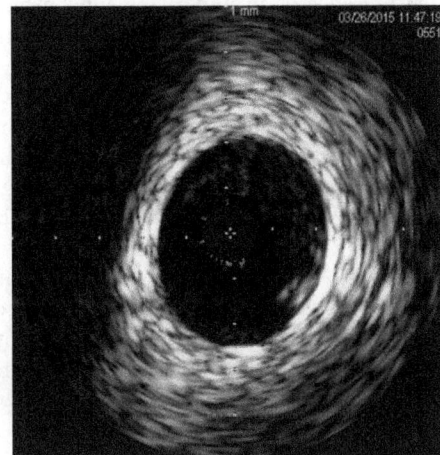

FIGURE 3: Intravascular ultrasound (IVUS) showing thrombus in proximal LAD, no evidence of dissection.

intervention, there have been several reports of AMI due to total epicardial thrombotic occlusion following blunt trauma and its successful treatment by percutaneous intervention [13–17]. Proposed mechanisms for AMI in this setting have included intimal injury due to shear forces imparted by the blunt trauma [18, 19], plaque rupture, coronary artery dissection, and coronary vasospasm [20]. In several reports, the presence of coronary artery dissection has been documented as the underlying pathophysiologic trigger for thrombosis [4–8]. In recent years, IVUS has become an increasingly routine adjunctive imaging modality in coronary revascularization. For a 40 MHz IVUS transducer the typical resolution is 80–100 microns axially and 200–250 microns laterally [21]. IVUS is extremely sensitive for the detection of coronary disease involving the vessel wall, including the presence of underlying atherosclerosis or dissection. All previous reports of blunt trauma-associated acute STEMI that included IVUS interrogation of the occluded epicardial vessel have identified the presence of a coronary dissection as the underlying pathophysiologic substrate triggering thrombosis. Coronary dissection presumably occurs in association with deceleration trauma, in some cases involving the aorta. It is not known whether affected individuals carry a genetic predisposition to vascular dissection; however, spontaneous coronary dissection has been associated with fibromuscular dysplasia [22]. The mechanism of thrombosis in the case presented here remains obscure. Acute psychological stress has been implicated in AMI, following diverse stressors, including earthquakes [23], missile attacks [24], and international soccer matches [25], but these primarily involved patients having underlying atherosclerotic disease, whereas the patient in the current case was a 25-year-old female with no coronary risk factors and no atherosclerosis by angiography or by IVUS interrogation of the vessel wall. It appears most likely that thrombosis in this case was the result of endothelial injury, possibly caused by direct compression of the proximal left anterior descending artery by the force of the blow or via shock waves [26]. A mathematical model for blunt injury leading to hemodynamic shade zone formation with high and low shear stress and hyperviscosity has been developed by Ismailov [27]. In addition, the presence of an underlying subclinical thrombophilic state that might interact with such an injury to produce thrombosis cannot be excluded. Park et al. demonstrated that patients with blunt trauma have greater numbers of circulating procoagulant microparticle and increased in vitro thrombin generation that correlated with injury severity despite normal values for standard clotting assays. Response to injury though appears to be variable between individuals [28].

The treatment approach to myocardial infarction (STEMI) following blunt chest trauma is immediate coronary angiography and revascularization with percutaneous intervention and continuation of dual antiplatelet therapy. We felt that use of GpIIb/IIIa inhibitor was contraindicated in our patient because of liver laceration and increased risk of bleeding.

In conclusion, we present a case of proximal left anterior descending artery thrombosis precipitated by blunt force

trauma to the chest in a 25-year-old woman with no history or risk factors for coronary disease and with no associated atherosclerosis or coronary artery dissection. The patient was successfully treated by primary PCI. Although significant chest pain would not be unexpected following severe blunt trauma injury to the chest, the possibility that ongoing pain represents myocardial ischemia should be considered, and a screening ECG should be considered to identify rare cases of STEMI.

Conflict of Interests

The authors report no financial relationships or conflict of interests regarding the content herein.

References

[1] A. R. Vasudevan, G. S. Kabinoff, T. N. Keltz, and B. Gitler, "Blunt chest trauma producing acute myocardial infarction in a rugby player," *The Lancet*, vol. 362, no. 9381, p. 370, 2003.

[2] J. E. Moore, "Acute apical myocardial infarction after blunt chest trauma incurred during a basketball game," *Journal of the American Board of Family Practice*, vol. 14, no. 3, pp. 219–222, 2001.

[3] E. Ginzburg, J. Dygert, E. Parra-Davila, M. Lynn, J. Almeida, and M. Mayor, "Coronary artery stenting for occlusive dissection after blunt chest trauma," *The Journal of Trauma—Injury, Infection and Critical Care*, vol. 45, no. 1, pp. 157–161, 1998.

[4] J. D. Adler and T. M. Scalea, "Right coronary artery dissection after blunt chest trauma," *Injury Extra*, vol. 41, no. 8, pp. 77–79, 2010.

[5] R. Moreno, J. Pérez del Todo, M. Nieto et al., "Primary stenting in acute myocardial infarction secondary to right coronary artery dissection following blunt chest trauma. Usefulness of intracoronary ultrasound," *International Journal of Cardiology*, vol. 103, no. 2, pp. 209–211, 2005.

[6] N. Gottam, S. Salami, M. Othman, J. Torey, H. Rosman, and A. Boguszewski, "Sealed with a kick: a case of posttraumatic coronary artery dissection and cardiomyopathy," *Case Reports in Vascular Medicine*, vol. 2012, Article ID 208985, 3 pages, 2012.

[7] X. Li, Y. Lei, and Q. Zheng, "Myocardial infarction caused by coronary artery dissection due to blunt injury: is thromboaspiration an appropriate treatment?" *Hellenic Journal of Cardiology*, vol. 55, no. 1, pp. 61–64, 2014.

[8] J. H. Chun, S.-C. Lee, H.-C. Gwon et al., "Left main coronary artery dissection after blunt chest trauma presented as acute anterior myocardial infarction: assessment by intravascular ultrasound: a case report," *Journal of Korean Medical Science*, vol. 13, no. 3, pp. 325–327, 1998.

[9] B. J. Maron, T. E. Gohman, S. B. Kyle, N. A. M. Estes III, and M. S. Link, "Clinical profile and spectrum of commotio cordis," *The Journal of the American Medical Association*, vol. 287, no. 9, pp. 1142–1146, 2002.

[10] E. Atalar, T. Açil, K. Aytemir et al., "Acute anterior myocardial infarction following a mild nonpenetrating chest trauma—a case report," *Angiology*, vol. 52, no. 4, pp. 279–282, 2001.

[11] E. G. Murray, K. Minami, H. Körtke, H. Seggewiß, and R. Körfer, "Traumatic sinus of Valsalva fistula and aortic valve rupture," *The Annals of Thoracic Surgery*, vol. 55, no. 3, pp. 760–761, 1993.

[12] M. Esmaeilzadeh, H. Alimi, M. Maleki, and S. Hosseini, "Aortic valve injury following blunt chest trauma," *Research in Cardiovascular Medicine*, vol. 3, no. 3, Article ID e17319, 2014.

[13] A. Salmi, M. Blank, and C. Slomski, "Left anterior descending artery occlusion after blunt chest trauma," *Journal of Trauma—Injury Infection & Critical Care*, vol. 40, no. 5, pp. 832–834, 1996.

[14] M. L. James, B. C. David, and S. M. Peter, "Acute myocardial infarction caused by blunt chest trauma: successful treatment by direct coronary angioplasty," *American Heart Journal*, vol. 132, no. 6, pp. 1275e–1277e, 1996.

[15] S. Thorban, A. Ungeheuer, R. Blasini, and J. R. Siewert, "Emergent interventional transcatheter revascularization in acute right coronary artery dissection after blunt chest trauma," *Journal of Trauma*, vol. 43, no. 2, pp. 365–367, 1997.

[16] E. Altekin, A. Er, C. Oktay et al., "Acute anterior myocardial infarction after being struck on the chest by a soccer ball," *Hong Kong Journal of Emergency Medicine*, vol. 18, no. 2, pp. 120–124, 2011.

[17] R. R. Patil, D. Mane, and P. Jariwala, "Acute myocardial infarction following blunt chest trauma with intracranial bleed: a rare case report," *Indian Heart Journal*, vol. 65, no. 3, pp. 311–314, 2013.

[18] J. L. Marcum, D. C. Booth, and P. M. Sapin, "Acute myocardial infarction caused by blunt chest trauma: successful treatment by direct coronary angioplasty," *American Heart Journal*, vol. 132, no. 6, pp. 1275–1277, 1996.

[19] S. J. Yoon, H. M. Kwon, D. S. Kim et al., "Acute myocardial infarction caused by coronary artery dissection following blunt chest trauma," *Yonsei Medical Journal*, vol. 44, no. 4, pp. 736–739, 2003.

[20] M. Imamura, Y. Tsuchiya, H. Tahara et al., "Acute myocardial infarction in a patient with primary coronary dissection and severe coronary vasospasm: a case report," *Angiology*, vol. 46, no. 10, pp. 951–955, 1995.

[21] E. E. van der Wall, F. R. de Graaf, J. E. van Velzen, J. W. Jukema, J. J. Bax, and J. D. Schuijf, "IVUS detects more coronary calcifications than MSCT; matter of both resolution and cross-sectional assessment?" *International Journal of Cardiovascular Imaging*, vol. 27, no. 7, pp. 1011–1014, 2011.

[22] M. S. Tweet, S. N. Hayes, S. R. Pitta et al., "Clinical features, management, and prognosis of spontaneous coronary artery dissection," *Circulation*, vol. 126, no. 5, pp. 579–588, 2012.

[23] K. Ogawa, I. Tsuji, K. Shiono, and S. Hisamichi, "Increased acute myocardial infarction mortality following the 1995 Great Hanshin-Awaji earthquake in Japan," *International Journal of Epidemiology*, vol. 29, no. 3, pp. 449–455, 2000.

[24] M. Zubaid, C. G. Suresh, L. Thalib, and W. Rashed, "Could missile attacks trigger acute myocardial infarction?" *Acta Cardiologica*, vol. 61, no. 4, pp. 427–431, 2006.

[25] U. Wilbert-Lampen, D. Leistner, S. Greven et al., "Cardiovascular events during world cup soccer," *The New England Journal of Medicine*, vol. 358, pp. 475–483, 2008.

[26] M. Hosseini, A. Hedjazi, and M. Bahrani, "Missed opportunities for diagnosis of post-traumatic thrombosis: a case series and literature review," *Journal of Forensic Sciences*, vol. 59, no. 5, pp. 1417–1419, 2014.

[27] R. M. Ismailov, "Mathematical model of blunt injury to the vascular wall via formation of rouleaux and changes in local hemodynamic and rheological factors. Implications for the mechanism of traumatic myocardial infarction," *Theoretical Biology and Medical Modelling*, vol. 2, article 13, 2005.

[28] M. S. Park, B. A. L. Owen, B. A. Ballinger et al., "Quantification of hypercoagulable state after blunt trauma: microparticle and thrombin generation are increased relative to injury severity, while standard markers are not," *Surgery*, vol. 151, no. 6, pp. 831–836, 2012.

54

Midventricular Hypertrophic Cardiomyopathy with Apical Aneurysm: Potential for Underdiagnosis and Value of Multimodality Imaging

Archana Sivanandam[1] and Karthik Ananthasubramaniam[2]

[1]University of California, Los Angeles, 405 Hilgard Avenue, Los Angeles, CA 90024, USA
[2]Heart and Vascular Institute, Henry Ford Hospital, 2799 W. Grand Boulevard, Detroit, MI 48322, USA

Correspondence should be addressed to Karthik Ananthasubramaniam; kananth1@hfhs.org

Academic Editor: Ertuğurul Ercan

We illustrate a case of midventricle obstructive HCM and apical aneurysm diagnosed with appropriate use of multimodality imaging. A 75-year-old African American woman presented with a 3-day history of chest pain and dyspnea with elevated troponins. Her electrocardiogram showed sinus rhythm, left atrial enlargement, left ventricular hypertrophy, prolonged QT, and occasional ectopy. After medical therapy optimization, she underwent coronary angiography for an initial diagnosis of non-ST segment elevation myocardial infarction. Her coronaries were unremarkable for significant disease but her left ventriculogram showed hyperdynamic contractility of the midportion of the ventricle along with a large dyskinetic aneurysmal apical sac. A subsequent transthoracic echocardiogram provided poor visualization of the apical region of the ventricle but contrast enhancement identified an aneurysmal pouch distal to the midventricular obstruction. To further clarify the diagnosis, cardiac magnetic resonance imaging with contrast was performed confirming the diagnosis of midventricular hypertrophic cardiomyopathy with apical aneurysm and fibrosis consistent with apical scar on delayed enhancement. The patient was medically treated and subsequently underwent elective implantable defibrillator placement in the ensuing months for recurrent nonsustained ventricular tachycardia and was initiated on prophylactic oral anticoagulation with warfarin for thromboembolic risk reduction.

1. Introduction

Hypertrophic cardiomyopathy (HCM) is an inherited disorder of the cardiac muscle and is well known as the most common cause of sudden cardiac death in individuals less than 35 years of age in North America. It is an autosomal dominant condition with reported prevalence of 1 in 500. HCM is caused by a genetic defect which results in the mutation of the sarcomere or its associated proteins resulting in dysfunction of the myocardium. Most HCM patients (90%) are diagnosed with asymmetric septal hypertrophy, with the less common variations being midventricular/apical (1%) and posteroseptal and isolated lateral wall hypertrophy (1%). Although only 25–35% of the patients demonstrate obstruction at rest, provocable gradients can be demonstrated in up to 75% of HCM patients [1].

Pathophysiology of HCM includes left ventricular outflow tract obstruction, diastolic dysfunction, myocardial ischemia, autonomic dysfunction, and mitral valve regurgitation [2].

We present a case where initial diagnosis of apical ballooning (Takotsubo cardiomyopathy) was suspected at coronary angiography, but subsequent multimodality imaging with echocardiography and magnetic resonance established the unique entity of midventricular HCM with apical aneurysm.

2. Case Report

A 75-year-old African American female with stage 4 chronic kidney disease presented with a 3-day history of atypical chest

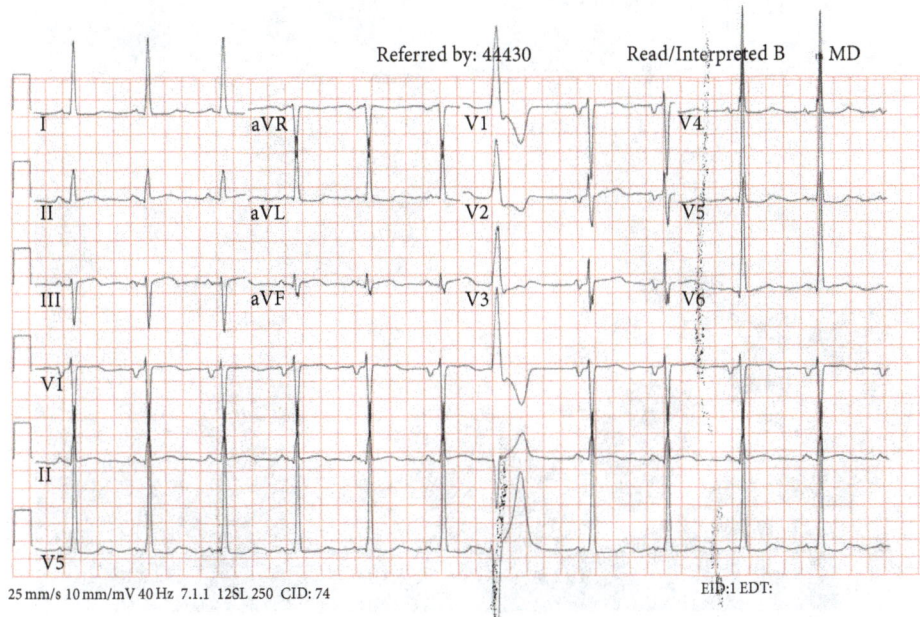

FIGURE 1: 12-lead electrocardiogram.

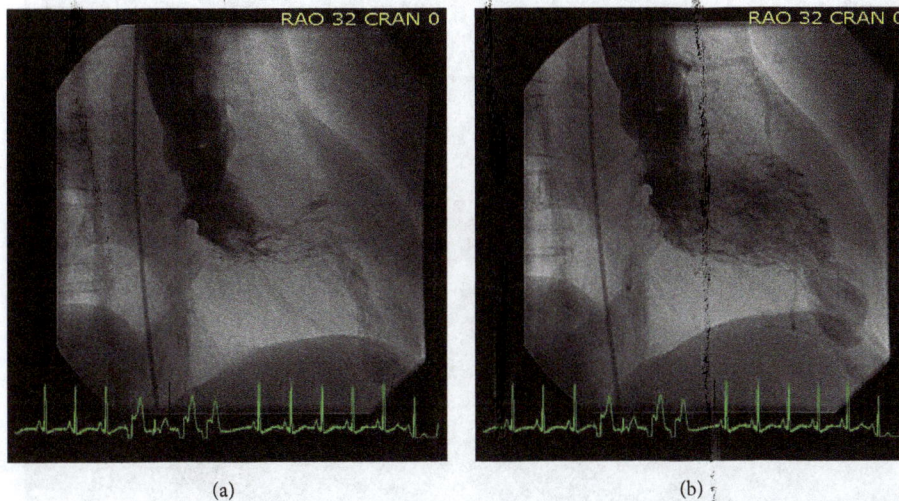

FIGURE 2: Left ventriculogram demonstrating midventricular obstruction with large aneurysmal apical pouch (diastole and systole).

pain and dyspnea. She had a long standing history of hypertension. At presentation, she was hypertensive with blood pressure of 180/100 mm Hg. The electrocardiogram ordered showed sinus rhythm (heart rate: 85 beats/min), ST depression, and deep T wave abnormality (Figure 1). Initial troponin I level was 1.5 ng/mL, and she was diagnosed with non-ST segment elevation myocardial infarction. She was started on aspirin, clopidogrel, heparin, and beta-blockers and underwent coronary angiography. The angiogram showed nonobstructive mild coronary artery disease.

Left ventriculogram was done and showed a hyperdynamic midportion of the ventricle with a large aneurysmal dyskinetic sac with stasis of contrast (Figures 2(a) and 2(b)). Given her acute coronary syndrome-like presentation, it was suspected that she had possible Takotsubo cardiomyopathy (apical ballooning) and was admitted for further evaluation.

She underwent transthoracic echocardiogram the next day, and the noncontrast image shown in Figure 3(a) displayed moderate left ventricular hypertrophy including asymmetric septal hypertrophy but poor visualization of the apex and no definite dyskinetic cavity as shown on the left ventricular angiogram. However, to define the apex better, echocardiographic contrast was utilized and the contrast images clearly demonstrated midventricular narrowing, a hyperdynamic zone, and apical aneurysmal zone similar to coronary angiogram (Figure 3(b)). There was flow acceleration demonstrable with paradoxic Doppler flow between

(a)

(b)

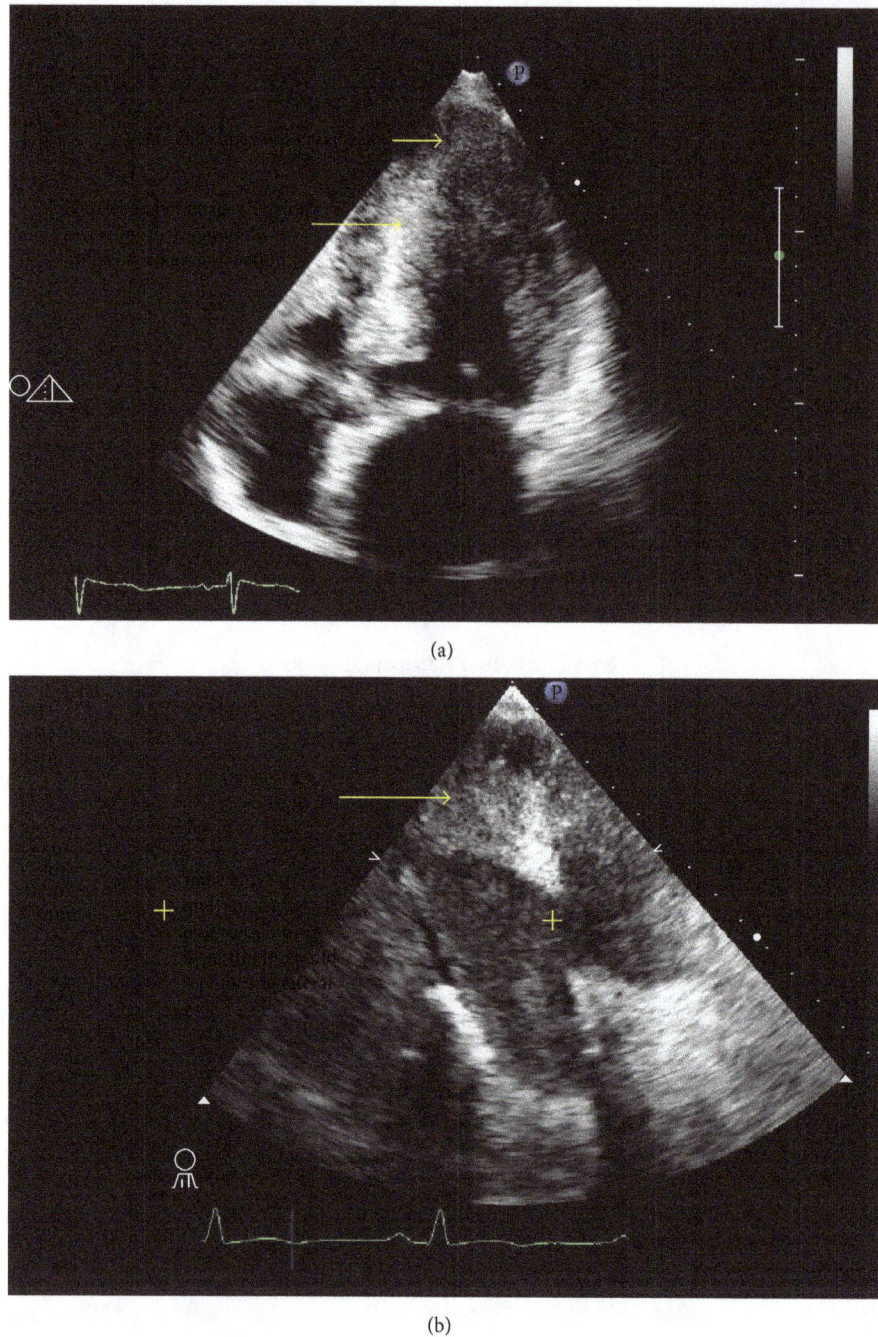

FIGURE 3: (a) Noncontrast transthoracic echocardiographic 4-chamber image demonstrating left ventricular hypertrophy and inability to visualize apical pouch. (b) Contrast transthoracic echocardiographic image demonstrating midventricular narrowing with aneurysmal apex.

the mid cavity narrowing and the apical aneurysmal zone (Figure 4).

Based on the constellation of findings, she was diagnosed with midventricular HCM with apical aneurysm formation. She underwent cardiac magnetic resonance imaging (MRI) with gadolinium contrast that confirmed the diagnosis and further illustrated concomitant outflow tract obstruction and significant septal hypertrophy with moderate to severe secondary mitral regurgitation (Figures 5(a) and 5(b)). During her hospital course, she had multiple bouts of

nonsustained ventricular tachycardia. She subsequently underwent implantable cardioverter defibrillator placement and was initiated on warfarin for stroke prevention.

3. Discussion

This case represents an uncommon variant of HCM, namely, midventricular obstructive variant with apical aneurysm formation, which occurs in only 1-2% of HCM patients [1]. Although a different diagnosis was entertained initially,

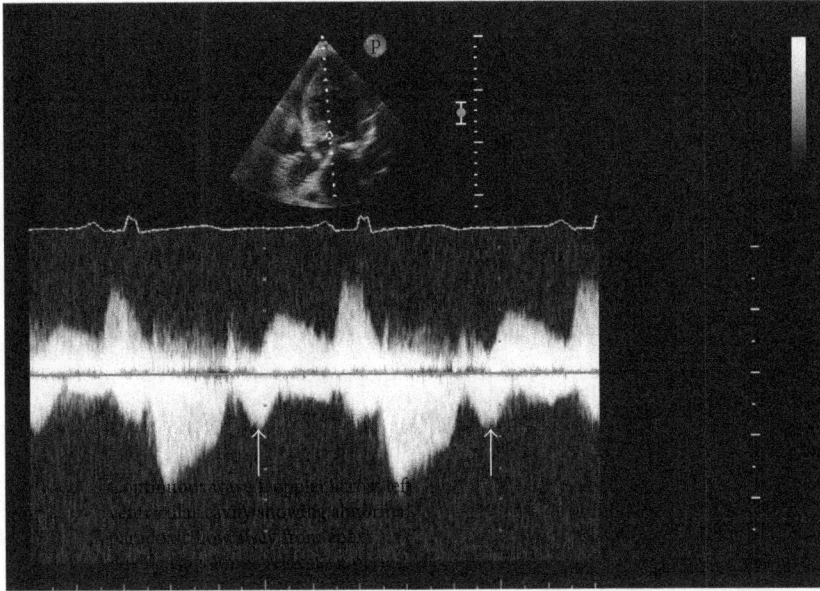

FIGURE 4: Doppler flow pattern across midventricular obstructive ventricle.

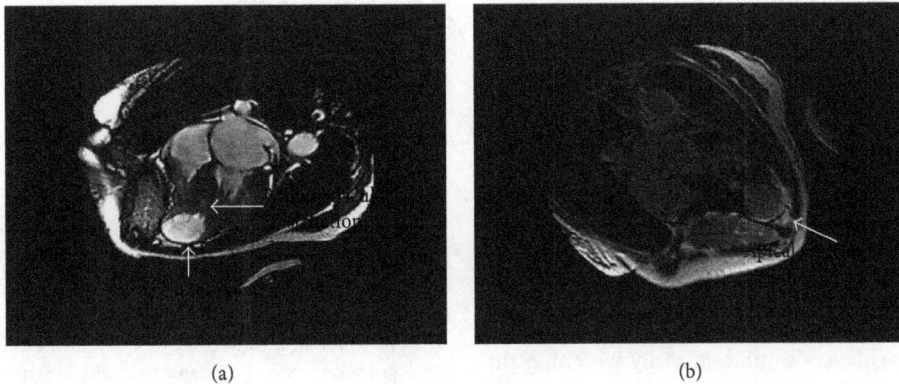

(a)   (b)

FIGURE 5: (a) Cine 4-chamber image of cardiac MRI done with steady state free precession imaging (SSFP) demonstrating diffuse hypertrophy with aneurysmal apex. (b) Delayed enhancement 4-chamber MRI image demonstrating thinned apex and apical scarring.

strengths of multimodality imaging performed appropriately in this case clinched the final diagnosis and significantly impacted patient management.

The pathophysiology of apical aneurysm formation is fascinating. The midventricular variant of HCM involves hypertrophy of the midventricle, which can be exacerbated by hypertension. The hypertrophy creates 2 adjacent cavities on either side of the obstruction during systole. The proximal cavity develops a low pressure zone and the distal cavity forms a high pressure zone leading to necrosis due to chronic subendocardial ischemia. This subsequently leads to scarring, thinning, and apical aneurysm formation in the infarcted tissue [1].

Apical aneurysm formation and the decrease in cardiac output are attributed to a higher risk of small vessel disease and increase the chances for sudden cardiac arrest or acute myocardial infarction from ventricular arrythmias and thrombus formation due to stasis of blood [3, 4].

Of note, noncontrast echocardiography did not correctly delineate this apical aneurysmal zone well. It is well known that foreshortening of the apex is a limitation of transthoracic echocardiograms. However, the addition of contrast imaging highlighted the apical dyssynergic zone very well. Unique Doppler patterns first described in midventricular HCM by Nakamura et al. (paradoxic jet flow) were also noted in our patient with Doppler echocardiography [5]. These unique Doppler flow patterns are often the clue towards concealed apical asynergy/dyssynergy, as was seen in our case. The paradoxic jet flow is from the apex to the base and is likely related to higher diastolic pressure at the apex moving blood to the lower pressure proximal zone, and in the original description by Nakamura et al., it was observed in 20/198 patients with midventricular HCM. Interestingly, such patients were found to have higher incidence of systemic embolism, ventricular arrhythmias, and thallium perfusion defects in their study. It is possible that persistent high diastolic pressure compromises subendocardial perfusion and contributes to apical necrosis and the development of aneurysmal deformation. Importantly, as Doppler is independent of image quality, such unique Doppler patterns can alert clinicians of apical pouch/midventricular obstructive physiology.

Cardiac MRI carries unique value in the workup of HCM as it helps to detect more atypical variants of HCM such as apical HCM and anterolateral wall variant HCM, which seems to be underrecognized by echocardiography due to limitations in adequately imaging these areas.

Cardiac MRI is also recommended as an adjunctive test by the 2011 guidelines for evaluating the anatomy when the decision regarding septal ablation versus myectomy is not clear [2]. Mitral valve morphologic variations, anomalous location of papillary muscles, multiple papillary muscle heads, and myocardial crypts are numerous additional findings that can be better demonstrated by cardiac MRI. More recently, cardiac MRI with delayed enhancement imaging with gadolinium has been shown to have increasing prognostic value with regard to assessment of myocardial scarring, which is noted in a majority of patients with HCM. In our patient, myocardial scarring was demonstrated in the infarcted apical zone, and such areas increase the risk for ventricular arrhythmias. Recent data suggest that the extent of scarring demonstrated on cardiac MRI greater than or equal to 15% of the total myocardium may be associated with an increased risk of cardiac events in HCM patients [6].

Treatment of midventricular HCM is targeted at reducing the symptoms, such as the intraventricular gradient, and the risk of complications, such as heart failure and sudden cardiac death. Beta-blockers and calcium blockers can contribute to reduction of obstructive gradients with negative inotropic effect, decreasing outflow obstruction and restoring cardiac output [2]. Septal myectomy, through resection of a portion of the septum, can achieve a similar effect by widening the outflow tract if concomitant outflow obstruction is present but may not be applicable to the midventricular variant [1].

For patients with midventricular HCM and apical aneurysm, treatment options are controversial. Relief of obstruction at the mid- and basal ventricle follows standard recommendations as in the guidelines for HCM [2, 7], but this subset of patients is at a higher risk for ventricular arrhythmias and has been identified as one of the anatomic substrates in decision-making towards a primary prevention implantable cardioverter defibrillator (ICD). Anticoagulants are not normally given to patients with traditional HCM unless concomitant atrial fibrillation is noted; however, the midventricular HCM with apical aneurysm variant may represent a higher risk variant due to apical stasis of the blood and high risk of thrombus formation and resulting embolization and warrant anticoagulation [2].

4. Conclusion

This report outlines a clinical presentation of obstructive midventricular HCM with apical aneurysm formation as identified by multimodality imaging. Clinicians should be aware of the manifestations of this entity to avoid misdiagnosis or underdiagnosis, to use multimodality imaging appropriately to delineate the anatomic substrate, to recognize the challenges in management of these patients, and to consider prophylactic anticoagulation and implantable cardioverter defibrillator placement to decrease adverse cardiac events in this subset.

Conflict of Interests

Archana Sivanandam and Karthik Ananthasubramaniam report no relevant conflict of interests in the preparation of this paper.

Authors' Contribution

Archana Sivanandam collected the case report data and was involved in paper writing and critical revision of the paper. Karthik Ananthasubramaniam was involved in the case report concept, paper writing, gathering of images, and critical revision of the paper.

Acknowledgment

The authors thank Stephanie Stebens, MLIS, AHIP, from Sladen Library, Henry Ford Hospital, for her expertise in this paper's preparation.

References

[1] K. Ananthasubramaniam, "Hypertrophic cardiomyopathy," in *Current Diagnosis & Treatment: Cardiology*, M. H. Crawford, Ed., pp. 301–313, McGraw-Hill Education, New York, NY, USA, 4th edition, 2014.

[2] B. J. Gersh, B. J. Maron, R. O. Bonow et al., "2011 ACCF/AHA guideline for the diagnosis and treatment of hypertrophic cardiomyopathy: executive summary: a report of the American College of Cardiology Foundation/American Heart Association Task Force on Practice Guidelines," *Circulation*, vol. 124, pp. 2761–2796, 2011.

[3] T. F. Cianciulli, M. C. Saccheri, I. V. Konopka et al., "Subaortic and mid-ventricular obstructive hypertrophic cardiomyopathy with an apical aneurysm: a case report," *Cardiovascular Ultrasound*, vol. 4, article 15, 2006.

[4] B. J. Maron, "Hypertrophic cardiomyopathy," *Circulation*, vol. 106, no. 19, pp. 2419–2421, 2002.

[5] T. Nakamura, K. Matsubara, K. Furukawa et al., "Diastolic paradoxic jet flow in patients with hypertrophic cardiomyopathy: evidence of concealed apical asynergy with cavity obliteration," *Journal of the American College of Cardiology*, vol. 19, no. 3, pp. 516–524, 1992.

[6] M. S. Maron and B. J. Maron, "Clinical impact of contemporary cardiovascular magnetic resonance imaging in hypertrophic cardiomyopathy," *Circulation*, vol. 132, no. 4, pp. 292–298, 2015.

[7] P. M. Elliot, A. Anastasakis, M. A. Borger et al., "2014 ESC guidelines on diagnosis and management of hypertrophic cardiomyopathy: the Task Force for the diagnosis and management of hypertrophic cardiomyopathy of the European Society of Cardiology (ESC)," *European Heart Journal*, vol. 35, no. 39, pp. 2733–2779, 2014.

55

Pulmonary Hypertension Secondary to Partial Anomalous Pulmonary Venous Return in an Elderly

Stefan Koester, Justin Z. Lee, and Kwan S. Lee

University of Arizona, Tucson, AZ 85714, USA

Correspondence should be addressed to Kwan S. Lee; klee@shc.arizona.edu

Academic Editor: Ramazan Akdemir

Background. Partial anomalous pulmonary venous return (PAPVR) is an uncommon congenital abnormality, which may present in the adult population. It is often associated with sinus venosus defect (SVD). The diagnosis and therapy for this condition may be challenging. *Case Presentation*. We describe a case of an elderly woman who presented with NYHA Class IV dyspnea and was suspected to have symptomatic pulmonary hypertension. She was later found to have anomalous right upper pulmonary vein return to the superior vena cava and associated SVD with bidirectional shunting. Therapeutic options were discussed and medical management alone with aggressive diuresis and sildenafil was adopted. Follow-up visits revealed success in the planned medical therapy. *Conclusions*. PAPVR is a rare congenital condition that may present during late adulthood. The initial predominant left-to-right shunting associated with this anomaly may go undetected for years with the gradual development of pulmonary hypertension and right heart failure due to right heart volume overload. Awareness of the condition is important, as therapy is time-sensitive with early detection potentially leading to surgical therapy as a viable option.

1. Introduction

Partial anomalous pulmonary venous return (PAPVR) is an uncommon congenital abnormality, which may present in the adult population. We describe a case of an elderly woman who presented with symptomatic pulmonary hypertension and was found to have PAPVR associated with sinus venosus defect (SVD). We also discuss the diagnostic and therapeutic challenges encountered.

2. Case Presentation

A 77-year-old Hispanic lady with a history of asthma and elevated pulmonary pressures attributed to respiratory disease presented with increased dyspnea at rest and worsening lower extremity swelling over a week. Prior to this, she had been independent and was able to walk without symptoms. Her past medical history was otherwise significant for hypertension and hypothyroidism. Her home medications included albuterol, amlodipine, levothyroxine, loratadine, and metoprolol. She was not a smoker and consumed no alcohol. Systems review was otherwise unremarkable.

Physical exam showed an irregular rhythm with a rate in the 130 s. Blood pressure was 147/88 mmHg; she was afebrile, tachypneic with O_2 sats. of 93%. She was a thin, elderly woman who was alert and cooperative. Her JVP was elevated at 15 cm H_2O. She had mild, diffuse wheezing bilaterally with bibasal fine, inspiratory crackles. Heart sounds were present with fixed splitting of the second heart sounds and a 2/6 pan-systolic murmur in the right parasternal base. Abdomen was soft and nontender. She had 2+ bilateral lower extremity edema.

A 12-lead ECG showed atrial fibrillation with a rate of 133 bpm. A chest X-ray showed cardiomegaly and prominence of the pulmonary arteries with a small right pleural effusion.

Lab tests including a complete blood count and complete-metabolic panel were unremarkable. Troponin was borderline elevated and B-type Natriuretic Peptide was moderately elevated at 626 pg/mL. TSH was normal.

A chest CT with pulmonary angiography showed no pulmonary emboli. There was right heart cardiomegaly and dilation of the main pulmonary artery with calcifications seen in the proximal pulmonary arteries (Figures 1 and 2). Small

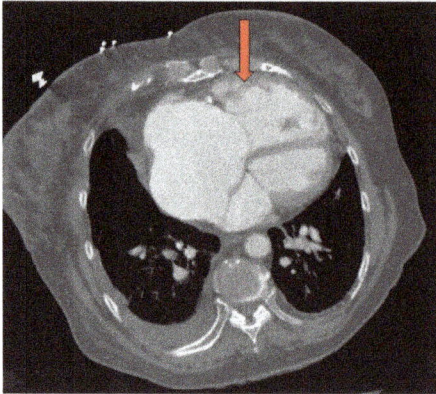

FIGURE 1: CT-scan showing right ventricular enlargement (red arrow).

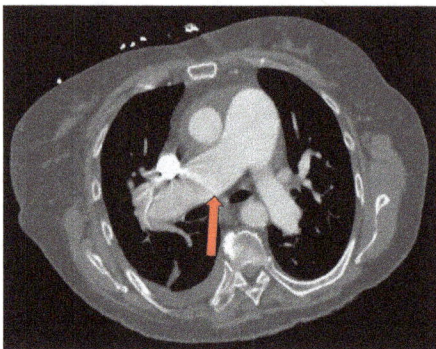

FIGURE 2: CT-scan showing enlarged pulmonary artery (red arrow).

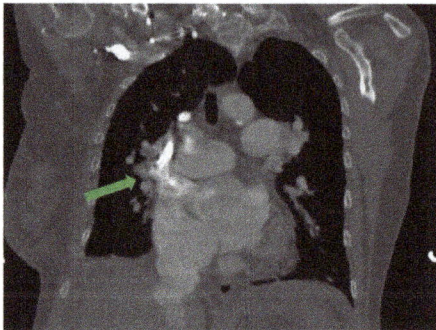

FIGURE 3: CT-scan showing anomalous right upper pulmonary venous return to superior vena cava (green arrow).

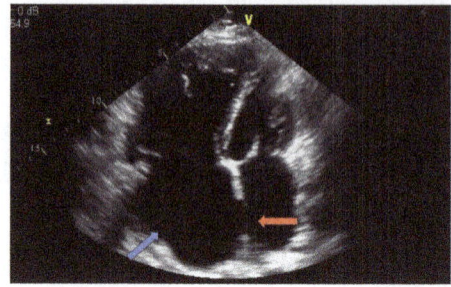

FIGURE 4: Echocardiography showing enlarged right ventricle and right atrium (blue arrow) with sinus venosus defect (red arrow).

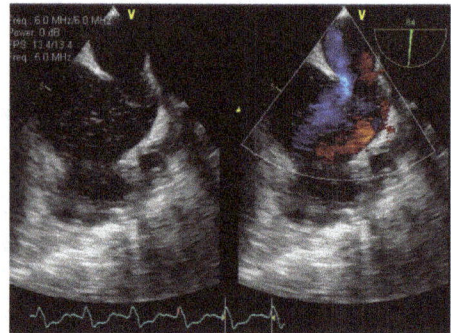

FIGURE 5: Color Doppler displaying sinus venosus defect.

bilateral pleural effusions were noted. A possible anomalous right upper pulmonary vein to lateral superior vena cava just above the right atrium to superior vena cava junction was also seen (Figure 3), with a possible associated interatrial septal defect. Compression ultrasonography with Doppler flow study revealed a nonocclusive deep venous thrombosis that was seen in the mid right superficial femoral vein.

Transthoracic echo showed left ventricular ejection fraction (LVEF) of 45%. The right heart was severely dilated with severe reduction in systolic function associated with systolic and diastolic ventricular septal flattening (Figure 4). Moderate mitral regurgitation and severe tricuspid regurgitation were noted with right ventricular systolic pressure (RVSP) estimated at 50 mmHg + CVP. Her IVC was dilated with minimal inspiratory change. Severe, resting right-to-left shunting was seen with saline bubble study.

Transesophageal echocardiography (TEE) guided cardioversion was performed. The TEE confirmed a sinus venosus (SV) atrial septal defect measuring 3.1 cm in maximum diameter (Figure 5). No left atrial appendage thrombus was seen. The right upper anomalous pulmonary venous return to the SVC was seen with no additional anomalous venous drainage. She was successfully cardioverted. Following atrial fibrillation cardioversion, her LVEF normalized with persistent right heart dilatation.

Right heart cardiac catheterization was performed with inhaled nitric oxide reactivity testing after several additional days of diuresis, initiation of digoxin, and the commencement of oral sildenafil. This showed a normal CVP of 2 mmHg, left atrial pressure of 6 mmHg, high-flow pulmonary hypertension of 74/15, and mean 37 mmHg. Pulmonary cardiac output was 12.5 L/min with systemic cardiac output of 8.7 L/min, resulting in a Qp/Qs of 1.4. Effective cardiac output was 5.1 L/min. Pulmonary vascular resistance was minimally elevated at 2.3 Wood units. Bidirectional shunting was present with predominant left to right shunt of 60% and right to left shunt of 40%. She had no significant response with inhaled nitric oxide and her systemic oxygen saturation corrected on a 100% O_2 nonrebreather.

Initial anticoagulation with iv heparin and warfarin was initiated for the DVT, which also prepared her for TEE-guided cardioversion. Rate control of her atrial fibrillation was initially achieved with oral digoxin. Beta-blockers and nondihydropyridine calcium channel blockers were not used secondary to her severe right heart failure. Oral sildenafil was initiated at this point at the recommendation of the pulmonary hypertension service. Aggressive IV diuresis was initiated.

After several days of initial stabilization, she was then scheduled for a TEE. This showed no left atrial appendage thrombus, and she was loaded with iv amiodarone. Elective biphasic cardioversion of her atrial fibrillation was performed. Two liters/min of home oxygen supplementation was started.

She improved over the course of therapy from NYHA Class IV symptoms to NYHA Class II symptoms by discharge. On follow-up in pulmonary hypertension clinic a month later, she remained symptomatically improved with good INR follow-up and atrial fibrillation free.

3. Discussion

We describe a case of late clinical presentation of symptomatic pulmonary hypertension secondary to PAPVR and a SVD with bidirectional shunting. PAPVC is a rare congenital heart disease, with a prevalence of 0.1 to 0.2% in the adult population [1, 2]. Anomalous right sided pulmonary veins could return to the right atrium, superior vena cava, inferior vena cava, azygos vein, hepatic vein, or portal vein. Anomalous left sided pulmonary veins might drain into the innominate vein, coronary sinus, and hemiazygos vein. Studies based on the pediatric population identified the most common form of PAPVR to be the right upper pulmonary vein connecting to the SVC which is most often associated with a SVD [3]. Interestingly, retrospective reviews of adults receiving CT imaging identified that only half of the anomalies were right sided, with the only case of right upper lobe PAPVR being associated with atrial septal defect [2]. This may be an indication that the pediatric and adult populations with PAPVR may be significantly different. Our patient was found to have PAPVR associated with right upper anomalous pulmonary venous return to the SVC with associated SVD.

In PAPVR, the persistent systemic venous connection acts similarly to a left-to-right shunt, where a portion of the right ventricular output is continuously recirculated and oxygenated blood is returned to the right heart without traveling to the systemic circulation. The initial predominance of left-to-right shunting causes the condition to be clinically undetected. Over time, the increase in pulmonary blood flow can lead to progressive remodelling of the pulmonary circulation and increased pulmonary vascular resistance, leading to pulmonary arterial hypertension [4]. This leads to gradual negative right heart remodelling occurring over the years due to right heart volume overload. As volume related pulmonary hypertension develops, severe tricuspid regurgitation often occurs associated with right atrial arrhythmias which may lead to sudden clinical decompensation. Over time, worse right failure occurs and may lead to reversal of the bidirectional shunting into predominant right-to-left shunting, systemic cyanosis and Eisenmenger's syndrome.

The diagnosis of PAPVC is challenging. The typical presenting clinical features such as shortness of breath, right heart failure, and pulmonary hypertension are not specific to PAPVC. Therefore, patients may be misdiagnosed initially as having primary pulmonary hypertension [5]. In our patient, diagnosis was made after CT pulmonary angiogram was performed to exclude thromboembolic disease (Figures 1, 2, and 3). This is similar to other cases where PAPVR was diagnosed following CT-angiogram to exclude pulmonary embolism [6, 7].

Awareness of the condition is important, as early recognition can lead to successful surgical correction which involves surgical redirection of the anomalous vein into the left atrium [8]. In our patient, her severe pulmonary arterial hypertension and elevated pulmonary vascular resistance preclude her as a good surgical candidate. It is not likely that surgery is going to alter the disease course, as the extensive vascular remodelling is unlikely to be reversible. Catheter embolization of the anomalous vein was also considered. However, this was not a viable option in our patient as there was no concomitant connection from the anomalous vein to the left atrium, which can accommodate the venous drainage after the anomalous vein has been embolized [9]. In our patient, given her high surgical risk, medical therapy alone was adopted. There have been small retrospective and observational studies of patients with pulmonary arterial hypertension secondary to congenital heart diseases, including PAPVR, having clinical and hemodynamic improvements with prostaglandins, phosphodiesterase inhibitors, and bosentan [10]. However, close monitoring of response to treatment is important in the event that the pulmonary hypertension progresses.

In conclusion, PAPVR is a rare congenital condition that may present during late adulthood. The predominant left-to-right shunting associated with this anomaly can go undetected for years with the gradual development of pulmonary hypertension and right heart failure due to right heart volume overload. There should be a high index of suspicion, especially in patients with unexplained pulmonary hypertension. Awareness of the condition is important, as therapy is time-sensitive with early detection potentially leading to surgical therapy as a viable option.

Conflict of Interests

Dr. Kwan Lee receives honoraries from St. Jude Medical and Maquet Medical Systems. All other authors have reported that they have no relationships relevant to the contents of this paper to disclose.

References

[1] L. B. Haramati, I. E. Moche, V. T. Rivera et al., "Computed tomography of partial anomalous pulmonary venous connection in adults," *Journal of Computer Assisted Tomography*, vol. 27, no. 5, pp. 743–749, 2003.

[2] M.-L. Ho, S. Bhalla, A. Bierhals, and F. Gutierrez, "MDCT of partial anomalous pulmonary venous return (PAPVR) in adults," *Journal of Thoracic Imaging*, vol. 24, no. 2, pp. 89–95, 2009.

[3] F. Senocak, S. Ozme, A. Bilgic, S. Ozkutlu, S. Ozer, and M. Saraclar, "Partial anomalous pulmonary venous return. Evaluation of 51 cases," *Japanese Heart Journal*, vol. 35, no. 1, pp. 43–50, 1994.

[4] G.-P. Diller and M. A. Gatzoulis, "Pulmonary vascular disease in adults with congenital heart disease," *Circulation*, vol. 115, no. 8, pp. 1039–1050, 2007.

[5] M. A. Gatzoulis and G. Giannakoulas, "Sinus venosus atrial septal defect in a 31-year-old female patient: a case for surgical repair," *European Respiratory Review*, vol. 19, no. 118, pp. 340–344, 2010.

[6] H. Wang, H. Guan, and D. Wang, "Partial anomalous pulmonary venous connection to superior vena cava that overrides across the intact atrial septum and has bi-atrial connection in a 75-year-old female presenting with pulmonary hypertension," *BMC Cardiovascular Disorders*, vol. 14, article 149, 2014.

[7] E. H. Sears, J. M. Aliotta, and J. R. Klinger, "Partial anomalous pulmonary venous return presenting with adult-onset pulmonary hypertension," *Pulmonary Circulation*, vol. 2, no. 2, pp. 250–255, 2012.

[8] T. Hijii, J. Fukushige, and T. Hara, "Diagnosis and management of partial anomalous pulmonary venous connection. A review of 28 pediatric cases," *Cardiology*, vol. 89, no. 2, pp. 148–151, 1998.

[9] L. W. Forbess, M. P. O'Laughlin, and J. K. Harrison, "Partially anomalous pulmonary venous connection: demonstration of dual drainage allowing nonsurgical correction," *Catheterization and Cardiovascular Diagnosis*, vol. 44, no. 3, pp. 330–335, 1998.

[10] M. A. Gatzoulis, R. Alonso-Gonzalez, and M. Beghetti, "Pulmonary arterial hypertension in paediatric and adult patients with congenital heart disease," *European Respiratory Review*, vol. 18, no. 113, pp. 154–161, 2009.

Permissions

List of Contributors

Anne Munch
Department of Oncology, Aarhus University, Nørrebrogade 44, 8000 Aarhus C, Denmark

Jens Sundbøll
Department of Cardiology, Aarhus University Hospital, Palle Juul Jensens Boulevard 99, 8200 Aarhus N, Denmark

Søren Høyer
Institute of Pathology, Aarhus University Hospital, Nørrebrogade 44, 8000 Aarhus C, Denmark

Manan Pareek
The Cardiovascular and Metabolic Preventive Clinic, Department of Endocrinology, Centre for Individualized Medicine in Arterial Diseases, Odense University Hospital, 5000 Odense C, Denmark

Fumiaki Nakao, Masashi Kanemoto and Takashi Fujii
Department of Cardiology, Yamaguchi Grand Medical Center, 77 Ohsaki, Hofu, Yamaguchi 747-8511, Japan

Jutaro Yamada
Division of Cardiology, Department of Medicine and Clinical Science, Yamaguchi University Graduate School of Medicine, 1-1-1 Minami-kogushi, Ube, Yamaguchi 755-8505, Japan

Kazuhiro Suzuki and Hidetoshi Tsuboi
3Department of Cardiovascular Surgery, Yamaguchi Grand Medical Center, 77 Ohsaki, Hofu, Yamaguchi 747-8511, Japan

Abhinav Agrawal, Martin Miguel Amor and Manan Parikh
Department of Medicine, Monmouth Medical Center, Long Branch, NJ 07740, USA

Deepa Iyer
Department of Cardiology, Robert Wood Johnson University Hospital, New Brunswick, NJ 08901, USA

Marc Cohen
Department of Cardiology, Newark Beth Israel Medical Center, Newark, NJ 07712, USA

Rose Tompkins, William J. Cole, Barry P. Rosenzweig, Sripal Bangalore and Anuradha Lala
Department of Cardiology, New York University Langone Medical Center, New York, NY 10016, USA

Leon Axel
Department of Radiology, New York University School of Medicine, New York, NY 10016, USA

Mahesh Anantha Narayanan and Toufik Mahfood Haddad
Department of Internal Medicine, CHI Health Creighton University Medical Center, 601 North 30th Street No. 5800, Omaha, NE 68131, USA

Christopher DeZorzi and Aiman Smer
Creighton University School of Medicine, 2500 California Plaza, Omaha, NE 68102, USA

Abhilash Akinapelli and William P. Biddle
Cardiac Center of Creighton University, 3006 Webster Street, Omaha, NE 68131, USA

Janani Baskaran
Sri Venkateshwaraa Medical College Hospital and Research Center, Puducherry 605102, India

Timothy Glew, Dennis Finkielstein and Susan Hecht
Department of Cardiology, Mount Sinai Beth Israel, New York, NY 10003, USA

Migdalia Feliciano
Department of Medicine, Mount Sinai Beth Israel, New York, NY 10003, USA

Daryl Hoffman
Department of Cardiothoracic Surgery, Mount Sinai Beth Israel, New York, NY 10003, USA

Nathalie Jeanne Magioli Bravo-Valenzuela
Pediatrics Department, University of Taubaté, 12020-130 Taubaté, SP, Brazil

Guilherme Ricardo Nunes Silva
University of Taubaté, 12020-130 Taubaté, SP, Brazil

Cem Sahin and Esmail Kirli
Department of Internal Medicine, School of Medicine, Mugla Sıtkı Kocman University, Orhaniye Mahallesi İsmet Catak Caddesi, Merkez, 48000 Mugla, Turkey

Fatih AkJn and Ebrahim Altun
Department of Cardiology, School of Medicine, Mugla Sıtkı Kocman University, Orhaniye Mahallesi İsmet Catak Caddesi, Merkez, 48000 Mugla, Turkey

Nesat Cullu
Department of Radiology, School of Medicine, Mugla Sıtkı Kocman University, Orhaniye Mahallesi İsmet Catak Caddesi, Merkez, 48000 Mugla, Turkey

Burak Özseker
Department of Gastroenterology, School of Medicine, Mugla Sıtkı Kocman University, Orhaniye Mahallesi İsmet Catak Caddesi, Merkez, 48000 Mugla, Turkey

Aasim M. Afzal and Jamil Alsahhar
Department of Internal Medicine, Baylor University
Medical Center, 3600 Gaston Avenue, Dallas, TX 75246,
USA

Varsha Podduturi
Department of Pathology, Baylor University Medical
Center, 3600 Gaston Avenue, Dallas, TX 75246, USA

Jeffrey M. Schussler
Division of Cardiology, Jack and Jane Hamilton Heart
and Vascular Hospital, 621 N. Hall Street, Dallas, TX
75246, USA
Department of Medicine, Texas A&M College of Medicine,
Dallas Campus, 3600 Gaston Avenue, Dallas, TX 75246,
USA

Melissa Dakkak, Khyati Baxi and Ambar Patel
Departments of Cardiovascular Diseases and Internal
Medicine, University of Florida Health, Jacksonville, FL
32209, USA

Juan Mieres, Marcelo Menéndez, Carlos Fernández-Pereira, Miguel Rubio and Alfredo E. Rodríguez
Cardiac Unit and Cardiovascular Surgery Department,
Otamendi Hospital, Azcue`naga 870, C1115AAB Buenos
Aires, Argentina

Adnan Kaya
Cardiology, Suruc State Hospital, Sanliurfa, Turkey

Emine Caliskan
Radiology, Suruc State Hospital, Sanliurfa, Turkey

Mustafa Adem Tatlisu, Mert Ilker Hayiroglu, Ahmet Ilker Tekessin, Yasin Cakilli, Sahin Avsar, Ahmet Oz and Osman Uzman
Cardiology, Dr. Siyami Ersek Cardiovascular and
Thoracic Surgery Hospital, Istanbul, Turkey

Rhanderson Cardoso, Carlos E. Alfonso and James O. Coffey
Miller School of Medicine, University of Miami, Miami,
FL 33136, USA

Caglayan Geredeli
Department of Medical Oncology, Konya Training and
Research Hospital, 42090 Konya, Turkey

Melih Cem Boruban, Mehmet Artac and Lokman Koral
Department of Medical Oncology, Meram Medical
Faculty, Necmettin Erbakan University, 42080 Konya,
Turkey

Necdet Poyraz
Department of Radiology, Meram Medical Faculty,
Necmettin Erbakan University, 42080 Konya, Turkey

Alpay Aribas
Department of Cardiology, Meram Medical Faculty,
Necmettin Erbakan University, 42080 Konya, Turkey

Mario Enrique Baltazares-Lipp, Juan Ignacio Soto-González, Carlos Manuel Aboitiz-Rivera, Héctor A. Carmona-Ruíz and Benito Sarabia Ortega
Departamento de Hemodinamia y Ecocardiografía,
Instituto Nacional de Enfermedades Respiratorias "Ismael
Cosío Villegas", 14080 Mexico City, Mexico

Ruben Blachman-Braun
Facultad de Ciencias de la Salud, Universidad Anáhuac
México Norte, 52786 Estado de México, Mexico

Nikolay Yu. Mironov, Natalia A. Mironova and Sergey P. Golitsyn
Department of Clinical Electrophysiology, Russian
Cardiology Research Center, Russia

Marina A. Saidova
Department of Sonography, Russian Cardiology Research
Center, Russia

Olga V. Stukalova
Department of Tomography, Russian Cardiology Research
Center, Russia

Tereza Augusta Grillo
Electrophysiology Department, Hospital Universita´rio
Sa˜o Jose´-INCOR Minas, 30140-073 Belo Horizonte, MG,
Brazil
Interventional Cardiology Department, Hospital
Universita´rio Sa˜o Jose´-INCOR Minas, 30140-073 Belo
Horizonte, MG, Brazil

Guilherme Rafael S. Athayde
Division of Cardiology and Cardiovascular Surgery,
Hospital das Cl´ınicas, Universidade Federal de Minas
Gerais, 30130-100 Belo Horizonte, MG, Brazil
Electrophysiology Department, Universidade Federal de
Minas Gerais, 30130-100 Belo Horizonte, MG, Brazil

Ana Flávia L. Belfort
School of Medicine, Universidade Federal de Minas
Gerais, 30130-100 Belo Horizonte, MG, Brazil

Andrea Z. Beaton
Children's National Health System, Washington, DC
20010, USA

Bruno R. Nascimento
Interventional Cardiology Department, Hospital
Universita´rio Sa˜o Jose´-INCOR Minas, 30140-073 Belo
Horizonte, MG, Brazil
Division of Cardiology and Cardiovascular Surgery,
Hospital das Cl´ınicas, Universidade Federal de Minas
Gerais, 30130-100 Belo Horizonte, MG, Brazil
School of Medicine, Universidade Federal de Minas
Gerais, 30130-100 Belo Horizonte, MG, Brazil
Interventional Cardiology Department, Hospital das
Cl´ınicas, Universidade Federal de Minas Gerais, 30130-100 Belo Horizonte, MG, Brazil

Reynaldo C. Miranda
Electrophysiology Department, Hospital Universita´rio
Sa˜o Jose´-INCOR Minas, 30140-073 Belo Horizonte, MG,
Brazil
Electrophysiology Department, Universidade Federal de
Minas Gerais, 30130-100 Belo Horizonte, MG, Brazil

**Shahzad Khan, Athanasios Smyrlis, Dmitry Yaranov,
David Oelberg and Eric Jimenez**
Danbury Hospital, Western Connecticut Health Network,
187 Willow Springs, New Milford, CT 06776, USA

George Kassimis and Athanasios Manolis
Department of Cardiology, Asklepeion General Hospital,
Athens, Greece

Jonathan N. Townend
Department of Cardiology, Queen Elizabeth Hospital,
Birmingham, UK

**Candice Baldeo, Abdul wahab Hritani, Robert Ali and
Sana Chaudhry**
Department of Internal Medicine, University of Florida,
Jacksonville, FL 32209, USA

Fawad N. Khawaja
Department of Cardiothoracic Surgery, University of
Florida, Jacksonville, FL 32209, USA

Shahbaz A. Malik and Sarah Malik
Department of Internal Medicine, University of North
Dakota School of Medicine and Health Sciences, Fargo,
ND 58102, USA

Taylor F. Dowsley
Department of Cardiology, Sanford Health, Fargo, ND
58102, USA

Balwinder Singh
Department of Psychiatry and Behavioral Science,
University of North Dakota School of Medicine and
Health Sciences, Fargo, ND 58102, USA

**Jeong-Woo Choi, Kyehwan Kim, Min Gyu Kang, Jin-
Sin Koh, Jeong Rang Park and Jin-Yong Hwang**
Division of Cardiology, Department of Internal Medicine,
Gyeongsang National University Hospital, Jinju 52727,
Republic of Korea

**Fady Y. Marmoush, Mohamad F. Barbour and Mazen
O. Al-Qadi**
Memorial Hospital of Rhode Island, Alpert Medical
School, Brown University, Pawtucket, RI 02860, USA

Thomas E. Noonan
Memorial Hospital of Rhode Island, Alpert Medical
School, Brown University, Pawtucket, RI 02860, USA
Harvard Medical School, USA

**Braghadheeswar Thyagarajan, Lubna Bashir Munshi
and Martin Miguel Amor**
Department of Internal Medicine, Monmouth Medical
Center, Long Branch, NJ 07740, USA

**Luigi Fiocca, Micol Coccato, Vasile Sirbu, Angelina
Vassileva, Giulio Guagliumi, Giuseppe Musumeci,
Amedeo Terzi, Gianluca Canu, Diego Cugola and
Orazio Valsecchi**
Cardiovascular Department, Papa Giovanni XXIII
Hospital, 24127 Bergamo, Italy

Elisa Cerchierini
Anesthesia and Intensive Care Department, Papa
Giovanni XXIII Hospital, 24127 Bergamo, Italy

Gaurav Rao
Division of Internal Medicine, Montefiore Medical
Center, Albert Einstein College of Medicine, Bronx, NY
10467, USA

James Tauras
Division of Cardiology, Weiler Hospital, Albert Einstein
College of Medicine, Bronx, NY 10461, USA

Daniel Angeli
Department of Medicine, Montefiore Medical Center,
Bronx, NY, USA

Stephen J. Angeli
Holy Name Medical Center, USA

Glenmore Lasam, Gina LaCapra and Roberto Ramirez
Department of Internal Medicine, Overlook Medical
Center, Summit, NJ 07901, USA

Roberto Roberti
Section of Cardiology, Overlook Medical Center, Summit,
NJ 07901, USA

Sachin Diwadkar and Aarti A. Patel
Division of Cardiovascular Medicine, University of South
Florida, 2 Tampa General Circle, Tampa, FL 33606, USA

Michael G. Fradley
Division of Cardiovascular Medicine, University of South
Florida, 2 Tampa General Circle, Tampa, FL 33606, USA
H. Lee Moffitt Cancer Center & Research Institute, 12902
Magnolia Drive, Tampa, FL 33612, USA

**Fadi J. Sawaya, Henry Liberman and Chandan
Devireddy**
Department of Medicine, Division of Cardiology, Emory
University School of Medicine, Atlanta, GA 30308, USA

**Angela Pimenta Bento, Renato Gil dos Santos Pinto
Fernandes, David Cintra Henriques Silva Neves, Lino
Manuel Ribeiro Patrício and José Eduardo Chambel de
Aguiar**
Hospital do Espirito Santo, Largo Senhor da Pobreza,
7000-811 E´vora, Portugal

Erwin E. Argueta and Menfil A. Orellana-Barrios
Department of Internal Medicine, Texas Tech University, Lubbock, TX 79430, USA

Teerapat Nantsupawat, Alvaro Rosales and Scott Shurmur
Department of Cardiovascular Medicine, Texas Tech University, Lubbock, TX 79430, USA

Archana Sinha and Rajan Kumar
Division of Cardiology, Saint Luke's University Health Network, Bethlehem, PA 18015, USA

Sri Lakshmi Hyndavi Yeruva
Division of Hematology and Oncology, Howard University Hospital, 2041 Georgia Avenue NW, Washington, DC 20060, USA

Bryan H. Curry
Division of Cardiology, Howard University Hospital, 2041 Georgia Avenue NW, Washington, DC 20060, USA

Kenichi Sakakura, Yusuke Adachi, Yousuke Taniguchi, Hiroshi Wada, Shin-ichi Momomura and Hideo Fujita
Division of Cardiovascular Medicine, Saitama Medical Center, Jichi Medical University, 1-847 Amanuma, Omiya, Saitama 330-8503, Japan

Manan Parikh, Martin Miguel Amor, Isha Verma and Madhu Paladugu
Department of Internal Medicine, Monmouth Medical Center, 300 2nd Avenue, Long Branch, NJ 07740, USA

Jeffrey Osofsky
Department of Cardiology, Monmouth Medical Center, 300 2nd Avenue, Long Branch, NJ 07740, USA

Tasuku Higashihara, Nobuo Shiode, Tomoharu Kawase, Hiromichi Tamekiyo, Masaya Otsuka, Tomokazu Okimoto and Yasuhiko Hayashi
Cardiovascular Center, Division of Cardiology, Akane Foundation, Tsuchiya General Hospital, 3-30 Nakajima-cho, Naka-ku, Hiroshima 730-8655, Japan

Vistasp J. Daruwalla and Hassan Tahir
Conemaugh Memorial Hospital/Temple University, USA

Keyur Parekh, Jeremy D. Collins and James Carr
Department of Cardiovascular Radiology, Northwestern University Feinberg School of Medicine, USA

Dayan Zhou, Zongjie Qu, Hao Wang, Zhe Wang and Qiang Xu
Department of Cardiology, Fifth People's Hospital of Chongqing, Renji Road No. 24, Nanan District, Chongqing 400062, China

Marcos Danillo Peixoto Oliveira, Fernando Roberto de Fazzio, José Mariani Junior, Carlos M. Campos, Luiz Junya Kajita, Expedito E. Ribeiro and Pedro Alves Lemos
Department of Interventional Cardiology, Heart Institute(InCor) of the University of São Paulo, Avenida Dr. Enéas de Carvalho Aguiar 44, 05403-900 São Paulo, SP, Brazil

Ata Bajwa, Udit Bhatnagar, Amit Sharma, Hani El-Halawany and Randall C. Thompson
Saint Luke's Mid America Heart Institute, University of Missouri-Kansas City School of Medicine, Kansas City, MO, USA

Chui Man Carmen Hui
Department of Medicine, Albany Medical Center, Albany, NY 12208, USA

Santosh K. Padala, Mandeep S. Sidhu and Mikhail T. Torosoff
Department of Medicine, Division of Cardiology, Albany Medical Center, Albany, NY 12208, USA

Michael Lavelle
Albany Medical College, Albany, NY 12208, USA

Xinjun Cindy Zhu
Department of Medicine, Division of Gastroenterology, Albany Medical Center, Albany, NY 12208, USA

Fumiaki Nakao
Department of Cardiology, Yamaguchi Grand Medical Center, 77 Ohsaki, Hofu, Yamaguchi 747-8511, Japan

Sherif Ali Eltawansy
Internal Medicine Department, Monmouth Medical Center, Long Branch, NJ 07740, USA

Andrea Bakos
Drexel University College of Medicine, Philadelphia, PA 19129, USA

John Checton
Internal Medicine Department, Monmouth Medical Center, Long Branch, NJ 07740, USA
Cardiology Department, Monmouth Medical Center, Long Branch, NJ 07740, USA

Shivesh Goberdhan
Department of Internal Medicine, Queens University, Kingston General Hospital, 76 Stuart Street, Kingston, ON, Canada K7L 2V7

Soon Kwang Chiew and Jaffer Syed
Department of Cardiology, McMaster University, St. Catharines Hospital, 1200 4th Avenue, St. Catharines, ON, Canada L2S 0A9

Budi Yuli Setianto, Anggoro Budi Hartopo, Putrika Prastuti Ratna Gharini and Nahar Taufiq
Department of Cardiology and Vascular Medicine, Faculty of Medicine, Universitas Gadjah Mada and Dr. Sardjito Hospital, Yogyakarta 55281, Indonesia

Karan Wats
Internal Medicine, Maimonides Medical Center, Brooklyn, NY 11219, USA

On Chen, Syeda Atiqa Batul, Norbert Moskovits, Vijay Shetty and Jacob Shani
Department of Cardiology, Maimonides Medical Center, Brooklyn, NY 11219, USA

Nupur Nippun Uppal
Department of Nephrology, North Shore Long Island Jewish Hospital, New Hyde Park, NY 11040, USA

Archana Sinha and Rajan Kumar
Division of Cardiology, Saint Luke's University Health Network, 801 Ostrum Street, Bethlehem, PA 18015, USA

O'Dene Lewis
Division of Pulmonary Medicine, Howard University Hospital, 2041 Georgia Avenue, Washington, DC 20060, USA

Sri Lakshmi Hyndavi Yeruva
Division of Hematology-Oncology, Howard University Hospital, 2041 Georgia Avenue, Washington, DC 20060, USA

Bryan H. Curry
Division of Cardiology, Howard University Hospital, 2041 Georgia Avenue, Washington, DC 20060, USA

Fahad Almehmadi
Schulich Heart Center, Sunnybrook Health Sciences Center, University of Toronto, 2075 Bayview Avenue, Toronto, ON, Canada M4N 3M5
King Saud Bin Abdulaziz University of Health Sciences, Jeddah, Saudi Arabia

Mark Davis and Sheldon M. Singh
Schulich Heart Center, Sunnybrook Health Sciences Center, University of Toronto, 2075 Bayview Avenue, Toronto, ON, Canada M4N 3M5

Mariana Faustino
Cardiology Department, Hospital Fernando Fonseca, IC 19, Amadora, 2720-276 Lisbon, Portugal

Inês Carmo Mendes and Rui Anjos
Pediatric Cardiology Department, Hospital de Santa Cruz, Avenida Professor Reinaldo dos Santos, Carnaxide, 2790-134 Lisbon, Portugal

Mustafa Cetin, Emrullah Kiziltunc, Harun Kundi, Birsen Gulkan and Hülya Cicekcioglu
Cardiology Department, Numune Education and Research Hospital, Cardiology Department, 06100 Ankara, Turkey

Zehra Güven Cetin
Cardiology Department, Dr. Nafiz Korez State Hospital, 06100 Ankara, Turkey

Emre Gürel
Department of Cardiology, Ordu State Hospital, 52200 Ordu, Turkey

Zeki Yüksel GünaydJn, Osman BektaG and Adil BayramoLlu
Department of Cardiology, Ordu University Hospital, 52200 Ordu, Turkey

Ahmet Karagöz and AslJ Vural
Department of Cardiology, Giresun University Hospital, 28200 Giresun, Turkey

Abdullah Çelik
Department of Cardiovascular Surgery, Giresun University Hospital, 28200 Giresun, Turkey

Rui Plácido, Susana Robalo Martins, Ana G. Almeida and Fausto Pinto
Hospital Santa Maria, Cardiology Department, Lisbon Academic Medical Centre, CCUL, Lisbon, Portugal

Ana Filipa Martins, Sónia do Vale and João Martin Martins
Hospital de Santa Maria, Avenida Professor Egas Moniz, 1649-035 Lisboa, Portugal

Archana Sinha, Francis Burt and Peter Puleo
Division of Cardiovascular Disease, Saint Luke's University Health Network, Bethlehem, PA 18015, USA

Michael Sibel and Keith Baker
Department of Emergency Medicine, Saint Luke's University Health Network, Bethlehem, PA 18015, USA

Peter Thomas and James Cipolla
Department of Trauma Surgery, Saint Luke's University Health Network, Bethlehem, PA 18015, USA

Archana Sivanandam
University of California, Los Angeles, 405 Hilgard Avenue, Los Angeles, CA 90024, USA

Karthik Ananthasubramaniam
Heart and Vascular Institute, Henry Ford Hospital, 2799 W. Grand Boulevard, Detroit, MI 48322, USA

Stefan Koester, Justin Z. Lee and Kwan S. Lee
University of Arizona, Tucson, AZ 85714, USA